Health Services

POLICY AND SYSTEMS FOR THERAPISTS

Robert W. Sandstrom, PhD, PT
Chair, Department of Physical Therapy
School of Pharmacy and Affiliated Health Professions
Creighton University
Omaha, Nebraska

Helene L. Lohman, OTR/L, OTD
Department of Occupational Therapy
School of Pharmacy and Affiliated Health Professions
Creighton University
Omaha, Nebraska

James D. Bramble, PhD
Department of Pharmaceutical and Administrative Sciences
School of Pharmacy and Affiliated Health Professions
Center for Practice Improvement and Outcomes Research
Creighton University
Omaha, Nebraska

Prentice Hall

Upper Saddle River, New Jersey

Library of Congress Cataloging-in-Publication Data

Sandstrom, Robert, 1957-
  Health services : policy and systems for therapists / Robert
Sandstrom, Helene Lohman, James D. Bramble.
      p. ; cm.
Includes bibliographical references and index.
  ISBN 0-13-028344-4
  1. Medical policy—United States. 2. Public health—United States.
3. Physical therapy—Practice. 4. Occupational therapy—Practice.
  [DNLM: 1. Health Services Accessibility—organization &
administration—United States. 2. Occupational Therapy—organization &
administration—United States. 3. Physical Therapy
(Specialty)—organization & administration—United States. 4. Health
Policy—United States. W 76 S221h 2003] I. Lohman, Helene. II.
Bramble, James D. III. Title.
  RA395.A3 S366 2003
  362.1'0973—dc21
                        2002004458

Production Director: Bruce Johnson
Production Liaison: Alex Ivchenko
Manufacturing Manager: Ilene Sanford
Art Director: Cheryl Asherman
Full Service Management: Russell Jones, Pine Tree Composition
Cover Designer: Joseph DePinho
Editorial Assistant: Mary Ellen Ruitenberg
Buyer: Pat Brown

This book was set in 10/12 New Baskerville by Pine Tree Composition, Inc.,
and was printed and bound by R.R. Donnelley and Sons.
The cover was printed by Phoenix Color Corp.

© 2003 by Prentice Hall, Inc.
Upper Saddle River, New Jersey 07458

Printed in the United States of America
10 9 8 7 6 5 4 3 2 1

ISBN: 0-13-028344-4

Pearson Education Ltd.
Pearson Education Australia PTY, Ltd.
Pearson Education Singapore, Pte. Ltd.
Pearson Education North Asia Ltd.
Pearson Education Canada, Ltd.
Pearson Educación de Mexico, S.A. de C.V.
Pearson Education—Japan
Pearson Education Malaysia, Pte. Ltd.
Pearson Education, Upper Saddle River, New Jersey

Notice: The author[s] and the publisher of this volume
have taken care that the information and technical recommendations contained herein are based on research
and expert consultation, and are accurate and compati-
ble with the standards generally accepted at the time of
publication. Nevertheless, as new information becomes
available, changes in clinical and technical practices become necessary. The reader is advised to carefully consult manufacturers' instructions and information
material for all supplies and equipment before use, and
to consult with a healthcare professional as necessary.
This advice is especially important when using new
supplies or equipment for clinical purposes. The author[s] and publisher disclaim all responsibility for any
liability, loss, injury, or damage incurred as a consequence, directly or indirectly, of the use and application
of any of the contents of this volume.

Contents

Preface vii
Acknowledgments xi

I PRINCIPLES OF HEALTH AND DISABILITY POLICY

1 Disablement, Policy and Systems 1

Introduction 1
Policy and Power 2
Sources of Power 4
Ethics and Values 5
Experience of Disablement 7
Conclusions 11

2 Access to Health Care 14

Introduction 14
Conceptualizing Access to Health Care Services 15
The Relationship of Access and Health Insurance 19
Access to Therapists 24
Conclusion 26

3 Economics/ Cost of Health Care 29

Introduction 29
Health Care Financing: Where It Comes From 30
Health Care Expenditures: Where It Goes 32

Reasons for the Growth of Health Care Expenditures   34
Efforts to Contain Health Care Expenditures   36
Health Care Financing: An International Comparison   37
Conclusion   39

4   Quality of Health Care   43

Introduction   44
Challenges to Health Care Quality   44
Perspectives on Health Care Quality   46
Structure, Process, and Outcome   49
Accreditation   53
Legal Issues and Quality   54
Conclusion   55

5   Public Policy and Disability   60

Introduction   60
Public Policies Supporting Youth   63
Work-Related Policy Acts   70
Technology and Persons with Disabling Conditions   79
Working with Disability Policies   81
Conclusion   83

**II   REIMBURSEMENT POLICY:
FINANCING THERAPY SERVICES**

6   Fundamentals of Insurance   87

Introduction   88
Why Have Health Care Insurance?   88
Organization and Administration of Health
Care Insurance   89
Basics of an Insurance Contract   90
Types of Insurance   94
Sponsorship   95
Method of Cost Sharing   96
Covered Events/Services   97
Regulation of Insurance   100
Conclusion   102

7   Managed Care   105

Introduction   106
Defining Managed Care   107
Managed Care Principles   107
Managed Care Products   111

Managed Care Provider Structures   113
Effect of Managed Care on Physical Therapy
and Occupational Therapy   114
Adapting to the Changes Brought about by Managed Care   116
Conclusion   118

8   Medicare   122

Introduction   123
History of Medicare   124
Scope and Organization of Medicare   126
Part A: Hospital Insurance   128
Part A: Payment Structures   135
Part A Medicare Reform and Prospective Payment   144
Part B: Supplementary Medical Insurance (SMI)   144
Medicare Part B: Payment Structure   146
Medicare Part C   148
Private Health Insurance and Medicare   149
Quality and Medicare   149
Fraud and Abuse   150
Medicare Reform   151
Conclusion   152

9   Medicaid, SCHIP, and Military/Veterans Medical Insurance   156

Introduction   157
Medicaid   157
State Children's Health Insurance Program (SCHIP)   164
Veterans Administration and Military Health Insurance Programs   165
Conclusion   167

III   THERAPISTS AND THE HEALTH CARE SYSTEM

10   The Acute Medical Care System   171

Introduction   171
Hospitals   172
Levels of Care   179
Hospital Integration   180
Conclusion   184

11   The Post-Acute Health Care System   187
Introduction   188
Informal Care   189
Formal Care   191
Conclusion   201

12   Health Care Personnel   209
      Introduction   210
      The Health Care Labor Force   211
      Occupational Therapists   212
      Occupational Therapist Assistants and Aides   213
      Physical Therapists   213
      Physical Therapist Assistants and Aides   214
      The Rehabilitation Team   215
      Medicine   216
      Nursing   218
      Exercise-Related Occupations   219
      Complementary and Alternative Medicine Providers   220
      Future of Health Care Personnel   222
      Conclusion   223

13   Mental Health Practice and Public Policy   229
      Introduction   229
      Historical and Policy Aspects of Mental Health Practice   230
      Practice Sites for Mental Health   234
      Conclusion   238

14   Public Health   242
      Introduction   242
      What Is Public Health?   243
      Organization of Public Health Services   246
      Assessment   248
      Policy Development   249
      Assurance   250
      Public Health and Therapy Services   251
      Conclusion   252

IV   ADVOCACY

15   Effecting Policy Change: The Therapist as Advocate   255
      Introduction   256
      Advocacy and Ethics   256
      Therapist Skills for Advocacy   257
      Sequence for Advocacy   264
      Conclusion   271
      Advocacy Resources   271
      Internet Advocacy Resources   273
      National Organizations for Disease and Disability Conditions   274

Glossary   279

Index   285

Preface

Policy makes a difference. Each day, occupational therapists and physical therapists alleviate pain, prevent and treat conditions, and improve the functioning of people with temporary or permanent disabilities. Therapists examine, evaluate, diagnose, establish goals, plan, and implement interventions to improve the lives of those they serve. All of this professional activity is supported by policies and systems that define what therapists do and provide the resources to get the job done.

This book is about policy and practice. Policy is not only for administrators and politicians. Policy is for all therapists. If you are a new practitioner, a measure of your effectiveness will be your understanding of the system in which you work and how you professionally socialize yourself within it. As an experienced therapist, one measure of your effectiveness will be your understanding of how you can help your patients receive affordable, necessary services when they need them. As an expert practitioner or administrator, one measure of your effectiveness is to anticipate policy change and proactively make effective choices to advance the quality of care in your work group.

The changes in health care during the 1990s were enormous. Managed care contracting, consolidation and mergers of health care providers, slow growth of government spending on health care, growing disparities between the health of different segments of the population, and the large number of uninsured or underinsured persons reflect some of these momentous events in American health care. For occupational therapists and physical therapists, the 1990s brought significant change, including weakened demand for therapists in traditional settings, the closing and restructuring of outpatient and long-term care businesses, increasing documentation requirements, and increased attention to therapist fraud and abuse of insurance programs. The working environment of therapists is significantly different in 2002 than it was in 1992. But for all of the turmoil and change, we believe that the outlook for the professions of physical therapy and occupational therapy remains positive. The population of Americans who will be retiring and experiencing disablement and need for rehabilitation services will mushroom in the next decade. Advances in medical research (e.g., gene therapy) promise new treatments for conditions that today are fatal. With these new treatments that extend life will come a new demand for improved quality of life for a growing population of persons with disabilities. The development of new practice opportunities in fitness centers and wellness clinics provides new growth potential for the rehabilitation professions. While these changes and others bode well for the long-term future of the rehabilitation professions, the achievement of success will require hard work and an understanding of policy, systems, and advocacy.

This book is about helping therapists to understand the forces and policies that shape the future of health care for people with disabilities. In order to survive and excel in the future health care environment, occupational therapists and physical therapists will need to understand the effect of policy on their work and advocate for the changes necessary to reduce or eliminate their disabling conditions of their patients/clients. Physical therapy and occupational therapy exist for a social purpose: namely, to address the problems created by disablement and to assist patients/clients to self-directed and more complete independence and participation in society. We believe that it is imperative for occupational therapists and physical therapists to understand the policies that support their professions so that they can effectively advocate for their patients and clients to reduce disablement and fulfill the societal purpose of their professions.

The idea for this book originated in courses for physical therapists and occupational therapists at Creighton University on *health services*, including health care policy, disability policy, and rehabilitation care systems. This book is not a substitute for the content taught in a traditional administration or management course. Rather, it is a complement to the textbooks and courses in this area. The intent of this book is to support the development and implementation of similar courses in other entry-level professional curricula and to stimulate faculty scholarship in this area.

We encourage the flexible use of this book in professional curricula. We recognize that a health services course is not included in many entry-level curricula and that these issues are often covered in a variety of courses, such as professional issues and seminars. We encourage faculty to make maximal use of the information contained in the book that can be easily incorporated into existing courses of study. Obviously, we hope that this book will stimulate faculty to offer a health services course in their curriculum. We believe that this content is important information for entry-level practitioners in both professions. We also hope that the book will inform policymakers and analysts of the issues facing people with disabilities and the rehabilitation therapists who daily work to improve their lives.

We have designed the book for maximal interest and use by both physical therapists and occupational therapists. There is content overlap between the professions, but we recognize that some content areas will not be appropriate for one or the other field (see, for example, Chapter 13). We also believe that this book will be very useful for practicing clinicians who would like to understand the policies, forces, and issues affecting their practice. Many of us have learned most of this information "on the job" and have yearned for a comprehensive textbook covering the basic information about the environments where we work and interact with patients. We hope that we have organized the book in a manner that will facilitate the user's understanding of the content in an efficient and effective manner.

The book is divided into four parts. Part I introduces and explores the fundamental principles of health policy and disability policy. Chapter 1 discusses the basic political concepts that drive policymaking, several conceptualizations of disablement, and how different views of disablement and politics have affected the policies and systems that therapists experience each day. Chapters 2, 3, and 4 address the fundamental concepts of health policy: access, cost, and quality. Chapter 5 concludes the first section of the book by explaining public policies that address social disability.

Part II focuses on the financing and reimbursement of health care, specifically physical therapy and occupational therapy services. Insurance and managed care (Chapters 6 and 7), Medicare (Chapter 8), Medicaid and veterans affairs health care programs (Chapter 9) are all introduced. Policies that finance therapy services are among the most potent forces that shape and direct contemporary practice on a daily basis for all therapists.

Part III of the book examines the structure and organization of the health care system that delivers therapy services. The acute health care and post–acute health care systems (Chapters 10 and 11) have developed in response to policy decisions and community needs for treatment of illness, injury, and chronic disease. Chapter 12 discusses the types and roles of the practitioners who work in this health care system and with whom occupational therapists and physical therapists interact on a regular basis. Chapter 13 introduces the mental health care system, an important site for occupational therapy services. Part III concludes with a chapter on public health (Chapter 14).

Part IV concludes the book with a chapter on advocacy. This chapter provides information on policy formation and how therapists can be active now and in the future, in ensuring effective policy for therapy services for persons with disabilities. We have included a glossary of all of the key words that are introduced at the beginning of each chapter.

We welcome comments, suggestions, and criticisms from our readers. Policy is a "contact sport." Improvements in this textbook will come from the people who read and utilize it. We encourage you to contact us (and to get involved in policy), and we look forward to considering and responding to your input as the book is utilized.

Acknowledgments

We wish to recognize the many people who educated and supported us throughout this endeavor. The government affairs staffs of our professional associations—have been mentors and exemplars for us of policymaking and advocacy. Mark Cohen, Melissa Kerian, and Laura Mann of Prentice-Hall have been available with wise counsel and support throughout this project. Our colleagues who reviewed the initial draft of this book provided important input, and we have striven to incorporate their comments and recommendations:

Elizabeth M. Kanny. PhD. OTR/L
Associate Professor and Head
Division of Occupational Therapy
University of Washington
Seattle, Washington

Kathleen Lewis, MAPT, JD
Associate Professor
Department of Physical Therapy
Witchiata State University
Witchita, Kansas

We also wish to thank our colleagues in the School of Pharmacy and Allied Health Professions at Creighton University for their daily encouragement of our scholarship. Thanks to the students who have listened and provided feedback to us about health policy/ systems in our classrooms. Finally, special thanks to Lori, Spencer, Mitchell, Nicolas (JDB), Mike, Ben, Lee (HLL) and Susie, Scott, and Amy (RWS) for their love, encouragement, and patience always.

Robert W. Sandstrom, PhD, PT
Helene L. Lohman, OTR/L,OTD
James D. Bramble, PhD
Omaha, Nebraska
March 2002

1

Disablement, Policy and Systems

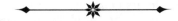

CHAPTER OBJECTIVES

At the conclusion of this chapter, the reader will be able to:

1. Explain the interaction between policy, systems, and everyday practice in occupational therapy and physical therapy.
2. Define power and describe how policy is used to create and distribute power in a society.
3. Compare and contrast the uses of private policy and public policy as a method to effect social change.
4. Discuss the experience of disablement using the medical disablement, social disability, and universalism models.
5. Differentiate medical care and human services systems as components of the health care system for persons with disabilities.

KEY WORDS: Biomedical Model, Disablement, Dualism, Health Services, Marginalization, Social Disability, Universalism

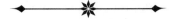

Introduction

Policies and systems are established to improve the lives of people and the overall community. This book is about an important and complex set of policies and systems in the United States: **health services.** Health services include the organizational, financing, and operational delivery of medical care and certain human services to persons who experience disease, illness, injury, and **disablement.** We are most interested in the health services that affect disablement because this book is intended for physical therapists and occupational therapists. Specifically, we are going to explore the policies that support and direct therapy care as well as the systems that organize these services. It is our intent that as you become better informed about health services, you will become a better advocate for your patients and profession in order to improve existing policies and systems.

This chapter will introduce broad concepts regarding the development and implementation of health services affecting both occupational therapy and physical therapy. While our two professions are different, we are often similarly affected by policy. The next three chapters will introduce and explore the three foundational principles of health care policy: access (Chapter 2), cost (Chapter 3), and quality (Chapter 4). As you will see in Parts II and III of this book, these issues have profound effects on the financing and organization of health care, including therapy services. First, we begin in this chapter by discussing the social structures that generate the policy and systems affecting therapists and persons with disabling conditions. Second, we will discuss different theoretical models of disablement and how they can explain different policies and systems. This will set the foundation for understanding the specific policies and systems discussed in Chapter 5.

We begin this chapter by introducing and discussing the issue of power as it affects health services. Specifically, we will discuss how power is distributed in American society through two policy-creating mechanisms: government (public) and private enterprise. Next, we will study different viewpoints about what it means to experience disablement. One's perspective on disablement affects the type of policy that is created and how its effectiveness is evaluated. Finally, we will integrate the concepts of a medical care system and human services system into our discussion. All of these systems affect the organization of health services for persons who are experiencing temporary or permanent disablement.

Policy and Power

In the twentieth century, many policies and systems were established to improve the health and well-being of the population. Not all of these health services were provided equally or comprehensively. Some of these health services were very effective. For example, the Medicare program virtually guaranteed access to medical care for people over age 65 and for people with permanent disablement. Other health services policies were ineffective; for instance, an insurance system that permitted a large number of working Americans to be without health insurance (see Chapter 2). Other policies have not yet been developed, such as a financing system for long-term care of the growing population of elderly Americans. Our policy-making system is unique in the world.

The lack of uniformity in health services in the United States can be traced to our system of policy **dualism** (see Table 1–1). Both the government and private enterprise are involved in the financing, organization, and delivery of health services, including occupational and physical therapy. In addition, the government has a large regulatory role (e.g., licensure of providers). The sources of these two forms of health services policy-making are the core documents of our republic and the dominant economic system, free market capitalism. Physical and occupational therapy services are shaped by each source.

As noted in Table 1–1, health services originate from two sources of *power* in the United States: public and private. The allocation of resources and the organizational ability of government and the free enterprise system create the foundation for health services in the United States. As we will discuss in later chapters, government uses its taxing and regulatory authority to create access to medical and rehabilitation services, and, in some cases, to provide them to persons in need. Health services are also large economic enterprises (see Chapter 3). Both not-for-profit and for-profit enterprises have privately invested in the delivery and financing of health care, including therapy services. The generation of profit from this investment creates economic power that influences the health services system. The tension and interplay between private policy and public policy affecting health services are dynamic and political.

While policy is often affected by government decisions and economic investment, effective and fair health services policy must consider those who are powerless. The lives of many persons who experience disablement are characterized by poverty, unemployment, lack of adequate housing and transportation, impaired access to medical care services, and barriers to equal social and economic opportunity in the broader society. Policies reflect the distribution of power in the decision-making process and the values and ethics of the broader society. Just policy considers the life and circumstances of the powerless and creates opportunities for empowerment and advancement in the entire society (Purtilo 1995; Bonja and DeJong 2000).

In summary, policies are expressions of power that allocate and organize resources to address identified needs in a society. As we will discuss later, systems are established that respond to policy decisions. Just policies affirm the human rights of those who are powerless and provide a pathway for advancement. In the next section, we will discuss in more detail the sources of power that drive health services: government, private enterprise, and moral/ethical principles.

Table 1–1. Dualism and American Health Services Policy

	Government	*Free Enterprise*
Source of power	Constitution	Capitalistic markets
Role	Financing	Financing
	Regulation	Organization and delivery
	Organization and delivery	

Sources of Power

Government

In the United States, the power of the government is established in the Constitution and other core documents. The United States was founded in a revolt against the authority of central government, based on the idea of promoting individual liberty. In general, the American democratic republic is a system of limited and distributed government. The American system distributes power among three branches: executive, legislative, and judicial. Government authority is further divided between the national government and the states. Laws enacted by legislative bodies require executive approval and are reviewable by the courts. All of these decisions are reported, analyzed, and commented upon by a free press to the governed citizenry. American citizens have a right to address their government, and public policymakers are held responsible for their decisions by election on a regular basis. As a result, government power is expected to be used cautiously, for understood reasons, and only when necessary.

When it does act, government power is coercive (Weiner and Vining 1992). Government has the power to unilaterally ascertain, restrict, permit, or direct resources of private individuals and organizations. Through the establishment and enforcement of laws and regulations, government can force behavior change on individuals and organizations that may not agree with the policy or that would not implement the same policy on their own. When and under what circumstances can government use this power?

We can summarize two reasons for this type of government action: failure of the private market to work as expected and a consensus among the governed populace for government action (Weiner and Vining 1992). In certain circumstances, private markets are perceived to be ineffective in meeting individual or community needs. For example, government provides the resources and ensures that roads and bridges are available to meet the transportation needs of society. It is accepted that it would be ineffective for each individual or community to privately organize and maintain a system of roads and bridges that permit people to work, shop, trade, or use recreational resources. It is a government responsibility to perform this responsibility.

Government action is also expected to address concerns raised by the will of the people. For example, the Americans with Disabilities Act of 1990 (see Chapter 5) was enacted to improve the civil rights of all Americans with disabilities and reflected the social consciousness that this was the "right thing to do." It would be very difficult, if not impossible, for civil rights to be achieved in all communities unless government power was used. Often, a combination of free market failure and a consensus of the population in favor of change is needed to enable the use of government power to address social concerns.

We also need to consider the important role of government in establishing the "playing field" for private enterprise. Laws are government policies that establish private property and regulate markets that help to create the conditions that allow competition and the efficient, effective allocation of economic resources, including health services.

Private Enterprise

Private enterprise creates power by the investment of capital and the organizational ability of individuals and institutions that create systems each day to exchange economic resources in a marketplace. The American system of capitalism provides opportunities for individual success and allows unsuccessful enterprises to fail. In this economic system, private enterprises accept the risk of failure, create strategy, innovate, and implement services that meet the needs of consumers. People who successfully do this have a proprietary advantage, a form of economic power. This proprietary advantage creates business activity, initiates competition, allocates economic resources efficiently, and creates wealth.

Decisions that meet the demands of the marketplace in an efficient manner result in rewards to the owner of the resources, that is, a profit. Profits are used to pay creditors, create new investment, and provide for the personal well-being of the owners (Helfert 1997). Profits create economic power. Investment and the incentive to invest provide the economic resources to build hospitals and clinics, hire therapists, educate the next generation of providers, and deliver critical medical care services to the ill or injured.

The generation of economic resources also finances the government. Individuals and businesses pay taxes that support governmental action. While government and private sources of power are different, we must recognize that they are symbiotic and, at times, complementary. This relationship fuels the reality of interest group politics, the necessary advocacy of specialized, private groups for governmental action, and political action committees, groups that privately finance the candidates for government office who support their perspectives. The American Physical Therapy Association (APTA) and the American Occupational Therapy Association (AOTA) have long recognized this reality at all levels of government and expend considerable time and resources to involve members in the process.

Ethics and Values

As we have already indicated, many people experience disenfranchisement from the mainstream of society. Socioeconomic disadvantage, discrimination, and isolation from opportunities affect the lives of people who are "different" from the majority in the community. Persons with disabilities have historically experienced these circumstances (Bonja 1997). Policies that affect everyone, including the powerless, should be fair and equitable. The debate of the federal government on a Patient's Bill of Rights demonstrates the importance of ethics and values in health services policy-making.

Laws and private policies reflect the basic values and ethics of the society and must be considered along with economic power and government authority in any debate on health services. Long (1994) describes four values that form the ethical base for health policy in the United States: freedom, equality, rewards, and treatment of the poor. Table 1–2 outlines the four principles and provides an example of a contemporary health services policy issue that is an application of the principles developed by Long.

Freedom is a social construct that describes our relationship to one another and our ability to make and act upon individual decisions. Related to the ethical principle of autonomy, the ability to make choices about health care and have access to services are examples of policy matters related to the principle of freedom. Should people have the freedom to choose their health care provider without interference from a managed care plan? This was one important question in the 2001 Patient's Bill of Rights debate in Congress.

Related to the ethical principle of beneficence, the principle of equality defines the sharing and disbursement of rewards and responsibilities in society. Who is entitled to receive health care services? How will health care services be distributed to people? The large number of Americans without health care insurance illustrates that we do not have a system that guarantees equal access to health care (see Chapter 2).

The principle of rewards addresses this question: Is health care a basic right, or is it payment for contributions to the greater social good? Our core government documents do not define health care as a basic right of citizenship. Over the last half century, certain groups have advocated several proposals (most recently in 1994) to create a basic right to health care. Despite these efforts, a universal, national health insurance plan for all Americans has not been enacted.

Finally, according to Long (1994), health care policy must address the issue of the powerless and the poor. Treatment of the poor is an issue of social justice. A civil and just society will have policies and systems that provide for the care and treatment of all people, not only the economically advantaged or socially elite. Government intervention in health care has often been predicated on meeting the needs of historically disadvantaged groups (see Chapters 8 and 9).

In summary, health services are affected by competing and complementary sources of power in society: government, private enterprise, and moral/ethical val-

TABLE 1–2.   Ethical Considerations of Health Services Policy

Ethical Principle	Contemporary Issue
1. Freedom	Patient's Bill of Rights
2. Equality	40+ million uninsured Americans
3. Rewards	Universal or employment-based health insurance
4. Treatment of the poor	SCHIP program

Adapted from: M. Long, *The Medical Care System: A Conceptual Model* (1994).

ues. This is a dynamic and changing situation that is created by multiple stakeholders making independent decisions each day. This system reflects the American decision to distribute power widely on important issues like health care. Unlike other industrialized nations, the United States has not decided to centralize its health care system. Health care in the United States is, however, political, and the decisions made in private enterprises and government affect the experience of disablement for millions of Americans. We will have more to say about how therapists can be effective in this political process in Chapter 15. Let us now turn our attention to the experience of disablement and discuss how changing perspectives on this issue have affected the development of health services for persons with disabilities.

Experience of Disablement

The special interest of this book is how policy and systems affect people with disabilities and the people who care for them. Physical therapy and occupational therapy exist as professions to serve a societal need. The incidence and prevalence of temporary and permanent disablement creates a human and social need for assistance, new opportunities for independence, and community.

The experience of disablement creates foundational paradigms for the understanding of what needs to be done and the organization of rehabilitation health services. Disablement is experienced as a biomedical problem, an economic challenge, and a sociopolitical issue. Disablement is a major social problem. It is estimated that disablement affects 49 million Americans at an annual cost of $300 billion to the American economy (Brandt and Pope 1997). The size and prevalence of disablement means that solutions require the involvement of major social institutions.

Disablement is common to the human experience and has existed since antiquity. It is only in the last 150 years, however, as Western society has industrialized, that formal attempts have been made to define disablement and to develop a major, organized, social response beyond the family unit. In the United States, a fundamental principle for defining and determining this social response is the individual's ability or inability to work (Alson 1997; Kennedy and Minkler 1998). The inability of a person to work jeopardizes the ability of the person and family unit to be self-sustaining. As a result, a broader social response is needed to provide the individual and family unit with support. At odds with this idea is the societal expectation that everyone capable of self-support and work will do so. Society can ill afford a policy that provides generous benefits to individuals and family units that are capable of working for self-support.

Ability to work as an establishing principle for defining disablement creates three new questions for policymakers: Who can work or not work? What types of services are needed by people who cannot work? What can society afford to provide to those who are unable to support themselves and their social unit? The first two questions have been addressed to medical care providers. The third question is a matter of continuing contention within and between private and public policy-makers.

Answers to these questions are affected by the prevailing definition of the disablement experience. The basic characteristics of three major perspectives of disablement are summarized in Table 1–3. Historically, the biomedical model has been the dominant model of thinking about disablement in the United States. The social disability model has arisen in complement to and, in some cases, opposition to the biomedical model. Universalism challenges the notion that disablement is a special or separate policy issue. All three models affect the organization and delivery of therapy services to persons with disability in the United States.

Biomedical Model

In order to determine eligibility for benefits, policymakers have turned to health care providers to determine the type and extent of disablement. Since the late nineteenth century, medical doctors have been granted power to determine and certify who is disabled and who, within the guidelines of the policy, can receive benefits. This policy decision resulted in the "medicalization" of disablement (Craddock 1996a; Williams 1991). As the scientific rationale for medical practice grew exponentially in the twentieth century, disablement became increasingly viewed as a biomedical problem.

The focus of the biomedical model is to explain the patient's experience by understanding the source of the problem in terms of basic science and cellular pathology. This perspective emphasizes the role of the physician. The expansion of science and the acceptance of the biomedical model fostered a sophisticated and expensive medical care system with an emphasis on the identification and cure of pathology. Disablement was understood as a problem of medical pathology.

The biomedical model has limits, however, in its ability to explain disablement. Disablement is not "curable." Disablement often begins at the point where medical practice has limited effectiveness to eliminate disease or reverse injury. The manifestations of the pathology are not acute. Instead, they are usually chronic. A definition of disablement and the ultimate determination of success in

TABLE 1–3.   Disablement Models

	Medical Rehabilitation	*Social Disability*	*Universalism*
Source of disablement	Person	Social attitudes and policies	Both
Experience of disablement	Structure and function of body	Discrimination and isolation	All persons have potential
Response	Medical care	Human services	Integrated system

treating disablement goes beyond the terms used in treating acute illness, that is, morbidity and mortality. By the mid-1960s and thereafter, with the emergence of the Nagi model (Nagi 1965), new biomedical models emerged to explain the experience of disablement.

These models of "medical disablement" broaden our understanding of the manifestations of disease and injury. Impairments, functional limitations, and disability define the organ/tissue, whole person, and societal role effects of chronic illness and disablement (Brandt and Pope 1997). The philosophy of medical disablement supports policies that develop systems to address these concerns. Physical therapy and occupational therapy services that improve function and address pain, weakness, contracture, and similar problems, can be defined as "medically necessary" and, therefore, are reimbursed through medical care insurance. This policy supports the provision of necessary services for those who are recovering from recent or recurring illness or injury.

The definition of "medical necessity" also limits independent therapist action and direct access to therapy services by the public. Many insurance plans, including public plans, require physician certification of therapy services in order for persons with disablement to access therapy care. We will discuss these issues in depth in Part II of this text. The medicalization of therapy services has also organized complex systems that employ therapists within the medical care system, typically dominated by physicians. We will explore this system in detail in Chapter 10. In summary, the medicalization of disablement has made it possible for many people to receive therapy services funded through medical care insurance. The dominance of the medical model, however, has also limited direct access to rehabilitation therapy care for persons with medically stable, disabling conditions. While providing many employment opportunities, the medical rehabilitation model also constrains the distribution of therapists to the medical care system.

While the medical disablement model broadens the understanding of disablement to include more than pathology, the focus of the disablement experience remains on the individual. This conceptualization reinforces the importance of the patient-provider relationship to the exclusion of broader societal influences on the experience of disablement. As a result, some theorists reject the biomedical model as an inadequate explanation of disablement. Since medicine has limits to its effectiveness in treating chronic and disabling conditions, they argue, improvements in lifestyle and the barriers that affect people with disabling conditions must be addressed by different mechanisms.

Social Disability Model

Social disability thinking has developed as "a dynamic social phenomenon that has as much to do with cultural norms and socioeconomic status as it is due to the individual's physiologic condition" (Kennedy and Minkler 1998). Social disability theory can be traced to the responses of people with chronic disease and illness to the limits of the biomedical model in explaining their experience and to the American civil rights movement of the 1960s (Craddock 1996b). The social disability movement has instigated the development and study of disability as a culture and caused the rethinking of the policy response to disablement.

From the perspective of social disability theory, medical disablement models are ineffective in explaining the situation of people who are physiologically stable but have ongoing disablement, social, and human services needs. Social disability theorists argue that the focus of medical disablement models on the person as the source of disability reinforces three negative stereotypes (Kennedy and Minkler 1998; Williams 1991). First, there is an excessive reliance on the health care provider as a source of solutions for disablement. Second, the biomedical model emphasizes a continual need for the person with a disabling condition to assume a "sick role" in order to receive services. Finally, the understanding of the disablement experience from a pathophysiologic perspective ignores other powerful social influences. From the social disability perspective, the source of disablement is not the pathophysiologic condition of the person but the sociopolitical environment.

Rather than originating as a pathologic event, disablement is created as the result of a social process of **marginalization** of persons with disabilities by the larger society and its policies. Marginalization of the disabled results in stigmatization by others (Williams 1991; Zola 1989). The inability to work weakens the economic power of people with disabilities, and as a result, their political voice weakens. Those who are not disabled begin to view the expensive and special services required for full social participation by people with disabilities as a drain on other pressing social needs. Persons with disabilities are then forced to compete for limited social resources but experience barriers in their attempts to do so. In summary, one social disability theorist writes that disability "becomes a problem when it causes a person to consume rather than produce economic surplus" (Kennedy and Minkler 1998). From this perspective, disablement is not found in the person with physical or mental impairments. Disablement is created by a pattern of social and economic discrimination by the majority of the population against one group through a mechanism of isolation and exclusion.

The effect of the social disability model on policy has led to the enactment of numerous civil rights laws over the last twenty-five years that address discrimination against persons with disabilities. Policies have also been enacted to support a human services system that empowers persons with disabilities to live more full and productive lives in the community. For example, the Rehabilitation Act of 1973 created Centers for Independent Living and state vocational rehabilitation programs that provide services to address the issues of community integration and socioeconomic discrimination. We will cover many of these programs and laws in Chapter 5.

It is important to note that the medical rehabilitation system and the human services system are distinct systems. Although both serve persons with disability, there is little formal integration and varying levels of coordination of policies and services between them. As we have discussed, their philosophical foundations, policy histories, and organizations are quite different. The problem of division, experienced in both theory and practice, is addressed by the concept of **universalism.**

Universalism

The historical development of disablement policy in the United States has created two separate systems. The medical rehabilitation system is organized using the biomedical model focusing on the person as the source of disablement and directing interventions, including therapy services, at improving the quality of life from this perspective. The human services system is based on a social disablement model that identifies the policies and attitudes of the society as the source of disablement. Services that empower the person with disability through expanded civil rights, access to employment, improved housing, and transportation are provided by organizations supported by policies that address social disablement.

Both of these models and systems emphasize the experience of separation and difference for persons with disability. Universalism attempts to explain disablement not as a condition that affects a few individuals who require specialized medical or human services but rather as a situation to be recognized by the entire population at risk for disablement (Zola 1989). All of us live in a temporary state of non-disablement. The universalism philosophy advocates that most people will be affected by disability at some point during the aging process. As a result, policies should be developed to integrate all persons and to educate the population about living with a disability. Universalism addresses the fundamental problem of the marginalization of those with disabling conditions, whether on biomedical, social, economic, or political terms.

Universalism attempts to bridge the gap between the biomedical and social disability models. Integrated and coordinated policy that addresses the biologic, social, economic, and political reality of disablement is needed to truly address the experience of disablement. Ideally, an integration of medical and human services would be of the greatest benefit for persons who are experiencing disablement (Leutz, Greenlick, and Capitman 1994; Leutz 1999). There are few current examples of this form of pragmatic policy and systems development for persons with disabling conditions in the United States.

Conclusions

In this chapter, we have introduced the principles that affect the creation of policy and systems to deliver rehabilitation services to people with disabilities as well as the practice of occupational therapy and physical therapy. Policy is about distributing power to maintain the status quo or to effect needed social change. The power to develop health services policy has three sources: government, private enterprise, and ethics/values. Policy development and implementation is a political process. Much of the remainder of this book will discuss the effects of policy decisions made in both private and public forums. Chapter 15 will explore the rationale and need for therapists to be engaged in this process.

Health services policy that addresses disablement has developed in response to the dominant perspective that has defined the disabling experience. The medical model focuses on the person as the source of disablement. Important in determining eligibility for medical and social benefits, this model has reinforced the development of an acute and post-acute health care system (Chapters 10 and 11) and a financing system for the rehabilitation health care system (Part II) to address these needs. The social disability model finds the source of disablement in the community and society. This model has fostered the development of a community-based system of services for persons with disability that is explored in Chapter 5.

Access, cost, and quality are three foundational principles that drive all health policy, including policies that affect occupational therapy and physical therapy. An ideal system would maximize access to high-quality health care at a reasonable cost. In the upcoming chapters, we will review the successes and challenges for U.S. health services policymakers as they attempt to achieve these objectives. Our primary focus will be on the medical/rehabilitation health care system. We will close Part I of the book by returning to the human services system and related policies that exist to improve the lives of persons with disabling conditions.

CHAPTER REVIEW QUESTIONS

1. Define the relationship between power and policy.
2. What are the sources of power in the policy-making process?
3. Who is involved in policy formation, and how is policy formed?
4. Identify the uses and limitations of private policy and public policy in meeting social need and effecting social change.
5. How does "ability to work" affect policy toward persons with disabilities?
6. Compare and contrast the characteristics of the biomedical and medical disablement models.
7. Define the source of disablement according to the social disability model.
8. What is universalism?
9. How have perspectives on the experience of disablement affected the development of system responses to disablement?

CHAPTER DISCUSSION QUESTIONS

1. Some people advocate for government action to improve health care. Others believe that private market solutions are the choice for increasing access to quality and affordable health care for more Americans. What are the pros and cons of each of these philosophies on health services policy?
2. Compare and contrast the positions of the social disability and medical disability models of disablement. Which of these models do you believe is most effective in meeting the needs of persons with disability? Why?

3. Physical therapy practices primarily within the model of medical disablement. Occupational therapy also practices within the context of social disability. How does the orientation of each profession affect the type of services provided?

REFERENCES

Alston, R. J. 1997. Disability and health care reform: Principles, practices and politics. *J Rehabil* 63(3): 15–19.

Banja, J. D. 1997. Values, function and managed care: An ethical analysis. *J Head Trauma Rehabil* 12 (1): 60-70.

Banja, J. D. and G. DeJong. 2000. The rehabilitation marketplace: Economics, values, and proposals for reform. *Arch Phys Med Rehabil* 81: 233-39.

Brandt, E. N. and A. M. Pope, eds. 1997. *Enabling America: Assessing the role of rehabilitation science and engineering.* Washington DC: National Academy Press.

Craddock, J. 1996*a*. Responses of the occupational therapy profession to the perspective of the disability movement. Part 1. *Br J Occup Ther* 59(1): 17–21.

———. 1996*b*. Responses of the occupational therapy profession to the perspective of the disability movement. Part 2. *Br J Occup Ther* 59(2): 73–78.

Helfert, E. 1997. *Techniques of financial analysis: A modern approach.* 9th ed. Chicago: Irwin Press.

Kennedy, J. and M. Minkler. 1998. Disability theory and public policy: Implications for critical gerontology. *Int J Health Law* 28(4): 757–76.

Leutz, W. 1999. Five laws for integrating medical and social services: Lessons from the United States and the United Kingdom. *Milbank Q* 77(1): 77–110.

———, M. R. Greenlick, and J. Capitman. 1994. Integrating acute and long term care. *Health Affairs* 13(4): 59–74.

Long, M. J. 1994. *The medical care system: A conceptual model.* Ann Arbor: AUPHA Press.

Nagi, S. Z. 1965. Some conceptual issues in disability and rehabilitation. In *Sociology and Rehabilitation,* 110–113, ed. M. B. Sussman. Washington DC: American Sociological Association.

Purtilo, R. 1995. Revisiting the basics of professional life. *PT Magazine* 3: 81–82.

Weiner, D. L. and A. R. Vining. 1992. *Policy analysis: Concepts and practices.* Englewood Cliffs NJ: Prentice Hall.

Zola, I. 1989. Toward the necessary universalizing of a disability policy. *Milbank Q* 67 (suppl 2, pt. 2): 401–28.

2

Access to Health Care

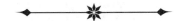

CHAPTER OBJECTIVES

At the conclusion of this chapter, the reader will be able to:

1. Distinguish and discuss the different components that define access to health care services.
2. Describe the role of health care insurance with regard to accessing health care services.
3. Explain the relationship of health care insurance, access to health care services, and a person's health status.
4. Explain the concept of direct access to health care services.

KEY WORDS: Access, Direct Access, Enabling Factors, Need Factors, Uninsured

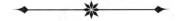

Introduction

Access, cost, and quality are three major constructs commonly used in describing and evaluating the health care system in the United States (Barton 1999). While cost refers to the expenditures for obtained services, and quality is how well those services are provided, access is the ability to obtain the appropriate health care services when needed. These concepts can be further illustrated through a set of relatively simple questions that have potentially complex answers. For example, when an individual is in need of medical attention, is the needed care for complete recovery available and accessible? Does the patient receive the necessary referrals to receive medical care from the appropriate provider? Is that care provided appropriately? How much will the care cost? How will the provider be paid, and who will pay for the care received? The latter questions address issues surrounding the cost and quality of health care services, which will be addressed in Chapters 3 and 4, respectively. The theme of the current chapter is centered on the issues surrounding access to health care services.

Unlike much of the industrialized world, access to health care in the United States is not a guaranteed right (Fuchs 1993). Thus, a person's ability to access needed health care services is a perennial issue for health care providers and policymakers. This chapter first conceptually defines access and discusses the various barriers that individuals and groups must overcome to access health services. We then focus on the largest barrier to access—the lack of adequate health insurance. Lastly, specifics are discussed regarding access to occupational and physical therapy services.

Conceptualizing Access to Health Care Services

There are many different dimensions worthy of consideration when conceptualizing access to health care services. Summarizing work done by various researchers on the utilization of health services, Barton (1999) grouped potential factors that may affect a person's access to health services into three groups: (1) predisposing factors, (2) need factors, and (3) enabling factors (see Table 2–1). The combination of these factors interactively working together, in various degrees of importance, influences the degree of access one has to health care services.

Table 2–1. Factors Affecting Access To Health Care Services

Predisposing Factors	Need Factors	Enabling Factors
Age	Perception of	Convenience
Sex	health status	Personal income
Race		System characteristics
Education		Health insurance
Socioeconomic status		
Occupation		

Source: P. B. Barton, *Understanding the U. S. Health Services System.* Chicago: Health Administration Press, 1999.

Predisposing factors include the person's demographic information, including age, sex, race, education, socioeconomic status, and occupation. Each of these variables influences the ability and need of an individual to access health care services. For example, the very young (e.g., infants) along with the elderly generally require more help to access appropriate medical care. Both of these populations are dependent on others to arrange and provide transportation to and from health care providers. Thus, the degree of access these individuals have to appropriate health care services is, in part, dependent on obtaining assistance from family, friends, or public programs (Taylor and Taylor 1996).

Gender and race also influence the ability and need to access health care services. A number of diseases and conditions are gender- or race-specific. For example, females of child-bearing age are likely to have a need to access services more frequently than their male counterparts. Certain diseases, such as sickle cell anemia, predominantly affect only a certain racial group, African-Americans. We must also recognize that racial groups may face cultural barriers or even discriminatory behavior that affects their ability to access health care services.

One's educational level and chosen occupation also influences access to medical care. People with higher levels of education frequently use health services more than those with less education (Barton 1999). An individual's occupation may influence access in many ways. First, some occupations are more hazardous than others and result in a greater number of injuries. Second, employers play an important role in providing financial access to health care services through voluntary, employer-based insurance—a topic that is more fully addressed in the following section. Thus, when analyzing the accessibility of health care services, the demographic makeup of the concerned population (i.e., predisposing factors) must be recognized.

Need factors refer to the decision an individual makes to seek health care services because a potential need exists. That is, it is one's perception of one's health status that influences whether one accesses health care services and seeks medical care. Given the financial means to do so, people who perceive their health as poor to fair are more likely to access care (Short and Lair 1995). Thus one's ability to interpret one's illness affects access to care. In the case of those who are dependent on others (e.g., infants or the elderly), it is the perception of the caretaker that is a determining factor in seeking out health care services.

Enabling factors are the last set of factors affecting potential access. Enabling factors include convenience, personal income, system characteristics of the local health care organizations, and health insurance coverage. Convenience factors include such concerns as the geographic, temporal, and physical dimensions of obtaining the appropriate level of medical care. System factors refer to the manner in which health care services are organized such that the population can use the services provided.

The last category of factors (i.e., enabling factors) is further captured by Penchansky and Thomas's (1981) conceptualization of access that examines the fit between the characteristics of health care providers and the expectations of patients (see Table 2–2). Penchansky and Thomas examine this fit along five dimensions: availability, accessibility, accommodation, acceptability, and affordability.

Table 2–2.   **Penchansky and Thomas Access Factors**

Availability
Accessibility
Accommodation
Acceptability
Affordability

Source: R. Penchansky and J. W. Thomas, (1981). The concept of access: Definition and relationship to consumer satisfaction. *Medical Care* 19, 2(1981):127–40.

Availability

Availability refers to the relationship between the amount and type of services provided by health care workers and the amount and type of services required by the population in need. The goal is to have the best possible match between the services provided and the services needed. For example, a community with a large elderly population would have more geriatric services than a younger community.

Accessibility

Many barriers to utilizing health care services derive from geographic factors; thus, the second dimension examines the accessibility of health care services. Accessibility describes the relationship between the location and supply of health care providers and services (e.g., therapy clinics) and the location and transportation resources of the population (i.e., potential patients). Health services tend to be located in population centers that are large enough to support them. People who live outside of these centers, such as in sparsely populated rural areas, may not have access to a full range of health care services regardless of their ability to afford those services. People who must travel great distances to reach the care that is needed may postpone or go without needed medical services. Thus, for all intents and purposes, certain medical services may not be accessible even if they are available. Rural communities across the country are some of the areas most at risk of having less than ideal access to health care services. Even in urban areas there are barriers to the accessibility of health services, including man-made barriers (e.g., freeway patterns) and natural barriers (e.g., rivers).

Accommodation

The third dimension, accommodation, addresses three related issues: (1) the manner in which health care providers, services, and facilities are organized, (2) the population's ability to use these providers, services, and facilities, and (3) the population's opinion of the appropriateness of the providers, services, and facilities. Accommodation is affected by temporal factors that can create barriers that may keep care seekers from accessing health care providers and services. One of these factors is the match between the schedules of providers and patients. The match of schedules may be inhibited by inflexible working hours, the ability to attain childcare, or a host of other factors. These issues need to be considered when organizing health care services so that they are "accommodating" to potential patients.

Acceptability

The fourth dimension, acceptability, examines the attitudes and perceptions that health service providers and the population have toward one another. For example, cultural differences, including language barriers, differing values on health, or conflicting customs or beliefs, may exist. All of these differences may prevent an individual from reaping the full benefits of available health care services even though the care may be available, accessible, accommodating, and affordable.

Affordability

The final dimension, affordability, is concerned with the price of health care services or the ability of the population to pay. Financial access to health care services is closely tied to health insurance and the ability to obtain insurance coverage. Health insurance is discussed more fully in Chapters 6 and 7. However, as has been discussed, health insurance coverage or one's ability to afford medical care is not the only factor to consider when examining access to health care services. Health insurance, by itself, does not guarantee access to care; for example, the necessary health care provider or therapy clinic may not be available where the patient lives.

As Penchansky and Thomas's conceptualization demonstrates, there are many factors that have a potential effect on the ability to access health care services. All of these dimensions (i.e., availability, accessibility, accommodation, acceptability, and affordability) along with the predisposing factors of potential patients need to be considered to fully understand the degree of access that defined populations have to health care services. Policymakers and health care practitioners must account for the many dimensions of access as they plan for the delivery of health care. However, it is difficult to determine which barrier is most important. Each person may have their own unique barriers to overcome; thus, the most problematic barrier to receiving care varies across individuals.

Though barriers vary across individuals, as a whole our country's biggest access-related problem is the affordability of health care services (Vistnes and Zuvekas 1999). Adequate health insurance is essential to overcome the affordability barrier and gain access to appropriate and timely medical care. Though health insurance, as has been argued, is only one of the dimensions of access, it is an important part of the financing and delivery of health care services in this country; the next section of this chapter takes a closer look at this barrier.

The Relationship of Access and Health Insurance

One key factor in making health care services accessible is health insurance coverage. The affordability of health care services is one of the greatest barriers we face as a nation with regard to access to the health care system (Stoddard 1994). It is one of the main reasons that almost every presidential administration has introduced some sort of health care reform. These reforms include President Johnson's Medicare and Medicaid legislation; the attempts by Presidents Ford, Nixon, and Reagan to reduce government expenditures; and President Clinton's introduction of legislation to provide some type of health care coverage for all Americans. Access to and the affordability of health care services continues to be an issue that policymakers and private citizens must address.

Financial access to health care services is mostly assured by means of securing some form of health care insurance. Over the years health insurance has provided the means for individuals to access the health care system and for health care providers to collect payment for services rendered. For those under 65 years of age, private-employer-sponsored coverage is the most common source of health care insurance. In 1998, 194.7 million persons under 65 years of age, or over 81.6 percent of nonelderly Americans, belonged to employer-based health plans (Fronstin 2000). While the majority of non-elderly persons are covered through private insurance, Medicare provides coverage for people over 65, and Medicaid pays for services for those eligible to receive funds from the Temporary Assistance to Needy Families or the Supplemental Security Income program. The specifics of health insurance will be discussed in Chapter 6 of this text. The focus of this section is the growing problem of the **uninsured** and how it relates to accessing health care services.

How Many People Are Uninsured?

The number of individuals without health insurance has steadily increased over time (see Figure 2–1) despite government efforts to plug the gaps in insurance coverage through various programs (Kuttner 1999). According to a 1999 report from the Agency for Healthcare Research and Quality, the total number of uninsured persons in the first half of 1997 was 44.2 million nonelderly Americans, or 18.9 percent of those under 65 years of age (Vistnes and Zuvekas 1999). In a more recent report by Fronstin (2000), 43.9 million people under 65 years of age were uninsured, or 18.4 percent of the nonelderly population in 1998. There are a number of factors to consider when examining the increasing trend of uninsured persons. Two of these factors are the declining trend of employer-based insurance benefits (Mishel, Bernstei, and Schmitt 1998) and rising premium costs for those who have access through their employer as well as those who buy health insurance individually (Freudenheim 1998; Kilborn 1998).

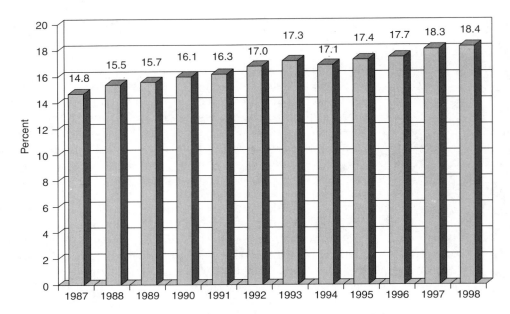

Figure 2–1.   Percent of Uninsured Nonelderly Americans, 1987–1998
Source: Employee Benefit Research Institute, Issue Brief Number 217, January 2000. Used
with permission.

Health insurance in the United States is tied to employment (Kuttner 1999),
but recent studies show that the number of Americans with employer-based health
care insurance has decreased over the last 10 years (Hoffman 1998). As outlined in
the Kaiser report on the uninsured, Hoffman suggests many plausible reasons for
this, including:

- The high and rising cost of health care service and insurance premiums (see
  Chapter 3).
- Shifts in the workplace to more low-income service sector jobs that do not
  offer health care insurance benefits.
- An increase in part-time jobs that have not historically offered health care
  insurance.
- A decrease in union activity.
- An increase in employees' contributions to their health benefits.

When discussing the number of people without health insurance, it is important to note that most statistics report the number of people without insurance on
any given day. This type of snapshot does not provide information on the number
of individuals who go through periods of time without any insurance. The Census
Bureau (1998) has estimated that 71.5 million Americans lacked insurance for at
least part of 1997. In a national survey that was conducted in 1997 for the Kaiser
Family Foundation and the Commonwealth Fund, researchers found that one of

every three adults between 18 and 64 were without health care insurance at some point in the previous two years (Schoen et al. 1998). These gaps in insurance coverage can be very problematic, especially if health services are needed during that time. One acute episode that requires medical attention (e.g., a limb fracture) can have far-reaching and devastating physical and financial effects on an individual.

Who Are the Uninsured?

This section examines the demographic makeup of people who are uninsured. In general, the majority of the uninsured are between the ages of 18 and 24, white, male, have lower incomes, and have at least one member of their family who works full-time. After examining these issues closer, we then discuss those at greatest risk for being uninsured.

In terms of age, almost everyone who is uninsured is under 65 years old because the elderly are receiving health care insurance under the Medicare program. Among those under 65 years of age, children are more likely than adults to have insurance coverage (Vistnes and Zuvekas 1999). This is in part due to the State Children's Health Insurance Program that Congress passed in 1997. As for adults, young adults aged 21–24 were the most likely not to have health care insurance (see Figure 2–2).

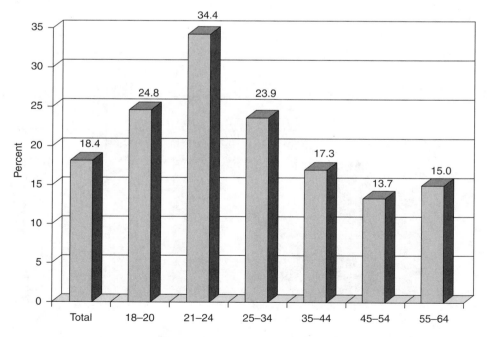

Figure 2–2.   Percentage of Nonelderly Uninsured Persons by Age, 1998
Source: Employee Benefit Research Institute, Issue Brief Number 217, January 2000. Used with permission

Over 34 percent of this age group did not have health care insurance in 1998 (Fronstin 2000). Fronstin also reported that more males did not have health care insurance than females during the same period, 21percent to 18.5 percent, respectively.

Race also appears to be associated with being uninsured (see Figure 2–3). Data indicate that there are significant disparities between the rate at which minorities are covered by health insurance as compared to white Americans. Though there are a far greater number of uninsured people that are white, Hispanics and African-Americans are disproportionately represented. Specifically, among those under age 65, over 37 percent of the Hispanic population and more than 23 percent of the African-American population are uninsured, while only 13.7 percent of the white population is without health care coverage (Fronstin 2000).

The link between income and health care insurance coverage is clear. Though public programs provide health insurance coverage for the poor, this is not universal. Among the nonelderly population, almost 36 percent of those below the poverty line lack insurance coverage (Fronstin 2000). Health insurance in the United States is closely tied to employment, but employment does not guarantee health insurance coverage. Indeed, studies have shown that many persons who are uninsured work. In 1997, 18 percent of the population that was employed did not have health care insurance (Vistnes and Zuvekas 1999). Those most at risk of being one of the working uninsured earned less than $20,000 per year, worked in small

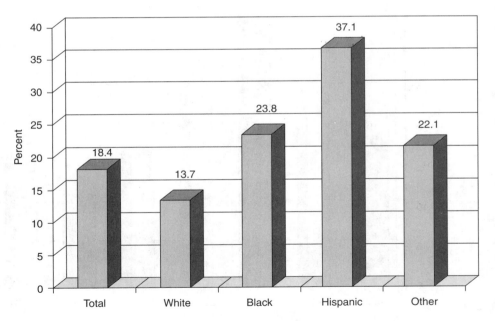

Figure 2–3. Percent of Nonelderly Uninsured Population by Race, 1998
Source: Employee Benefit Research Institute, Issue Brief Number 217, January 2000. Used with permission

businesses, and worked less than full-time (Fronstin 2000; Hoffman 1998). These findings are consistent with the findings of Fronstin (2000) shown in Figure 2–4.

Health Status and the Uninsured

Discussions of health care reform are often centered around the attainment of a sense of equity with regard to the delivery and accessibility of health care services (Seiden 1994). Currently, lack of insurance coverage results in large discrepancies between the health care services available to the insured and the uninsured. The amount and type of health care services that people who are uninsured can afford and obtain is severely limited. One common belief is that uninsured persons are able to get the medical care they need from doctors and hospitals, especially public hospitals. However, this is not supported in the literature.

Uninsured adults are reportedly four times more likely than insured adults to state that they did not receive care they believed was necessary (Hoffman 1998). In general, those who are uninsured are more likely to experience a reduction in access to health care services and more specifically a reduction of preventative services that may have an impact on health status (Franks, Clancey, and Gold 1993).

Davis, Rowland, Altman, Collins, and Morris (1995) showed that those without insurance were more likely to postpone seeking health care services compared to those with insurance coverage, 71 percent to 21 percent respectively. Moreover,

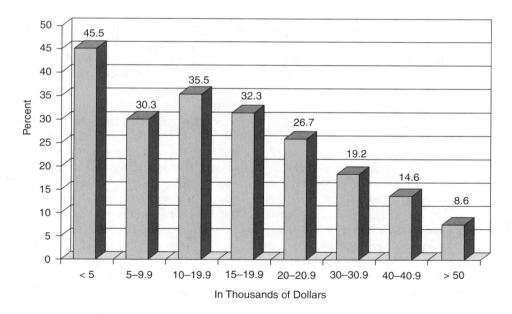

Figure 2–4.   Nonelderly Uninsured Americans by Family Income, 1998
Source: Employee Benefit Research Institute, Issue Brief Number 217, January 2000. Used with permission

34 percent of the uninsured population went without care because of financial reasons, as compared to only 7 percent of the insured population (Davis et al. 1995). Thus, the uninsured experienced an increase in avoidable hospitalizations and subsequent mortality independent of other risk factors in comparison to their insured counterparts (Franks et al. 1993). The postponement of seeking care can have catastrophic consequences. For example, Braveman, Schaaf, Egerter, Bennett, and Schecter (1994) found that uninsured patients with appendicitis were more likely to have their appendix rupture due to delaying surgical intervention than were insured patients.

People with no insurance or limited ability to pay out-of-pocket often receive care in public hospitals and clinics that provide care at greatly discounted rates or no cost at all. When the uninsured do get care, they are more likely to get it in the emergency department, where care is more expensive than in other ambulatory facilities (Spillman 1992), thus ultimately increasing the cost of health care. Because they receive the bulk of their care from the emergency department or other ambulatory care center, uninsured persons often do not have a regular source of health care. Having a regular doctor increases the continuity of services. One in five uninsured children and more than half of uninsured adults do not have a regular place or person where they receive care (Hoffman 1998).

Access to Therapists

Even when an individual has adequate health care insurance, access to health care practitioners may be limited. Historically, physicians have controlled access to physical and occupational therapy services. As will be discussed in Chapter 7, many insurers require those they insure to see a primary care doctor before visiting a specialist, including physical and occupational therapists. The primary care physician acts as a gatekeeper who must refer patients to more specialized care.

Both physical and occupational therapists are working to improve **direct access** to their services. Thus, patients would be able to bypass their primary care physician and go directly to a therapist. Providing patients with direct access to their services has been a goal of physical and occupational therapists for some time.

The current statement on this issue for the American Occupational Therapy Association (AOTA) states that referrals are not required for the provision of occupational therapy services. However, the AOTA maintains that occupational therapists must be aware of and adhere to the requirements of third-party payers, such as managed care organizations (American Occupational Therapy Association 2000).

Direct access to physical therapy services has been a major professional objective for the last two decades. Since regulation of health care providers is a state issue, this process has been long and arduous. Currently, 34 states permit direct access to physical therapy (see Table 2.3). Another thirteen states and the District of Columbia permit direct access only to a physical therapy evaluation. Three states prohibit patient contact with a physical therapist without a physician referral.

Table 2–3. States That Allow Direct Access to Physical Therapy Treatment or Evaluation

Treatment and Evaluation (with modifications in some states)	Evaluation Only	None
Alaska	Connecticut	Alabama
Arizona	Georgia	Indiana
Arkansas	Hawaii	Ohio
California	Kansas	
Colorado	Louisiana	
Delaware	Michigan	
Florida	Mississippi	
Idaho	Missouri	
Illinois	New Jersey	
Iowa	New York	
Kentucky	Oklahoma	
Maine	Pennsylvania	
Maryland	District of	
Massachusetts	Columbia	
Minnesota	Wyoming	
Montana		
Nebraska		
Nevada		
New Hampshire		
New Mexico		
North Carolina		
North Dakota		
Oregon		
Rhode Island		
South Carolina		
South Dakota		
Tennessee		
Texas		
Utah		
Vermont		
Virginia		
Washington		
West Virginia		
Wisconsin		

Adapted from: American Physical Therapy Association. Accessed October 2001 at *https://www.apta.org/pdfs/gov_affairs/directalaws.pdf*

Effects of Direct Access

The research evidence indicates that 9–12 percent of a physical therapist's practice may be by direct access. In a study of 1,580 patients with low back pain treated by 208 health care providers in North Carolina, Mielenz et al. (1997) reported that 12.6 percent of the patients received physical therapy through direct access. Additionally, one-third of responding physical therapists in Massachusetts used direct access, which accounted for 8.8 percent of their practice (Crout, Tweedie, and Miller 1998). In an early study of direct access to physical therapy, Domholdt and Durchholz (1992) reported that 45 percent of physical therapists utilized direct access, which accounted for 10.3 percent of their practice.

An argument against direct access to physical therapy services alleges that the cost and usage of therapy services both increase when there is no physician referral. However, recent evidence fails to demonstrate that direct access to physical therapy increases cost or utilization rates (Mitchell and deLissovy 1997).

Conclusion

Access to health care services is a complicated issue. Many interacting factors create an environment that promotes access to appropriate health care providers or, alternatively, places barriers in the way. Therapists must understand the many factors that influence access if they are to better help their patients navigate the barriers that make obtaining needed care more difficult.

CHAPTER REVIEW QUESTIONS

1. Recall the three foundational policy principles that define health policy.
2. Define predisposing factors, need factors, and enabling factors.
3. Define each of Penchansky and Thomas's five dimensions of access.
4. What is the relationship between health insurance and access to health care services?
5. Define the characteristics of the uninsured.
6. Describe the effect of direct access to therapy services on the cost and quality of health care.

CHAPTER DISCUSSION QUESTIONS

1. The development of a marketing plan for a therapy practice will benefit from a consideration of the principles of access. Discuss how you could use Penchansky and Thomas's model of access to determine whether to open a therapy practice.

2. Discuss how the unique American policy decision to support both private and public health insurance affects access to health care.
3. Is direct access to occupational and physical therapy essential? Do you think it will increase access for the population? Explain your answer.

REFERENCES

American Occupational Therapy Association (AOTA). 2000. Statement of occupational therapy referral (Approved 1994). AOTA FAX-on Request, FAX No. 907.

Barton, P. B. 1999. *Understanding the U. S. health services system.* Chicago: Health Administration Press.

Braveman, P., V. M. Schaaf, S. Egerter, T. Bennett, and W. Schecter. 1994. Insurance related differences in the risk of ruptured appendix. *N Engl J Med* 331(7):444–49.

Bureau of the Census. 1998. *Dynamics of economic well-being: Health insurance, 1993–1995.* Washington DC: Government Printing Office.

Crout K. L., J. H. Tweedie, and D. J. Miller. 1998. Physical therapists' opinions and practice regarding direct access. *Phys Ther* 78(1): 52–61.

Davis, K., D. Rowland, D. Altman, K. S. Collins, and C. Morris. 1995. Health insurance: The size and shape of the problem. *Inquiry* 32(2):196–203.

Domholdt, E. and A. G. Durchholz. 1992. Direct access use by experienced therapists in states with direct access. *Phys Ther* (8):569–74.

Franks, P., C. M. Clancey, and M. R. Gold. 1993. Health insurance and mortality. *JAMA* 270(6):737–41.

Freudenheim, M. 1998. Employees facing steep increases in health care. *New York Times,* November 27, A1.

Fronstin, P. 2000. *Sources of health insurance and characteristics of the uninsured: Analysis of the March 1999 current population survey.* Washington DC: Employment Benefit Research Institute (Issue brief no. 217).

Fuchs, V. R. 1993. National health insurance revisited. In *Debating health care reform: A primer from Health Affairs,* ed. J. K. Iglehart, 81–91. Bethesda MD: Project Hope.

Hoffman, C. 1998. *Uninsured in America: A chart book.* Kaiser Commission on Medicaid and the Uninsured. *http://www.kff.org.*

Kilborn, P. 1998. Premiums rising for individuals. *New York Times,* December 5, A7.

Kuttner, R. 1999. The American health care system: Health insurance coverage. *N Engl J Med* 340(2): 163–68.

Mielenz, T. J., T. S. Carey, D. A. Dyrek, B. A. Harris, J. M. Garrett, and J. D. Darter. 1997. Physical therapy utilization by patients with acute low back pain. *Phys Ther* (10):1040–51.

Mishel, L., J. Bernstein, and J. Schmitt. 1998. *The state of working America, 1998–99.* Washington DC: Economic Policy Institute.

Mitchell, J. M. and G. deLissovy. 1997. A comparison of resource use and cost in direct access versus physician referral episodes of physical therapy. *Phys Ther* 77(1): 10–18.

Penchansky, R. and J. W. Thomas. 1981. The concept of access: Definition and relationship to consumer satisfaction. *Med Care* 19(2):127–140.

Schoen, C., C. Hoffman, D. Rowland, K. Davis, and D. Altman. 1998. *Working families at risk: Coverage, access, cost and worries.* New York: Commonwealth Fund.

Seiden, D. J. 1994. Health care ethics. In *Health care delivery in the United States,* ed. A. R. Kovner 486–531. New York: Springer.

Short, P. F. and T. J. Lair. 1995. Health insurance and health status: Implications for financing health care reform. *Inquiry* 31(4): 425–37.

Spillman, B. C. 1992. The impact of being uninsured on utilization of basic health care services. *Inquiry* 29(4): 457–66.

Stoddard, J. J., R. F. St. Peter, and P. W. Newacheck. 1994. Health insurance status and ambulatory care for children. *N Engl J Med* 330(20):1421–25

Taylor, B. and A. Taylor. 1996. Social work with the transport disabled persons: A wayfinding perspective in health care. *Soc Work Health Care* 23(4): 3–19.

Vistnes, J. P. and S. H. Zuvekas. 1999. *Health insurance status of the civilian noninstitutionalized population: 1997.* MEPS Reseach Findings No. 8. AHRQ Pub. No. 99–0030. Rockville MD: Agency for Health Care Research and Quality.

Zuckerman, S., N. Brennan, J. Holahan, G. Kenny, and S. Rajan. 1999. *Snapshots of America's families: Variations in health care across states.* Washington DC: Urban Institute.

3

Economics/Cost of Health Care

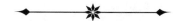

CHAPTER OBJECTIVES

At the conclusion of this chapter, the reader will be able to:

1.   Identify and discuss the major components of health care revenue in the United States.
2.   Discuss the major components of health care expenditures in the United States.
3.   Explain the economic, demographic, and systems reasons for the growth in health care costs.
4.   Discuss the effects of different payment mechanisms on health care costs.
5.   Compare and contrast the methods of financing for health care in the United States and several other countries.

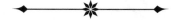

KEY WORDS: Capitation, Case Rate, Fee-for-Service, Financing, Global Budgeting, Gross Domestic Product, Markets

Introduction

As discussed in the preceding chapter, the major concepts used to describe health services in the United States are access, cost, and quality. This chapter focuses on the cost and economics of health care services. The goal of this chapter is to provide an overview of health care financing in the United States and not necessarily all the different complexities that may exist. We start with an overview of health care expenditures, where the money comes from and where it goes. After exploring the sources of revenues and expenses, we discuss the possible reasons for the unprecedented growth in health care spending, the role of government, and cost-containment mechanisms that have developed to slow the growth of health care spending here in the United States and internationally.

With both private and public resources developing a multitude of health care programs and health plans, the financing of medical care in the United States is very complex. The percentage of **gross domestic product** spent on health care represents millions of dollars in revenue for many businesses and industries (Foley 1993). Thus, the provision of health care services is big business. National health care expenditures in 1998 reached $1.1 trillion, which represented an increase of 5.6 percent from the previous year (Cowan et al. 1999). Translating this figure to a per person expense, health care spending reached a per capita level of $4,094. This level of spending represents 13.5 percent of the U.S. gross domestic product (GDP), or about one in seven dollars of all economic activity in the nation. Health care spending is expected to continue to grow into the foreseeable future. By 2008, it is estimated that health care expenditures will reach $2.2 trillion (Cowan et al. 1999).

Health Care Financing: Where It Comes From

As shown in Figure 3–1, in 1998, 54.5 percent of health care expenditures were funded by private sources, while public sources such as Medicare and Medicaid funded 45.5 percent of national health care spending (Cowan 1999). On the private side, private health insurance, obtained mostly through employers, accounted for just shy of 33 percent of expenditures, and out-of-pocket payments accounted for 17.4 percent. Out-of-pocket payments include payments for services not covered by private insurance as well as co-payments, co-insurance, and deductibles.

Private Health Insurance

Americans spent $375 billion for private health care insurance in 1998, representing an increase of 8.2 percent over the previous year, while the benefits paid during that time accounted for $337 billion, or a growth rate of 7.9 percent from 1997 (Cowan 1999). Managed care plans had generally kept premiums low during the mid-1990s. However, as profits began to wane and the cost of covering paid benefits increased, insurers raised premiums in 1998 (Meyer 1998; Mercer/Foster Higgins 1998).

An additional factor explaining the rising costs of private health insurance is consumer demand for more choices in their health care plans. A consumer backlash against restrictive managed care plans has resulted in an increase in enrollment in managed plans that tend to be less restrictive and offer patients more

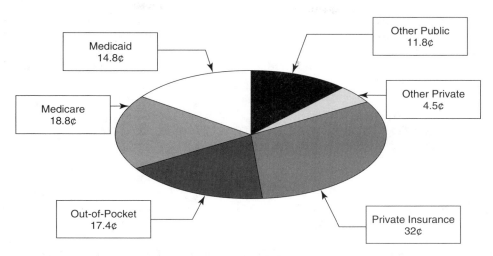

Figure 3–1. Where the Nation's Health Care Dollar Comes From
Source: C. A. Cowan et al. 1999, p. 159. Used with permission.

choice. However, in most cases health care plans offering more choice tend to be more expensive.

Medicare and Medicaid

Medicare spending for health care in 1998 grew to $216.6 billion, an increase of 2.5 percent, which was the slowest growth rate ever experienced by Medicare (Cowan 1999). The slower growth of Medicare spending is in large part due to mandates that were part of the Balanced Budget Act of 1997 (BBA). For example, efforts to control spending for free-standing and hospital-based skilled nursing facilities (SNF) worked to slow the growth of Medicare spending. This was accomplished by changing the method by which SNF services were reimbursed. Once paid on a cost-based reimbursement system, SNFs now are paid by a prospective-payment system that requires them to bundle the services they provide to be included in prospective payment. Also, the cracking down on fraud and abuse has helped to control the cost of Medicare spending. Efforts to detect and stop fraud and abuse have reportedly slowed these illegal activities (U.S. Government Accounting Office 1997). These and other mandates are discussed in more detail in Chapter 8.

Medicaid spending accounted for 14.8 percent of the total national health care expenditures, or $170.6 billion in 1998 (Cowan 1999). A number of policy changes in the Medicaid program have influenced Medicaid spending. Specifically, a decrease in the number of enrollees and an effort to enroll many Medicaid beneficiaries in managed care plans has reduced expenditures. A strong economy and welfare-to-work incentives provided by the Temporary Assistance to Needy

Families statute has also contributed to a decline in Medicaid enrollment (Cowan 1999). Additionally, through the BBA, states now have the ability to mandate enrollment in less expensive managed care plans without having to obtain a federal waiver. The Medicare and Medicaid programs are discussed in greater detail in future chapters.

Health Care Expenditures: Where It Goes

Figure 3–2 shows where health care expenditures went in 1998. Of the $1.1 trillion spent on health care, outpatient and inpatient hospital services accounted for one-third of all expenditures (Cowan et al. 1997). Hospital care, representing 33 percent of expenditures, is the largest single component of health care spending. The next largest component of expenditures is physician services, which account for 20 percent of the national expenditures. It is worth noting that though prescription drug costs accounted for less than 10 percent of all health care spending, these costs represented the largest increase in any category of spending, rising from 7.2 percent in 1997 to 7.9 percent in 1998.

Hospital Expenditures

Though the hospital sector is by far the largest consumer of health care spending, it has experienced a continual decrease in its share of national health care expenditures. Since 1993, when Medicare's prospective payment system was initiated, the

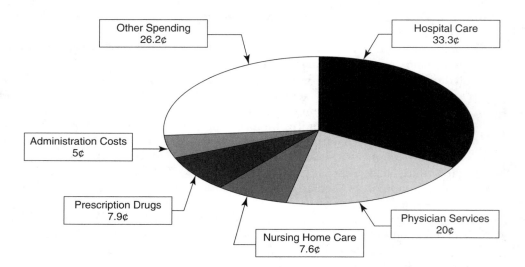

Figure 3–2.   Where the Nation's Health Care Dollar Goes
Source: C. A. Cowan et al. 1999, p. 179. Used with permission.

hospital share of national health expenditures has decreased from about 40 percent to 33 percent (Cowan et al. 1999). Incentives for hospitals to become more efficient in the delivery of care were introduced with the development of prospective
payment systems and managed care (Casey 1998). Many hospitals have responded
by forming strategic alliances with other hospitals and health care facilities to enhance their bargaining position with managed care organizations and become
more efficient (Luke, Olden, and Bramble 1998).

As payment incentives changed, community hospitals began to shift services
that once were considered inpatient services to outpatient departments. This has
resulted in outpatient revenue shares becoming an increasing portion of the community hospital's revenue. Outpatient revenues represent revenues generated by
outpatient departments, outpatient clinics, emergency departments, and hospital-
based home health agencies. In 1998, outpatient revenues represented 35.8 percent of total community hospital revenue (Cowan et al. 1999).

Physician Expenditures

As shown in Figure 3–2, physician expenditures in 1998 represented one-fifth of all
expenditures, or $229.5 billion. Since then, physician expenditure growth has in-
creased steadily, with private health insurance representing the major source of
this spending, 50.5 percent (Cowan et al. 1999). As more and more individuals became covered by health care insurance, the out-of-pocket share of physician expenditure has dropped off and private health insurance has accounted for most of the
spending. Private health insurance as a share of physician expenditures grew
steadily during the 1980s to the early 1990s, going from 37.9 percent to 50.5 percent. Since 1993 this rapid growth has stabilized, in large part because of the
greater number of enrollees in managed care plans (KPMG Peat Marwick 1998).

As more and more patients enrolled in managed care plans, physicians have
had to increase their participation in these plans. In 1998, 94 percent of physicians
had at least one managed care contract and 56 percent of their revenues resulted
from such contracts (Cowan 1996). This reliance on managed care and the introduction of other payment systems, such as Medicare's resource-based relative value
scale, have put increased pressures on physician incomes. Like hospitals, physicians are attempting to bolster their position with insurers by forming physician alliances and physician group practices (Burns et al. 2000; Gorey 1993).

Prescription Drug Expenditures

More than $90 billion was spent on prescription drugs in 1998, which was 15.4 per-
cent higher than the previous year and represents the highest growth rate relative
to other personal health categories (Cowan 1999). As a result, prescription drug
costs have received much attention in the ongoing debates regarding the Medicare
system. The reasons for the rapid increase in prescription drug use and spending
include increased consumer demand due to direct-to-consumer advertising, as well
as increases in the availability of pharmaceutical products and their ability to sub-

stitute for other forms of health care (Copeland 1999; Fine 1999). Though the rapid rise in prescription drug costs is alarming, some analysts believe that the use of prescription drugs is a more cost-effective way to treat certain conditions that would otherwise require more intense treatments, such as hospitalization (Copeland 1999; Strongin 1999).

Reasons for the Growth of Health Care Expenditures

As noted, health care expenditures in the United States have had almost uninterrupted growth over the past few decades. What factors are influencing this growth in expenditures? The list of potential reasons includes economic factors, demographic changes, and system factors (see Table 3–1). It is probably the complex interaction of all these factors and not one discrete event that has resulted in the growth of health care expenditures.

Economic reasons for the growth in health care spending include inflation, market structure, and insurance. Most experts would agree that of all the potential reasons, inflation (both general and medical care inflation) is the major driving force behind the increases in health care expenditures. Indeed, some researchers claim that inflation is responsible for up to 70 percent of the increase in expenditures (Levit et al. 1997). Health care markets are unique and different from other economic markets, such as commodity markets (Folland, Goodman, and Stano 1997). "Perfect" markets balance supply and demand at a price that is competitively determined by buyers and sellers in a marketplace. This marketplace has many informed buyers and sellers who exchange known economic resources. Buyers and sellers are free to enter and exit the market as conditions warrant. Perfect markets create competition that allows for the production of goods and services at an affordable price. Health care markets differ from perfect markets. As we discussed in Chapter 2, access to health care services is not uniform. As we will discuss in Chapters 8 and 9, price is not always competitively determined but rather is regulated and fixed. Consumers are often at an information disadvantage when making health care purchasing decisions. Providers are often prevented by regulation,

Table 3–1.   Reasons for Growth in Medical Care Expenditures

A. Economic
   1. Inflation
   2. Market structure
   3. Insurance
B. Demographic Change
C. System
   1. Provider behavior
   2. Technology

licensure, and tradition from entering high-cost markets in order to offer a comparable service at a lower cost. Finally, health care insurance has a unique effect on health care markets.

The role of health insurance is a major contributor to the growth in health care expenditures (Peden and Freeland 1995; Fuchs 1990). The protective role of health care insurance has acted to insulate consumers from the true costs of their health care purchases. Because of this, some observers cite market failure of health care insurance as a major cause of expenditure growth. In sum, inflation, market structure, and health insurance have prevented the forces of competition from working to restrain the growth of health care costs.

Demographic effects also play a role. As the baby boom generation ages, the elderly population (i.e., those over 64) will grow from just under 32 million in 1993 to an estimated 78.9 million in the year 2050 (Anzick 1993). The elderly population, due to the increase in the incidence of sickness with age, accounts for a large portion of health care expenditures. For example, studies show that persons over 75 have twice as many contacts with their health care provider as persons between the ages of 25 and 44 (U.S. Department of Health and Human Services 1991). Additionally, the same patients have more than five times as many hospital days than their younger counterparts (Health Insurance Association of America 1992). An aging population results in higher utilization and cost of health care.

System factors that affect growth in health care costs include administrative bureaucracy, provider behaviors, and the American affinity for high-technology health care. The complexity of administrating the multi-payer health care system has added to the growth rate of health care expenditures in this country. Woolhandler and Himmelstein (1991) compared the administrative costs for hospital, physician, and nursing services in Canada with those in the United States and found that on a per capita basis the United States spent significantly more on administrative costs than the single-payer system in Canada. However, it should be noted that others have stated that only a limited amount of savings might be achieved with a single-payer system in the United States, and it would not result in dramatic savings in total expenditures (Schwartz and Mendelson 1994).

Inefficiency is not only a result of complex administrative systems, but also a product of provider behavior. Some of the abuse is a result of physicians practicing "defensive medicine" in order to protect themselves from costly legal actions. The practice of defensive medicine is an expenditure-increasing activity, and some analysts believe that major savings would be produced if it could be stopped (Fuchs 1990). Again, others report that malpractice reform would only result in savings of $8 million annually, a small fraction of the total health care expenditures (Schwartz and Mendelson 1994). As we will discuss shortly, incentives in payment mechanisms also have powerful effects on provider utilization of health care services and overall costs. Finally, the American fascination with high-technology health care has resulted in the identification and treatment of more disorders (Sultz and Young 1999). The costs of delivering this technology are associated with higher overall costs to the system.

Efforts to Contain Health Care Expenditures

As a percentage of GDP, national health care spending has remained relatively stable over the last six years. This slower growth is in contrast to annual growth rates that exceeded 10 percent in the past and provided the stimulus for many cost-containment efforts and health care reform proposals (Levit et al. 1997).

Accounting for the slowing cost growth rates are the fundamental changes that are occurring in the health care delivery system. Managed care plans that control utilization of services and market factors that have allowed purchasers of health insurance to negotiate directly with providers have both contributed to the decline in the growth rate of national health care expenditures. Additionally, restrictions imposed by prospective payment programs and other restrictive fee schedules have slowed expenditure growth (Levit et al. 1997). The following sections briefly explain the various payment mechanisms for health care providers and the incentives that each of these mechanisms has created.

Payment Mechanism for Health Care Providers

Four major payment structures are discussed in this section: (1) fee-for-service, (2) case-based, (3) capitation, and (4) global budgeting. All four of these payment systems are currently used in the U.S. health care system (Reinhart 1993). Their basic features are summarized in Table 3–2.

After World War II, the increase in indemnity health insurance and the introduction of Medicare and Medicaid created a formal payment system for health care providers. While hospitals were paid either on a per day or a per stay basis, the primary payment mechanism for physicians was known as **fee-for-service** (FFS). This entailed charging the patient a separate fee for each service provided by the physician. If the patient had health care insurance, the insurer paid this fee either in full or at least in part. Some of the FFS charges depended on the physician's specialty and geographic region. Thus, variation existed in the charges for certain services across physicians. For this reason, some payers began to institute a more

Table 3–2. Characteristics/Incentives of Payment Mechanisms

Payment Mechanism	*Characteristics*	*Incentive on Risk/Costs*
Fee-for-service	Provider paid for each procedure rendered	Highest utilization/costs All risk borne by payer
Case rate	Provider paid for each episode of care	Shared risk with payer
Capitation	Provider paid flat rate	All risk borne by provider
Global budgeting	Flat, all-inclusive budget	Known, capped costs

uniform payment system that was still fee-for-service, but based on usual, customary, and reasonable charges for a given area.

This payment mechanism creates an incentive for providers to add additional days or tests. For example, physicians may add a test that will have results that are interesting but not essential. Similarly, hospitals may be inclined to keep a patient an extra day "just to be sure" it is safe and the patient is ready to leave the hospital. In this payment system, the patient bears all of the financial risk while the provider has no risk at stake. In cases when patients have health insurance, this payment mechanism drives up expenditures. Patients are not fiscally responsible because their insurance is handling all payment claims. Several observers have cited the inflationary effect of this type of payment structure (Reinhardt 1994).

As the shortfalls of the fee-for-service payment mechanism were exposed, alternative payment structures began to emerge. One of these changes was the enactment by Medicare in 1983 of a change from a fee-for-service payment system for hospitals to a **case-based payment.** This reimbursement system shifted payment from a retrospective reimbursement system to a prospective payment system (see Chapter 8). Reimbursement was predetermined based on the patient's diagnosis. This diagnostic-related group (DRG) payment system provided one payment for all services relating to a given diagnosis instead of paying separately for all the different services used in treating the patient. The DRG payment schedule included adjustments based on the teaching status of the hospital, its geographic location, and outlier cases (i.e., patients whose treatments significantly exceeded the norm). The incentive created by DRG payments was for hospitals to use resources more efficiently and avoid unnecessary procedures in treating patients. Prospective payment systems are a major part of financing health care services in the public and private sectors.

The third payment mechanism, the flat fee per patient per month is a feature of some types of health maintenance organizations. This payment mechanism is known commonly as **capitation.** In this payment system, providers are paid a monthly fee for each patient enrolled in their practice. If the cost of treating a patient is less than the capitation, greater profits are realized; however, if a patient's care is more than the monthly capitation, the health care provider loses money. This creates an incentive for the physician to keep the patient well to avoid costly care and thus keep most of the capitation as profit.

Global budgeting, the fourth payment mechanism, is used primarily for hospitals. It is used extensively in Canada for hospital care. Provinces provide a predetermined amount to the hospital to cover all of its operational expenses.

Health Care Financing: An International Comparison

Due to the shortcomings in financing the U.S. health care system, many researchers have looked at the health care systems in Canada and Western Europe as potential solutions to the American dilemma of how to pay for the nation's health care system (Danzon 1992; Hurst 1991). In this section, we explore the financing structure of some of these health care systems and how they differ from the financing structure of the U.S. system.

Although the United States does not have a national health care system, the role of the government in the financing of health care services is of major importance. As mentioned earlier in this chapter, the government, through a combination of public programs, most notably Medicare and Medicaid, accounts for more than 45 percent of health care expenditures. The government's outlays for health care services include support for U.S. Public Health Service hospitals, the Indian Health Service, Veterans Affairs hospitals, Department of Defense hospitals and health services, and various public health activities. Although the government accounts for a large portion of health care expenditures, it is important to remember that this does not constitute a national health care system. Additionally, the government works on a vendor-purchaser relationship. For example, in the Medicare program the government contracts with hospitals and other health care providers, whereas in Great Britain the government is both the payer and the operator of the health care system.

In terms of magnitude, Medicare reflects the government's biggest source of financing. Though Medicare is discussed in detail later in this book, we introduce some of its aspects now. Since Medicare's inception in 1965, Medicare spending has surpassed government projections for reasons that include the growing elderly population, growing hospital payroll expenses, and growing utilization of more expensive treatments using advanced medical technology (Sultz and Young 1999). Throughout the years, the government has made significant changes to the Medicare program, many of which were efforts to contain rising costs.

The other large government program is Medicaid. Unlike Medicare, Medicaid was designed as a jointly administered federal and state program to provide basic health care services to qualified members of the indigent population. Like Medicare, Medicaid has also experienced a rapid rise in costs. The reasons for this rapid rise include growth in the covered population, increases in payment rates, advances in medical technology, and an increase in those needing intense or long-term services. In response, states have tried numerous ways to control the rising costs, such as utilization reviews, prospective payment systems, and prepaid managed care approaches (Sultz and Young 1999).

Canada's 13 provinces and territories have separate plans that differ significantly with regard to the fee schedules used to pay providers. Though the provinces have different payment schedules, there is a single government-operated provincial health plan that is the sole payer for hospital and physician services in all provinces and territories (Savage, Hoelsher, and Walker 1999). Personal and corporate income taxes as well as a payroll tax, nonfederal sales and property taxes, and federal customs and excise taxes provide the money for the federal and provincial portions of health care expenditures (Neuschler 1990). In 1996, Canada spent 9.2 percent of its gross domestic product on health care, or U.S. $2,002 per capita.

Unlike the United States, Sweden finances health care almost entirely through the public sector. Employers pay a general social insurance tax for each employee that, in part, goes to pay health insurance that covers ambulatory care, prescription costs, and lost wages due to illness. The majority of physicians in Sweden are public employees who work in primary care settings and are paid on a salary basis (Saltman 1990). The percentage of Sweden's gross domestic product devoted to health care expenditures is 7.2 percent, or $1,405 per capita.

The entire population of the United Kingdom is offered comprehensive care funded through general taxation. District hospital authorities, serving populations of about 250,000, act as the sole purchaser of health care services and administrators of physician contracts. Hospitals operate as free-standing facilities and compete, along with other health care providers, for contracts from the district hospital authority. Providers are accountable for the efficient and effective practice of medicine. Clinical managers, with the help of senior nurses and business managers, are responsible for the operating budgets of hospital departments (Day and Klein 1991; Enthoven 1991). The United Kingdom spends 6.9 percent of its gross domestic product on health care, or $1,304 per capita.

The purpose of this discussion was not to draw any conclusions about appropriate spending levels on health care or which method for financing a country's health care needs is best. Purposely omitted from this discussion were issues regarding quality of care. Methods of financing health care reflect broad social philosophies about the responsibility for people who are sick, injured, or disabled. As illustrated in these brief overviews, the organization and payment mechanisms of a health care system can have a large effect on the cost of health care services.

Conclusion

Devising a health care financing system that will distribute a finite set of resources in a way that is acceptable to health care professionals, employers, and consumers is a never-ending challenge for health care policymakers. Add to this challenge concerns about patient safety, quality of care, and improved quality of life, and the problem becomes more complex and compelling. All one can safely say is that approaches to financing health care will continually change. In the near future, the health care industry's response to managed care and other market forces will probably dictate how the United States pays for its health care.

In this chapter, we have discussed the extent of the United States health care economy and the forces that affect the size and growth of the system. About $1 trillion is spent on health care each year in the United States. This is anticipated to grow to more than $2 trillion before the end of the first decade of the twenty-first century. Changing demographics, inflation, market structure, insurance, provider behavior, and technology are among the factors that affect the cost of health care. A number of mechanisms have been used to create incentives to control costs, with mixed effects. The dualistic nature of financing the system creates a unique system for the United States in comparison to other industrialized nations. In Chapter 4, we will address the concept of quality and how this issue affects the nature of health care policy and the system.

CHAPTER REVIEW QUESTIONS

1. Identify the percentage of U.S. health care spending that comes from public sources and private sources.
2. What is the largest single category of U.S. health care spending? The next-largest?
3. What category of U.S. health care spending had the greatest rate of inflation in the late 1990s?
4. Identify three reasons for rising health care costs in the United States.
5. Define fee-for-service, flat fee per medical case, flat fee per person, and global budgeting. What is the effect of each of these payment systems on health care costs?
6. Define prospective and retrospective payment systems and their role in health care cost containment.
7. Review how health care is paid for in Canada, Sweden, and Great Britain. How do these systems differ from the systems that finance health care in the United States?

CHAPTER DISCUSSION QUESTIONS

1. The United States is the only major industrialized democracy without a system of national health care insurance. How would the development and implementation of national health care insurance in the United States affect the cost of health care?
2. It is estimated that more costs of health care may be transferred to the consumer from the employer/government in the form of higher premiums, deductibles, and co-payments. What would the effect of these changes be on the growth of the costs of health care? On occupational therapists and physical therapists?
3. Discuss the incentives of fee-for-service and capitated payment systems on the cost of health care. How do these systems promote or inhibit access to care?
4. Americans spend more money on specialized, high-technology medical care than people in other countries. This decision may affect the availability of resources for other worthwhile social goals (e.g., education, transportation). What effect do you believe this policy decision may have on persons with disabilities or with other forms of medically stable, chronic diseases?

REFERENCES

Anzick, M. 1993. Demographics and employment shifts: Implications for benefits and economic security. *EBRI Issue Brief* No. 140. Washington DC: Employee Benefit Research Institute.

Burns, L. R., G. J. Bazzoli, L. Dynan, and D. R. Wholey. 2000. Impact of HMO market structure on physician-hospital alliances. *Health Serv Res* 35(1 pt. 1):101–132.

Casey, M. 1998. Hospital mergers: Where have they gone? *Medical Industry Today*. Accessed at *http://www.medicaidata.com/mit.*

Copeland, C. 1999. Prescription drugs: Issues of cost, coverage, and quality. *EBRI Issue Brief* No. 208:1–21.

Cowan, C. A., H. C. Lazenby, A. B. Martin, P. A. McDonnell, A. L. Sensenig, J. M. Stiller, L. S. Whittle, K. A. Kotova, M. A. Zezza, C. S. Donham, A. M. Long, and M. W. Stewart. 1999. National health care expenditures, 1998. *Health Care Fin Rev* 21(2):165–210.

Danzon, P. M. 1992. Hidden overhead costs: Is Canada's system less expensive? *Health Affairs* 11(1):21–43.

Day, P. and R. Klein. 1991. Britain's health care experiment. *Health Affairs* 19(3): 22–38.

Enthoven, A. C. 1991. Internal market reform of the British health services. *Health Affairs* 10(3):60–70.

Fine, A. 1999. Increased direct-to-consumer advertising driving pharmaceutical costs, trends. *Executive Solutions for Healthcare Management* 2(1):2–3.

Foley, J. D. 1993. The role of the health care sector in U.S. economy. *EBRI Issue Brief* No. 142. Washington DC: Employee Benefits Research Institute.

Folland, S., A. C. Goodman, and M. Stano. 1997. *The economics of health and health care.* 2nd ed. Upper Saddle River NJ: Prentice Hall.

Fuchs, V. 1990. The health sector's share of the gross national product. *Science* 247(4942):534–38.

Gorey, T. M. 1993. Physician organizations and physician-hospital organizations. *Mich Med* 92(9):34–38.

Hurst, J. W. 1991. Reforming health care in seven European nations. *Health Affairs* 10(3):7–21.

KPMG Peat Marwick. 1998. *Health benefits in 1998.* Montvale NJ.

Levit, K. R., H. C. Lazenby, B. R. Braden, C. A. Cowan, A. L. Sensenig, P. A. McDonnell, J. M. Stiller, D. K. Won, A. B. Martin, M. L. Savarajan, C. S. Donham, A. M. Long, and M. W. Stewart. 1997. National health care expenditures, 1996. *Health Care Fin Rev* 19(1):161–200.

———, H. C. Lazenby, and L. Sivarajan. 1996. National health expenditures, 1994. *Health Care Fin Rev* 17(3):205–42.

Mercer/Foster Higgins. 1998. *National survey of employer-sponsored health plans, 1998.* New York: Mercer/Foster Higgins.

Meyer, M. 1998. Oh no, here we go again. *Newsweek* 44–47, December 14.

Moser, J. 1999. *Recent development in physician income: Physician socioeconomic characteristics 1999–2000.* Chicago: American Medical Association.

Neuschler, E. 1990. *Canadian health care: The implication of public health insurance.* Washington DC: Health Insurance Association of America.

Peden, E. A. and M. S. Freeland. 1995. A historical analysis of medical spending growth, 1960–1993. *Health Affairs* 14(2):235–47.

Reinhardt, U. E. 1993. Reorganizing the financial flows in American health care. *Health Affairs* 12:172–93.

————.1994. Planning the nation's workforce: Let the market in. *Inquiry* 31(3): 250–63.

Saltman, R. B. 1990. Competition and reform in the Swedish health system. *Health Care Fin Rev* 68(4): 597–618.

Savage, G. T., M. L. Hoelscher, and E. W. Walker. 1999. International health care: A comparison of the United States, Canada, and Western Europe. In *Health Care Administration: Planning, Implementing and Managing Organized Delivery Systems*, 3d ed., ed. L. F. Wolper, 3–52. Gaithersburg MD: Aspen Publishers.

Schwartz, W. B. and D. M. Mendelson. 1994. Eliminating waste and inefficiency can do little to contain costs. *Health Affairs* 13(1):224–38.

Scott, M. 1999. New drugs, managed care use pushes up prescription drug costs. Analyst Report. *Employee Benefit Plan Review.*

Strongin, R. 1999. The ABCs of PBMs. *Health Policy Forum Issue Brief No 749,* Washington DC: George Washington University.

Sultz, H. A. and K. M. Young. 1999. *Health care USA: Understanding its organization and delivery,* 2d ed. Gaithersburg MD.: Aspen Publishers.

U.S. General Accounting Office. 1997. Nursing homes: Too early to assess new efforts to control fraud and abuse. Publication No. GAO/T-HEHS-97-114. Washington DC: Government Printing Office.

U.S. Department of Health and Human Services. 1991. Current estimates from the National Health Interview Survey, 1990. Vital and Health Statistics, Series 10, No. 181. Washington DC: U.S. Government Printing Office.

Woolhander, S. and D. Himmelstein. 1991. The deteriorating administrative efficiency of the U.S. health care system. *N Engl J Med* 324(18): 1253–58.

4

Quality of Health Care

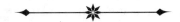

CHAPTER OBJECTIVES

At the conclusion of this chapter, the reader will be able to:

1. Define current challenges to the quality of health care in the United States.
2. Compare and contrast the population-based and personal-based conceptualizations of health care quality.
3. Describe the following basic components of a quality health care system:
    a. Adequate structure
    b. Effective processes
    c. Satisfactory outcomes
4. Review the mechanisms of measuring and reporting on the quality of the health care system:
    a. Peer review
    b. Accreditation
    c. Report cards
5. Discuss the legal foundations for quality in the health care system:
    a. Professional regulation
    b. Patient rights
    c. Medical negligence

KEY WORDS   Accreditation, Clinical Practice Guideline, Medical Negligence, Outcomes, Patient's Bill of Rights, Peer Review, Process, Professional Regulation, Standards, Structure

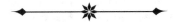

Introduction

Quality is the third foundational principle of health policy. As already explained, health policy establishes access to and finances the health care system. People and society want access to and are willing to pay only for a high-quality health care system. In this chapter, we will explore the meaning of quality health care. Recent studies have pointed out serious deficiencies in the health care system, such as the high rate of medical error (Institute of Medicine 1999). Depending on one's perspective, Americans are either receiving the highest-quality health care in the world or are not getting an adequate return on quality from the most expensive health care system in the world.

We will also discuss the basic components of a quality personal health care system: structure, process, and outcomes. We will introduce methods to measure the quality of each of these components. Finally, we will review the basic foundation of quality: the legal rights of patients to be protected and informed when interacting with the health care system.

Challenges to Health Care Quality

Physical therapists and occupational therapists are among the many professional and nonprofessional health care providers dedicated to quality patient care. To many observers, the United States has the finest and most technologically sophisticated health care system in the world. As we discussed in the preceding chapter, the United States devotes more public and private resources to health care than any other nation. Although this condition is not universal or uniform, most Americans have access to a safety net of health care services. The United States is a recognized leader in health professional education and research through a strong network of academic medical centers. New innovations are supported by this research, and many patients have benefited from such advances as organ transplantation, minimally invasive surgery, and joint replacements. Unlike the situation facing much of the world's population, rehabilitation services and long-term care are provided for insured persons and families faced with chronic disease and illness. The burden of long-term care is not borne solely by the extended family.

The emphasis in the last ten years on slowing the growth of health care expenditures, discussed in Chapter 3, has not been without adverse consequences on health care quality. Of most concern is the rate of serious errors being made in the system. In November 1999, the Institute of Medicine released *To Err Is Human: Building a Safer Health System,* a major report on the quality of health care in the United States. This report found that 44,000 deaths annually in the United States could be attributed to medical error. The report attributed more deaths to medical error than to highway accidents, breast cancer, or AIDS. A recent study of medical errors in Utah and Colorado found that nearly 5 percent of per person health care costs were spent on medical error cases, more than expenditures for HIV/AIDS

(Thomas et al. 1999). Of concern to physical therapists and occupational therapists, falls have been identified as one of the most common forms of adverse event experienced by elderly patients (Thomas and Brennan 2000; Rothschild, Bates, and Leape 2000). Most of these errors were attributed to the design of the health care system and not to individual provider practices (Leape 1997; Casarett and Helms 1999).

Continued work is needed to study and improve not just individual provider behavior but the decisions of many providers who work in an increasingly complex health care system. In 2001, the Institute of Medicine released *Crossing the Quality Chasm: A New Health System for the 21st Century.* This report advocates a redesign of the health care system to bolster the clinical information infrastructure, encourages the use of evidence-based practice by clinicians, and calls for the inclusion of clinical quality indicators as well as cost efficiency measures in determining the system's functioning. A second concern with the quality of the health care system has been the finding of regional differences in the utilization of expensive services without a corresponding difference in patient outcomes.

In 1989, Wennberg et al. reported significant differences in hospital utilization and mortality rates between Boston and New Haven for several surgical procedures. The lower utilization of hospital care in New Haven was not associated with an increased rate of mortality. In fact, mortality rates in Boston were significantly higher. This study has led other researchers to find similar discrepancies in the medical treatment offered to patients based on provider preferences, geographic variations, or socioeconomic factors, not medical reasons. Unlike pharmacological therapy, the outcomes of many medical and surgical procedures have not been well demonstrated, nor have the procedures themselves been closely peer-reviewed for evidence of effectiveness (Wennberg 1990; Wennberg 1998; Birkmeyer et al. 1998; Fisher et al. 2000). The same statement can be made for many rehabilitation interventions. These studies point out that many interventions have been based on tradition and individual provider decision-making. When evaluated in the light of evidence, it is clear that the quality of some interventions is markedly better than others.

Besides these concerns with error rates and the need for greater use of evidence-based practice paradigms, the health care system has been defined as a "1 trillion dollar industry without a definition of its product" (Kindig 1998). This comment is made by critics of the current health care system who point out that the health status of Americans is overall not better, and may be worse, than that of citizens in other nations who expend considerably less per person on health care. Policymakers, consumers, payers, and health care workers are confronting the problem of determining the expectations of a health care system that has grown to consume a large percentage of the nation's resources and economic output. They are asking the logical question: What are we receiving for this large investment in the health care system?

The gap in the health status of some citizens in the United States as compared to citizens in other industrialized nations has been well documented. Table 4–1 presents the findings of Starfield (2000), who concluded that the American

**Table 4–1.   Public Health Status of the United States Compared
to 13 Other Industrialized Nations**

A. Percentage of children born with low birth weight—13th
B. Overall neonatal and infant mortality—13th
C. Postneonatal mortality rate—11th
D. Years of potential life lost—13th
E. Life expectancy of a 1-year-old infant—11th if female, 12th if male
F. Life expectancy of a 15-year-old person—10th if female, 12th if male
G. Life expectancy of an 80-year-old person—3rd
H. Age-adjusted mortality rate—10th

Source: B. Starfield, Is U. S. health really the best in the world? (2000).

people "do not have anywhere near the best health in the world." As can be seen
by reviewing the results in the table, the United States ranks near the bottom in
basic indicators of public health for infants and young children, but near the top
of the public health rankings for the elderly population. Eliminating the traditional, population-based reasons of smoking, alcohol abuse, violence, and diet as
the cause of these discrepancies, Starfield points to social policy and health system
factors as being primarily responsible for the poor health status of Americans compared to people living in Canada or Western Europe. Poverty, a poorly developed
primary care delivery system, and medical errors occurring within the health care
system are identified as major causes of the gap in the health status of Americans
compared to their economic peer group. A deliberate investment in health care
for older Americans has resulted in improved health status. Social problems and
lack of access to primary care for women and children has resulted in poor health
for many of these Americans.

The issue of quality of the health care system is important to all Americans.
Does the health care system in the United States deliver a high-quality product?
How can we improve the quality of health care in America? The answers to these
questions are partly based on how one defines quality health care. In the next section, we will explore different ideas about what constitutes quality health care.

Perspectives on Health Care Quality

There are two fundamental paradigms with which to analyze the quality of health
care services in the United States: one is personal-based, and the other,
population-based. Each of these perspectives is influenced by the structure of the
current system, contemporary social expectations, and legal mandates to assure
quality health care. The personal-based perspective focuses on the patient-provider
relationship and the organization, delivery, and outcome of the services patients
receive. It is the perspective used most commonly by physical therapists, occupational therapists, and other providers. The population-based perspective analyzes

health care quality by examining the experiences and health status of populations and subgroups. The roots of the population-based perspective of health care quality can be traced to the public health philosophy (see Chapter 14). A definition of quality from this perspective includes not only medical care, but also socioeconomic status and the community environment. Table 4–2 compares and contrasts the population-based and personal-based concepts of quality.

The incorporation of a population-based quality perspective into the definition and measurement of the quality of the personal health care system is still evolving. One challenge in using the population-based perspective in the personal health care system is the need to develop a workable definition of quality. Providers are very used to considering and measuring health care quality in terms of the patient's experience within the personal health care system (e.g., hospitals, clinics, nursing homes). Population-based quality challenges providers to consider the patient's health both inside and, more important, outside the personal health care system. Health status and quality of life are critical concepts from the population-based quality perspective.

According to Dijkers (1999), quality of life is an important concept in population-based quality discussions but it is not clear what part(s) of the concept can be practically measured, given the current technology in quality assessment. Kindig (1998) notes that "population health" includes health and function and is affected not only by medical care but by socioeconomic status, the environment, and public health. Wan, Counte and Cella (1997) describe health-related quality of life as "a multidimensional construct that includes an individual's physical, functional, emotional and social well being relative to their actual and anticipated levels of functioning." These definitions of health broaden the traditional perspective of how to consider and measure the quality of services rendered to improve health care quality. These definitions are important to physical therapists, and occupational therapists, since the quality of life of persons with chronic disease and disability (and services for them) are often affected by nonmedical issues. In the future, therapists will need to develop and utilize measurements of the quality of rehabilitation interventions in both medical and nonmedical environments.

Table 4–2. Population-Based vs. Personal-Based Concepts of Health Care Quality

	Population-based	*Personal-based*
Theoretical Model	Public health	Medical
Key Components	Quality of life/health status	Patient-provider interaction
	Function	Structure, process, outcome
	Satisfaction	Satisfaction
How to measure?	Survey, interview	Peer review, accreditation
	Community-based	Within the health care system

For patients with chronic diseases and disabilities, the quality of their health entails much more than medical care. This is a challenge for occupational therapists and physical therapists. The population-based quality perspective needs to be increasingly used to determine the effectiveness of services for persons with temporary or permanent disabilities. As we will discuss later, outcomes and comparative databases currently provide a rich source of information for therapists to use when determining the quality of their interventions. However, the full utilization of population-based quality assessment in rehabilitation situations awaits an accepted definition of quality and the development of the methods to measure population-based quality standards.

A personal-based perspective is the more traditional view of what constitutes quality health care. This perspective is most common to the administration and practice of a physical therapy or occupational therapy practice. For example, the Institute of Medicine (1990) defines quality of health care as "the degree to which health services for individuals and populations increase the likelihood of desired health outcomes and are consistent with current professional knowledge." In contrast to population-based perspectives, this definition focuses on services: providers, organizations, processes, and knowledge. To further illustrate this perspective, Table 4–3 lists "seven pillars of quality" as defined by Avedis Donabedian (1990), a seminal thinker on the quality of the health care system. The quality of most clinical care prior to the age of managed care was defined and measured as to its acceptability, effectiveness, and efficacy. Today, in the cost-restraint period of health care, quality health care must also be efficient, optimal, legitimate, and equitable. Quality health care is no longer measured only in terms of the patient-provider relationship, irrespective of broader social concerns. Instead, quality health care must also be viewed as socially acceptable from a cost and justice perspective.

Both of these perspectives on quality health care are affected by the legal mandates to assure high-quality health care services. The tort system of law affects the ability of the system to measure and improve quality. Provider-caused medical error and negligent practice are harms that are remediated in the courts. Licensure and other forms of regulation ensure a base level of provider capability to

Table 4–3.   Seven Pillars of Quality Health Care

A. Efficacy—the best care provided under the best circumstances
B. Effectiveness—the best care provided under ordinary, everyday circumstances
C. Efficiency—care that considers the relationship of cost to the amount of improvement in health.
D. Optimality—care that is the best value between cost and amount of improvement in health
E. Acceptability—care that is accessible and meets patient preferences.
F. Legitimacy—care that meets societal perspectives of optimal services.
G. Equity—care that is fair and just for all people.

Source: A. Donabedian, The seven pillars of quality (1990).

serve the public and protect it from harmful practices. The law also establishes fundamental rights for patients in their interactions with the system. The basis for all of these governmental actions is the expectation that providers have a responsibility to provide the best care for the patients they serve.

Most health care providers—hospitals, nursing homes, clinics, individual providers—measure, assure, and improve quality based on a personal-based perspective of the meaning of quality. This is reinforced by legal mandates that hold providers accountable for their actions. The managed care revolution in health care financing has introduced population-based perspective on quality of health care services. This perspective forces a social perspective on utilization of resources into the patient-provider interaction.

The current discussion regarding the quality of health care in America was stimulated by the need to restrain the growth in health care costs. It is in some ways a struggle between the two competing perspectives on the quality of health services in America. Armstead and Leong (1999) illustrate the emerging challenge to the traditional, personal-based understanding of quality health care that is accepted by many health care providers: "The definition of the term 'quality' continues to be centered on health care providers and not the health of the community. Instead of only viewing health plan members as recipients of medical care services, health plans should also view members as a population group with subpopulations within them, needing both medical and nonmedical services to improve their health." This definition calls for the measurement and assurance of quality of health care not only by providers but also by health plans, that is, insurers. This statement reflects an initiative by payers to measure quality for themselves, something traditionally performed only by providers with direct treatment responsibilities. As we will discuss later, quality measurement by health plans typically focuses on the population-based perspective of quality, in contrast to the personal-based perspective held by many providers.

First, however, we will introduce in more detail the concept of personal-based quality and how it is measured and assessed. In the next sections, we will introduce and explore each component of Donabedian's model to determine the quality of health care. In addition, we will introduce accreditation, the predominant method of assuring quality in the health care system today. Finally, we will also discuss the legal issues that affect quality of health care: provider regulation, patient rights, and medical negligence.

Structure, Process, and Outcome

In 1966, Avedis Donabedian put forth a template that is widely accepted today as the basis for understanding the framework of quality in the health care system (see Figure 4–1). This template has three components: **structure, process,** and **outcomes.** Structure comprises the permanent features of the health care system—hospitals and the various health care providers. Process is the method of delivery of care. Outcomes are the results of the health care encounter. Over the years, the

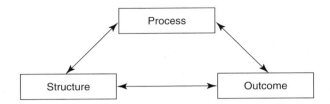

Figure 4–1.   Donabedian Quality of Health Care Framework

definition and measurement of quality have steadily developed from an initial focus on structure, then on how health care is delivered (process), to outcomes. Today, outcomes are very important to the examination of the quality of health care in America (e.g. medical error rates and functional outcomes). Let us consider each of these components of health care quality separately. The basic features of structure, process, and outcome are displayed in Table 4–4.

Structure

Structure is the basic foundation of the health care system. It comprises the services and the organization of the health care system, and as such is closely related to the health policy principle of access. A quality system has to have the physical and human resources with which to deliver services at locations that can be accessed by the public it serves. If a location or region lacks the facilities or provider types to provide appropriate care, it is defined as "medically underserved"; in other words, it lacks a proper structure to meet the needs of the population it serves. The Health Resources Services Administration (2000) maintains a database of health professional shortage areas and provides grant funding to alleviate structural problems of this kind. Health care systems with these problems are typically in rural areas or poor districts of urban areas. Besides impaired access, regulation of providers, whether they be therapists or long-term care facilities, is the basis for the determination of adequate structural quality.

Table 4–4.   Features of Structure, Process, and Outcome

	Structure	*Process*	*Outcome*
Key components	Physical facilities Human resources	Technical excellence Interpersonal excellence	Results
How measured?	Access to care Professional regulation	Standards Peer review	Survey Interview

Process

Process is the method by which health care is delivered. It has two components: technical excellence and interpersonal excellence (Donabedian 1988). Technical excellence is the ability of the health care provider to use informed decision-making and skill to improve the patient's situation. In essence, a quality health care intervention should shorten the length of time of a disabling condition, reduce its severity, or both. The measurement of technical excellence requires the utilization of accepted intervention protocols and a mechanism of review to determine the appropriateness of the actual intervention.

Technical excellence is determined by measuring provider performance against a set of **standards.** Standards are statements that describe either minimal or optimal actions that providers should take in a clinical situation, and as such they form the basis for the **accreditation** process. Standards are also incorporated into procedural documents called **clinical practice guidelines.** Clinical practice guidelines are "systematically developed statements to assist practitioner and patient decisions about appropriate health care for specific clinical circumstances" (Institute of Medicine 1990). When based on the professional literature, clinical practice guidelines are an example of evidence-based practice. An increasing number of guidelines have been developed in the last decade in response to the demonstrated variation in medical care practice across the country. The Agency for Healthcare Research and Quality maintains a database of clinical practice guidelines (see *www.guideline.gov*). In addition, many individual providers (including physical therapists and occupational therapists) have developed practice guidelines in order to standardize practice, improve outcomes, lower costs, and reduce the risk of potentially negligent activity.

Peer review is the primary mechanism for measuring provider performance against standards or a clinical practice guideline. The Institute of Medicine has defined medical review criteria as "systematically developed statements that can be used to assess the appropriateness of specific health care decisions, services and outcomes" (Institute of Medicine 1990). Peer review usually evaluates the activities of the provider by close examination and consideration of the documentation. It is widely used by providers and payers to determine the appropriateness of the care given. Quality-assurance and quality-improvement programs are standard managerial procedures used by therapists to measure and report clinical quality internally and to accrediting agencies.

A recent innovation in the reporting of quality is "report cards." These are documents intended to increase consumer awareness of the quality of the health care they are purchasing and receiving. One of the most well known quality report cards is the Health Plan Employer Data and Information Set (HEDIS) (National Committee for Quality Assurance 2000). HEDIS measures and compares the quality performance of managed care plans using fifty performance measures. Employers and others use HEDIS to report health plan performance to the public. Wicks and Meyer (1999) identify five features of a useful report card system for quality reporting: interested consumers, understandable report cards, a focus on outcomes and high-priority quality areas, utilization of accurate measures, and a reward system to encourage provider accountability based on the results of the report card. Fielding, Sutherland, and Halfon (1999) found a significant variation in the quality and usefulness of report cards. Consumer acceptance and utilization of report cards is just beginning and varies widely (Romano, Rainwater, and Antonius 1999; Schneider and Epstein 1998; Mukamel and Mushlin 1998; Fowles et al. 2000).

Interpersonal excellence relates to how the care is provided and considers the humanistic features of the process (Donabedian 1988). Patient satisfaction measurement is the form of process assessment most commonly used to determine interpersonal excellence. Measurement of interpersonal excellence is used both by providers and health plans.

Outcomes

Outcomes are a "technology of patient experience" (Ellwood 1988). As the results of the patient's care, outcomes are an important measure of the quality of the health care system. They are typically measured by examining the health status of the person, or in the case of a person with disability, the status of disablement. As we stated in Chapter 1, disablement consists of pathology, impairment, functional limitations, and disability. Measurement tools exist for each of these categories of disablement.

Improved function and a lowered need for external-care assistance is a critical outcome for the care of persons with temporary or permanent disablements. Contemporary outcomes measurement in rehabilitation settings includes patient-reported measures of health status, a report on interpersonal excellence, clinical measures of disablement, and a descriptive report of all patients served by a provider (Dobrzykowski 1997). A number of outcome measurement and reporting systems have been developed in the last twenty years. The Focus on Therapeutic Outcomes (FOTO), a commercially available outcomes management system, measures disablement in outpatient orthopedic settings (FOTO 2000). Studies of the FOTO database have demonstrated the effectiveness of outpatient orthopedic rehabilitation procedures (Dobrzykowski and Nance 1997; Amato, Dobrzykowski, and Nance 1997). In medical rehabilitation, the Uniform Data System for Medical Rehabilitation and its outcome measurement tool, the Functional Independence Measure (FIM™), has been the standard for functional-limitations outcomes assessment for a decade. The implementation of prospective payment system methodologies by the Medicare and Medicaid programs introduced new outcomes measurement systems for rehabilitation environments in 2001.

Each of these systems is an example of a disease-specific outcomes measurement program. These quality-measurement programs collect, analyze, and report data for specific pathologies or patient types. Generic health status assessment is another type of patient outcomes measurement. Generic health status surveys are especially valuable when a clinician wants to monitor the health status of an individual or a population. Tools have been designed to measure health status, quality of life, and global health outcomes. The Medical Outcome Study–Short Form (SF-36), developed by Ware et al. (1992, 1993) is a well-known global health status measure. The SF-36 is a quick, norm-referenced survey of eight domains of physical, social, emotional, and mental health status. It is widely used as a measure of outcomes for many types of medical pathologies.

Accreditation

Accreditation is the primary method by which institutional providers measure their structure, process, and outcomes against consensus quality standards. Most individual providers are not accredited. Payer review of provider documentation is the dominant method of quality determination of individual practitioner performance. Accreditation is a voluntary process by which an institutional provider allows a focused survey of its organization and operations using the accrediting body's standards. If the institution meets the accrediting body's standards, it receives a public proclamation of its quality for a period of time until the next accreditation is required. We will discuss three major accreditation processes of interest to occupational therapists and physical therapists: the Joint Commission on the Accreditation of Health Care Organizations, the Commission on the Accreditation of Rehabilitation Facilities, and the National Committee on Quality Assurance.

The Joint Commission on the Accreditation of Healthcare Organizations (JCAHO) is the oldest accrediting body of healthcare organizations in the United States (JCAHO 2000). Originally established in 1951 to accredit hospitals, JCAHO now accredits a full array of health care organizations, including skilled nursing facilities, home health agencies, and behavioral health organizations. JCAHO has developed performance standards for the structure, organization, and processes of the institutions it accredits. Surveys are conducted by teams of JCAHO employees who conduct on-site reviews and interview key leaders and workers. In 1997, JCAHO initiated the ORYX program, which requires most of the organizations it accredits to demonstrate an outcomes management system.

The Commission on the Accreditation of Rehabilitation Facilities (CARF) was created in the late 1960s to perform institutional quality-review assessment for organizations that serve persons with disabilities (CARF 2000). CARF accredits organizations that serve persons with physical and behavioral disabilities. Like JCAHO, CARF utilizes performance standards to determine quality, but unlike JCAHO, it utilizes part-time surveyors recruited from the clinical fields to conduct the surveys. The CARF accreditation process emphasizes patient rights and a provider commitment to quality improvement.

The National Committee on Quality Assurance (NCQA) was formed in the 1990s by business, labor, and the insurance industry as a body to accredit quality in health plans, specifically forms of managed care (NCQA 2000). NCQA assesses health plans in regard to access and service, provider qualifications, wellness and prevention activities, and care for people who are sick and who have chronic diseases and illnesses. NCQA utilizes a focused survey of health plans to make its accreditation decisions.

Each of these accrediting bodies has developed performance standards and survey processes that measure components of quality. The traditional emphasis has been on structure (leadership and organization) and processes (patient safety, quality assurance). All of these organizations are now emphasizing patient outcomes and health status as a key measure of the quality of health care.

Legal Issues and Quality

For certain health care quality issues, the government has set mandatory minimum, standards for medical care and mechanisms to enforce these standards. These issues include **professional regulation,** patient rights, and **medical negligence.**

The purpose of professional regulation is to protect the public from harm by poorly prepared practitioners. Professional regulation can take one of three forms: registration, certification, or licensure. Registration, the least rigorous process, is the voluntary registration of an individual with an association of practitioners. Certification is the process whereby a state or national board attests that an individual has met the minimum educational standards of the board. The National Board for Certification in Occupational Therapy is a certification body for occupational therapists (NBCOT 2000). Licensure is the most stringent form of professional regulation. It codifies into state law the scope of practice, educational qualifications, testing requirements, and disciplinary procedures for a profession. All 50 states require physical therapists to be licensed. Licensure laws vary from state to state. A model state practice act for physical therapy has been presented by the Federation of State Boards of Physical Therapy (see *www.fsbpt.org* for more information).

Informed consent and patient confidentiality during health care interactions are fundamental patient rights that have emerged in the law over the last half-century. Annas (1998) has identified five core patient rights in health care: the right to information, the right to privacy and dignity, the right to refuse treatment, the right to emergency care, and the right to an advocate. Occupational therapists and physical therapists are legally required to obtain informed consent prior to treatment. This means that the patient needs to be provided with information in order to decide whether to accept or refuse treatment. Specifically, the therapist needs to inform the patient of the type of procedures to be employed, any risks or hazards, the anticipated outcome of the intervention, whether alternatives to the treatment exist, and the consequences of not receiving treatment. Two other forms of informed consent are an advanced directive and a durable power of attorney. An advanced directive is a legal document that details what treatment a patient does or does not wish to be given when no longer able to make a decision about such matters. Examples of an advanced directive are a living will and a "do not resuscitate" order in a hospital setting. A durable power of attorney is a legal document that designates another person to make health care decisions if the patient becomes unable to do so.

Patient's Bill of Rights

In August 2001, a major compromise was struck between President Bush and the House of Representatives about **Patient's Bill of Rights** legislation (Pear 2001). The purpose of a Patient's Bill of Rights is to assure access to health care and provide legal remedies for patients who have been adversely affected by an insurer's decision to deny care. Specifically, this type of legislation guarantees access to emergency care and certain drugs while placing limits on insurance rules that restrict access to specialist services (e.g., obstetrics/gynecology medical care). There are legislative differences over the method and extent of remediation for claims under this law (e.g., lawsuits, independent review boards, caps on damage awards). At the time of this writing, the Patient's Bill of Rights legislation was scheduled for conference action between the Senate and House of Representatives in the fall of 2001. With the terrorist attacks of September 11, 2001, this legislation has stalled.

Remediation for medical error or negligence is achieved through civil court action. An action by a therapist that produces a wrong (called a tort) resulting in injury is termed medical negligence or malpractice. The law provides for relief from this wrong by suing the provider for damages caused by the action. Medical negligence is the failure by a provider to perform those duties and functions that would be done by a similarly trained provider in the same situation. The person suing the provider must demonstrate that the actions of the provider caused the harm and that damages or injuries were suffered by the patient. Standards of care, accreditation policies, organizational policies and procedures, clinical practice guidelines, expert opinion, and professional publications are all key measuring sticks to determine the ability and actions of the provider accused of medical negligence. Good patient communication skills, insurance, and legal representation are necessary for adequate protection of the therapist in a medical negligence situation (Scott 1991).

Conclusion

In this chapter, we have reviewed the fundamentals of determining and measuring quality in the health care system. In summary, Figure 4–2 depicts a "quality pyramid" describing the components of quality in the U.S. health care system. At its base are the fundamental patient rights to be informed and involved in decision-making and to have health conditions to be treated with privacy and respect. The next three levels of the pyramid define components of quality for the personal health care system. Structure is the fixed physical and human resource investment in health care quality. Process is the delivery of health care by this structure. Outcomes is the newest level of health care quality to be emphasized, the results of the intervention. The final level is population health. High-quality population health will be the final achievement of the U.S. health care system if it is to truly become the best in the world.

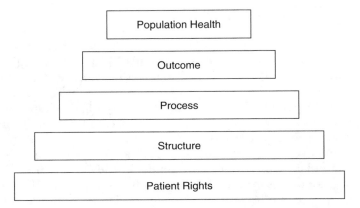

Figure 4–2.   The Quality Pyramid

In the last three chapters we have introduced and discussed the fundamental principles of health policy: access, cost, and quality. An ideal system would provide excellent access to high-quality services at an affordable cost. For many middle- and upper-income Americans, the elderly, and certain segments of the poor, this statement is a reality today. For many lower-income Americans, especially the working poor, this statement is an illusion. Future policymaking will, hopefully, maintain the characteristics of an ideal system and extend its reach to all Americans.

CHAPTER REVIEW QUESTIONS

1. Review and discuss the evidence for the quality of the U.S. health care system.
2. Define quality from the population-based and personal-based perspectives.
3. Define the legal foundation for quality in the health care system:
   a. provider regulation
   b. patient rights
   c. medical negligence
4. What are the features of each component of Donabedian's model of health care quality?
   a. structure
   b. process
   c. outcome
5. How is each component of Donabedian's model of quality measured?
   a. structure
   b. process
   c. outcome
6. What is the purpose of accreditation?
7. Compare and contrast the organizations that conduct accreditation functions in the health care system.

CHAPTER DISCUSSION QUESTIONS

1. A concern about utilizing the population-based perspective in determining the quality of health care is that providers do not have the resources or responsibility to affect concerns outside the health care system. Do you agree with this position? Why or why not?

2. One reason cited for the high rate of medical error in the U.S. health care system is the risk to providers of legal suits due to medical negligence. This risk acts as a barrier to the reporting and analysis of medical error. What effect do you believe this situation may have on medical error? How would you reconcile the competing claims of providers fearful of repercussions for openly discussing errors with the demands of some patients to recover through the courts for damages received at the hands of providers?

3. Report cards are one potential method to reduce the information barrier between provider and patient when making medical care decisions. From your perspective, what are the positives and negatives of report cards for health care quality? Would you use one to make a health care purchasing decision? Under what circumstances? What would you like to know about the quality of your health care provider?

REFERENCES

Amato, A., E. Dobrzykowski, and T. Nance. 1997. The effect of timely onset of rehabilitation on outcomes of outpatient orthopedic practice. *J Rehabil Outcomes Meas* 1(3): 32–38.

Annas, G. J. 1998. A national bill of patient rights. *New Engl J Med* 338(10): 695–99.

Birkmeyer, J., S. M. Sharp, S. M. Finlayson, E. S. Fisher, and J. E. Wennberg. 1998. Variation profiles of common surgical procedures. *Surgery* 124(5): 917–23.

Casarett, D. and C. Helms. 1999. Systems errors vs. physicians' errors: Finding the balance in medical education. *Acad Med* 74(1): 19–22.

Commission on the Accreditation of Rehabilitation Facilities. 2000. CARF mission, vision, core values, and purposes. Accessed at *www.carf.org/AboutCARF/Mission Purposes.htm* on December 4, 2000.

Committee on the Quality of Health Care in America. 2001. *Crossing the quality chasm: A new health system for the 21st century.* Washington DC: National Academy Press.

Dijkers. M. 1999. Measuring quality of life: Methodological issues. *Am J Phys Med Rehabil* 78(3):286–300.

Dobrzykowski, E. 1997. The methodology of outcomes measurement. *J Rehabil Outcomes Meas* 1(1): 8–17.

——— and T. Nance, 1997. The Focus on Therapeutic Outcomes (FOTO) outpatient orthopedic rehabilitation database: Results of 1994–1996. *J Rehabil Outcomes Meas* 1(1): 56–60.

Donabedian, A. 1966. Evaluating the quality of medical care. *Milbank Q* 44: 166–203.

———. 1988. The quality of care: How can it be assessed? *JAMA* 260(12): 1743–48.

———. 1990. The seven pillars of quality. *Arch Pathol Lab Med* 114(11): 1115–18.

Ellwood, P. 1988. Shattuck Lecture. Outcomes management: A technology of patient experience. *New Engl J Med* 318(23): 1549–56.

Field, M. J. and K. N. Lohr, eds. *Guidelines for Clinical Practice: From Development to Use.* Washington DC: National Academy Press.

Fielding, J. E., C. E. Sutherland, and N. Halfon. 1999. Community health report cards. Results of a national survey. *Am J Prev Med* 17(1): 79–86.

Fisher, E. S., J. E. Wennberg, T. A. Stokel, J. S. Skinner, S. M. Sharp, J. L. Freeman, and A. M. Gittelsohn. 2000. Association among hospital capacity, utilization and mortality of U.S. Medicare beneficiaries, controlling for sociodemographic factors. *Health Serv Res* 34(6): 1351–62.

Focus on Therapeutic Outcomes, Inc. (2000). About FOTO. Accessed at *http://www.fotoinc.com/htdocs/company.shtm* on December 18, 2000.

Fowles, J. B., E. A. Kind, B. L. Braun, and D. J. Knutson. 2000. Consumer responses to health plan report cards in two markets. *Med Care* 38(5): 469–81.

Guide for the Uniform Data Set for Medical Rehabilitation (including the F. I.M instrument), Version 5.1, Buffalo NY: State University of New York at Buffalo, 1997.

Health Resources Services Administration. Health Professional Shortage Areas. Accessed at *http://bphc.hrsa.gov/databases/newhpsa/newhpsa.cfm* on December 18, 2000.

Institute of Medicine. 1990. *Clinical practice guidelines: Directions for a new program,* Washington DC: National Academy Press.

Joint Commission on the Accreditation of Healthcare Organizations. 2000. Accessed at *www.jcaho.org/aboutjc/facts.html* on December 4, 2000.

Kindig, D. 1998. Purchasing population health: Aligning financial incentives to improve health outcomes. *Health Serv Res* 33(2 Pt 1): 223–42.

Kohn, L., J. M. Corrigan, and M. S. Donaldson, eds. *To Err Is Human: Building a Safer Health System.* Washington DC, National Academy Press. Accessed at *http://www.nap.edu/books/0309068371/html/* on December 4, 2000.

Leape, L. L. 1997. A systems analysis approach to medical error. *J Eval Clin Pract* 3(3): 213–22.

Lohr, K. N., ed. 1990. *Medicare: A Strategy for Quality Assurance.* Vol 1. Washington DC: National Academy Press. Accessed at *http://books.nap.edu/books/0309042305/html/R1.html* on December 15, 2000

McHorney, C. A., J. E. Ware, and A. Raczek. 1993. The MOS 36-item, short-form health survey (SF-36). II. Psychometric and clinical tests of validity in measuring physical and mental health constructs. *Med Care* 31(3): 247–63.

Mukamel, D. B. and A. I. Mushlin. 1998. Quality of care information makes a difference: An analysis of market share and price changes after publication of the New York State Cardiac Surgery Mortality Reports. *Med Care* 36(7): 945–54.

National Committee for Quality Assurance. An overview. Accessed at *www.ncqa.org/Pages/about/overview3.htm* on December 4, 2000.

Pear, R. 2001. House approves deal with Bush on suing HMOs. *New York Times,* August 3, A1, A16.

Romano, P. S., J. A. Rainwater, and D. Antonius. 1999. Grading the graders: How hospitals in California and New York perceive and interpret their report cards. *Med Care* 37(3): 295–305.

Rothschild, J. M., D. W. Bates, and L. L. Leape. 2000. Preventable medical injuries in older patients. *Arch Intern Med* 160(18): 2717–28.

Schneider, E. C. and A. M. Epstein. 1998. Use of public performance reports: A survey of patients undergoing cardiac surgery. *JAMA* 279(20): 1638–42.

Scott, R. W. 1991. The legal standard of care. *Clin Management* 11(2): 10–11.

Starfield, B. 2000. Is US health care really the best in the world? *JAMA* 284(4): 483–85.

Thomas, E. J., D. M. Studdert, J. P. Newhouse, B. I. Zbar, K. M. Howard, E. J. Williams, and T. A. Brennan. 1999. Costs of medical injuries in Utah and Colorado. *Inquiry* 36(3): 255–64.

———— and T. A. Brennan. 2000. Incidence and types of preventable adverse events in elderly patients: Population-based review of medical records. *BMJ* 320(7237): 741–44.

Wan, G. J., M. A. Counte, and D. F. Cella. 1997. A framework for organizing health–related quality of life research. *J Rehabil Outcomes Meas* 1(2): 31–37.

Ware, J. E. and C. D. Sherbourne. 1992. The MOS 36-item short-form health survey (SF-36) I. Conceptual framework and item selection. *Med Care* 30(6): 473–83.

Wennberg, J. E. 1998. Variation in the delivery of health care: The stakes are high. *Ann Int Med* 128(10): 866–68.

————. 1990. Better policy to promote the evaluative clinical sciences. *Qual Assur Health Care* 2(1): 21–29.

————, J. L. Freeman, R. M. Shelton, and T. A. Bubolz. 1989. Hospital use and mortality among Medicare beneficiaries in Boston and New Haven. *New Engl J Med* 321 (17): 1168–73.

5

Public Policy and Disability

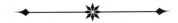

CHAPTER OBJECTIVES

At the conclusion of this chapter, the reader will be able to:
1. Discuss different societal perspectives about disabilities.
2. Describe the focus of key public policies for people with disabilities.
3. Explain how therapists can access each of the public policies about disabilities.

KEY WORDS: Assistive Technology, Barriers, Empowerment, Inclusion, Independent Living, Vocational Rehabilitation

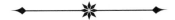

Introduction

In Chapter 1, we introduced the social disability model as an important paradigm with which to understand disablement. The social disability model defines disablement as a sociopolitical experience that is created as the result of the marginalization of people with disabling conditions by the policies, social structures, and attitudes of the nondisabled population. In this chapter, we will focus on public policies that have been developed to address the isolation and discrimination against people with disabling conditions.

United States citizens have historically held different perspectives about people with disabilities. For example, at the beginning of the twentieth century it was considered humane to place people with disabilities in institutions to be protected from society. Our current perspective is to encourage people with disabilities to be included in societal, school, work, and living activities. In current terminology this is called **inclusion,** integration, or mainstreaming. This philosophy is written into many policies and approaches. For example, the American Physical Therapy Association House of Delegates position on civil rights for persons with disabilities states that "It is a matter of civil rights that all citizens including the physically handicapped should share the same rights to free access and opportunities for full development economically, socially, and personally as all other citizens, and that in the Association through its members, committees, and officers take all actions necessary and possible to implement a **barrier**-free environment" (APTA 2000, 12). The American Occupational Therapy Association (AOTA) has developed several position papers related to disability and inclusion (AOTA 1992; AOTA 1993*a*; AOTA 1993*b*; AOTA 1995; AOTA 2000).

Thoughtful readers may question the different perspectives about disabilities that have been adapted from the beginning of the twentieth century until now. However, societal perspectives are never right or wrong; rather they reflect the beliefs and knowledge of what people thought was the best approach at the time. For example, in the United States a paradigm shift about disabilities occurred between 1968 and 1988. Several factors contributed to this different perspective. People with disabilities were living longer. There was more community exposure to people with disabilities. Disability organizations that advocated for the rights of people with disabilities emerged. In addition, a disability rights movement and an independent-living philosophy were strong contributing factors. The disability movement considered the civil rights of the "minority" group of people with disabilities (Bristo 1996). The independent-living philosophy was based on self-rule, and self-help, and political and economic rights (Bristo 1996). Therefore, a paradigm shift occurred, from viewing people with disabilities solely from a medical perspective to an inclusion model. With the medical model, people with disabilities were perceived as "sick" or "impaired" and needing a cure. The newer perspectives incorporated people with disabilities into a community-based model emphasizing inclusion. Thus, disability began to be seen as a larger societal problem needing societal intervention, and this is reflected in many of the recent disability laws, including the Americans with Disabilities Act (ADA) (Bristo 1997). Table 5–1 describes the paradigm switch from a medical model perspective to the current perspective.

The perspectives of a society about important issues like disability, are supported by policy, for public policy is the codification of the shared values of a society (McClain 1996). Policies about disabilities can also be perceived as regulatory and allocative tools mandated by the government (McGregor 2001). Therefore it is relevant for therapists to become aware of the different policies about disabilities, how they are regulated and allocated and the values influencing them. Therapists commonly work with some but not all of society's health care–related policies. For example, therapists working in school systems provide services to children through the Individuals with Disabilities Education Act (IDEA). IDEA supports the education of children and youth with disabilities. However, therapists may not be as fa-

Table 5–1.   Contrast of Paradigms

	Old Paradigms	New Paradigms
Definition of disability	The individual is limited by his/her impairment or condition	The individual with an impairment requires an accommodation to perform functions required to carry out life activities
Strategy to address disability	Fix the individual, correct the deficit	Remove barriers, create access through accommodation and universal design, promote wellness and health
Method to address disability	Provision of medical, vocational, or psychological rehabilitation services	Provision of supports, e.g., assistive technology, personal assistance services, job coach
Source of intervention	Professionals, clinicians, and other rehabilitation service providers	Peers, mainstream service providers, consumer information services
Entitlements	Eligibility for benefits based on severity of impairment	Eligibility for accommodations seen as a civil right
Role of disabled individual	Object of intervention, patient, beneficiary, research subject	Consumer or customer, empowered peer, research participant, decision-maker
Domain of disability	A medical "problem"	A socio-environmental issue involving accessibility, accommodations, and equity

Adapted by Betty Jo Berland from materials prepared for the NIDDR's Long-Range Plan by Gerben DeJong and Bonnie O'Day and reprinted with permission from NIDRR, Washington DC, (NIDDR 2000).

miliar with the Developmental Disabilities Act (DDA) or the Rehabilitation Act (RA). Yet these acts offer services that help similar clients.

The public policies presented in this chapter will be divided into three main themes based on the societal values they represent. The first theme represents policies that help the youth of our society. The second theme represents civil rights policies that focus on people who work, and the third theme represents a policy related to technology, which helps people of all ages with disabilities. We will consider the following public policy acts: the ADA, the **Assistive Technology** Act (AT), DDA, IDEA, and the RA. Table 5–2 overviews the main focus of each of these laws. The chapter presents the main considerations about each, and how these laws are relevant to helping therapy clients.

Table 5–2.   Focus of Disability Policies

Disability Policy	*Focus*
Americans with Disabilities Act (ADA)	A major civil rights act which provides protection not only in employment but in transportation and public accommodations, telecommunications, and with state and local governments for people with disabilities. Expanded coverage to areas not previously covered by other federal disability acts.
Assistive Technology Act	Supports state programs for public-awareness programming to increase access to technology.
Developmental Disability Act	Services those with mental retardation and other developmental disabilities. Provides protection and advocacy. Promotes "independence, productivity, integration and inclusion into the community."
Rehabilitation Act	Helps people with disabilities maximize their employment abilities and independent living abilities, and supports inclusion in society.

L. F. Rothstein, *Disability and the Law* (1992); K. Jacobs, Work assessments and programming (1996).

Public Policies Supporting Youth

Public policy supports the societal value of helping the future of our youth and children. In this section we will discuss the Individuals with Disabilities Education Act and the Developmental Disabilities Act.

The Individuals with Disabilities Education Act (IDEA)

IDEA is rooted in earlier legislation enacted in 1975 called the Education for Handicapped Act (EHA), or P.L. 99–142 (NICHCY 2000). This legislation resulted from the strong advocacy efforts of groups interested in children with disabilities receiving educational opportunities. Prior to this act, many children with disabilities did not get an education, and families had to find their own means for educational services (Bristo 1996; Mellard 2000). IDEA and its predecessor, EHA, are considered to be landmark legislative acts that have helped the integration of disabled youth into American society (Bristo 1997; Mellard 2000). IDEA supports spe-

Table 5–3.   History of the Individuals with Disabilities Education Act (IDEA)

1975: Public Law 94-142, 89 Stat. 773, Part B of the Education for All Handi–capped Children Act of 1975.	Authorized special education for children with disabilities.
1986: Public Law 99-457, 100 Stat. 1145, Education of the Handicapped Act Amendments of 1986	Authorized education for children with disabilities aged 3–5 (Part B) as well as early home-based intervention for families and toddlers 0–3 years (Part H). Included occupational and physical therapy as primary interventions.
1990: P.L.101-476, 104 Stat. 1103, Education of the Handicapped Act Amendments of 1990	Changed the name of the act to Individuals with Disabilities Education Act (IDEA). Added autism and traumatic brain injury. Strengthened guidelines for early intervention programs. Included rehabilitation and social services under related services. Added a transition plan to the IEP.
1997: P.L. 105-17, 111 Stat. 37, Individuals with Disabilities Education Act Amendments of 1997 (most current)	Maintained related services (occupational and physical therapy and others). Encouraged access to general curriculum for children with disabilities. Strengthened parental role. Changed evaluations to include discrepancies between child's performance and expectations of curriculum and general classroom. Insured usage of qualified state personnel. Included verbiage reflecting that utilization of paraprofessionals is consistent with state laws and regulations. Included related services in division of special education. Included participation of related service personnel in child's IEP if personnel are involved in education-provided services to child. Restructured IDEA into four parts: (a) general provisions, (b) assistance for education of all children with disabilities, (c) infants and toddlers with disabilities (d) national abilities to improve the education of children with disabilities.

From: APTA, 2000; Mellard, 2000; Nichcy, 2000; Stephens & Tauber, 1996; *www.caselink*

cial education in the least-restrictive environment for children and youth from birth though age 21. IDEA enables children with disabilities to receive a free and appropriate public education (NICHCY 2000). As with any legislation, it has been amended over the years. Table 5–3 outlines the history of IDEA and some of its key amendments. Many of these amendments have an impact on therapy, but of particular note are the 1986 amendments, which expanded age eligibility for interventions; with these amendments occupational therapy and physical therapy were identified as primary interventions.

Barriers and Concerns Related to the IDEA

IDEA has made great progress in helping children with disabilities access educational systems and services. Today, more youth with disabilities are completing high school. Yet children with disabilities are still behind their nondisabled peers with respect to educational outcomes. In addition, barriers related to the inclusion of children with disabilities into the general classroom remain (Bristo 1996). For even if children with disabilities are transitioned into the general classroom, regular teachers may not have the training and support that they need to work effectively with them (Bristo 1996). Another major problem is labeling of children with disabilities. With the current system there is some failure to identify children who are appropriate for IDEA services. In addition, there is over- and under-identification of minority children as disabled (Bristo 1996). Furthermore, some of the testing is not culturally sensitive. Informing parents of their rights under the law is another concern. Controversies that Congress considered during the most recent reauthorization in 1997 had to do with fair discipline of children with disabilities, holding high expectations and assuring successful long-term outcomes for children with special needs, streamlining paperwork, and involving parents (Bristo 1996; Muhlenhaupt 2000).

IDEA and Therapy

IDEA supports services for children with mental retardation, hearing impairments, speech or language impairments, visual impairments, emotional disturbances, orthopedic impairments, autism, traumatic brain injury, learning disabilities, deaf-blind or multiple disabilities, and other health impairments (IDEA, section 1401 3A). Under IDEA, therapists provide related services, which are defined as "those services necessary for the student to benefit from his or her special education program" (Muhlenhaupt 2000, 10). Related services can follow children with these conditions as long as the Individualized Education Program (IEP) process determines a need for occupational therapy and physical therapy interventions. The only therapy services that are provided under IDEA are those interventions required to help children benefit from their programs of special education. Therefore, therapy is not perceived as a medically based intervention. Thus, therapists trained in traditional medical settings will need to adapt to a different therapy focus.

All children followed by this law receive an IEP. This program has the following purposes: "1) To establish measurable annual goals for the child 2) to state the special education and related services and supplementary aides and services that the public agency will provide to, or on behalf of the child" (NICHY 2000, 13). Therapists and others, including parents, participate in the IEP process. The plan is therefore based on collaborative planning designed to integrate parent and school personnel (Muhlenhaupt 2000). There are very clear guidelines that therapists must follow to address the required areas of an IEP. However, again the focus for therapy services is that the student needs services related to occupational therapy or physical therapy.

Since the 1997 amendment revisions, numerous concerns related to therapy provision and evaluation have been documented (Mauhlenhaupt 2000) Although these concerns are mentioned in the occupational therapy literature, most of them also apply to physical therapists. For example, although procedures for school-based therapy have been published, there are concerns about lack of research support for them, and about inclinations toward objective standardized approaches over individualized approaches. The individual approach has been the focus since the 1997 amendments. In addition, in some situations there has been a dependence on a one-discipline viewpoint rather than the collaborative team perspective promoted with the 1997 IDEA amendments. For example, some IEP teams still support individual or several sets of discipline-focused IEP goals instead of one-set of unified collaborative team IEP goals. Concern has also been expressed about therapists basing their approach on individual performance components rather than a holistic approach, as this may not truly reflect a student's true functioning. Since there is no single assessment protocol that can provide the team with answers for all students, therapists will need to strongly consider the unique characteristics of each child as they plan and interpret assessment data and design interventions (Mauhlenhaupt 2000).

As the above discussion illustrates, therapists need to keep abreast of legislative changes and how they affect therapy. They need to take a pro-active stance before and when the act is reauthorized, especially since so much of school-based practice is defined and largely funded by this act.

The Developmental Disabilities Act (DDA)

In the United States, there has been a long history of people with mental retardation not getting adequate services. However, it was only in the 1960s, during President Kennedy's administration, that treatment of people with mental retardation became a high-priority societal concern. This concern corresponded with an overall societal interest in civil rights. During this time-period, the societal view of mental retardation changed from a congenital causation to one resulting from a societal problem related to poverty, prenatal care, and other social influences (Hightower-Vandamm 1979). Table 5–4 provides a concise history of the DDA.

The legislative roots of the modern-day Developmental Disabilities Act were established in 1963 with two federal laws. P.L. 88–156 was aimed at helping higher-risk mothers, and P.L. 88-164 provided federal funds for building facilities for peo-

Table 5–4.   History of Legislation Related to Developmental Disabilities

1963 P.L. 88-156, 77 Stat. 273, Maternal and Child Health and Mental Retardation Planning Amendments of 1963	Precursor to modern act. Established a federal program for maternity and infant care for high-risk mothers.
1963: P.L. 88-164, 77 Stat. 282 Mental Retardation Facilities and Community Mental Health Centers Construction Act of 1963	Precursor to modern act. First major federal initiative for building of facilities for mentally ill and mentally retarded.
1970: P.L. 91-517, 84 Stat. 1316, Developmental Disabilities Services and Facilities Construction Amendments of 1970	Used terminology "developmental disabilities" instead of "mental retardation" for first time. Expanded definition of individuals substantially handicapped to include those with mental retardation, cerebral palsy, epilepsy, and other neurological conditions. Changed focus from institutions to communities. Provided grant money to state designated agencies and for university-affiliated programs (UAFs).
1975: Developmental Disabilities Assistance and Bill of Rights Act (P.L. 94-103, 89 Stat. 486)	Expanded upon earlier legislation by adding more diagnostic conditions to include autism, learning disabilities, and other conditions related to mental retardation that affect intellectual functioning. Required that disability occur before age of 18 and would be chronic. Funded UAFs. Included with Title II a bill of rights for people with mentally retardation and other developmental disabilities. Established protection and advocacy programs.
1978 P.L.95-602, 92 Stat. 2455, Rehabilitation Comprehensive Services, and Developmental Disabilities Amendments of 1978	Expanded age requirement to 22. Changed definition of disability by making it general and based on functional limitations rather than specific handicaps. Established priority service areas to be done by states.
1984 Developmental Disabilities Act of 1984 Amendments and reorganized (P.L. 98-527, 98 Stat. 2662)	Insured that people with DD received appropriate services and established systems to monitor services. Added statement of purpose specifying that

(continued)

Table 5–4.   History of Legislation Related to Developmental Disabilities

	programs help people with DD achieve their maximal potential with integration into community. Established employment as a priority.
1987 Developmental Disabilities Assistance and Bill of Rights Amendments of 1987 (P.L.100-146, 101 Stat. 840)	Established focus on capacities, rather than limitations, for people with DD. Clarified and enhanced roles of state planning councils and protection and advocacy systems.
1990 Developmental Disabilities Assistance and Bill of Rights Act of 1990 (P.L.101-496, 104 Stat. 1191)	Clarified and enhanced roles of state planning councils.
1994 Developmental Disabilities Assistance and Bill of Rights Act Amendments of 1994 (P.L. 103-230, 108 Stat. 284)	Established language more consistent with other federal acts, such as the ADA, IDEA and the Technology Related Assistance Act. Established funding regulations for state grants. Strengthened and clarified state planning councils, protection and advocacy systems, and UAPs.
2000 Amendments (actually passed in 1999) Consolidated Appropriations Act, 2000 (P.L.106-113, 113 Stat. 1501)	Established guidelines for allocation of grants with the developmentally disabilities councils to bring about permanent improvements. Included new programs to assist states to strengthen family support and for development of curriculum with scholarship and availability for direct support workers.

K. Boyd et al., Developmental Disabilities Act (1996); J. Perinchief, Service management (1996); P. J. Graney, RS20194 (2000); K. L. Reed, History of federal legislation for people with disabilities (1992); Hightower-Vandamm, Nationally speaking (1979).

ple with mental retardation (Hightower-Vandamm 1979). Although, these legislative acts were important beginnings, they were very limited in their scope of coverage, as they addressed the physical institutions and not programming. Furthermore, these laws only covered people with mental retardation and disregarded other developmental disabilities. Therefore, by 1970 a new law, P.L. 91-517, expanded the definitions for conditions covered by the law and began to focus on community-based coverage. The focus on community-based care reflects the societal value of integration and deinstitutionalization of persons with mental disabilities. P.L. 91-517 provided the foundation for some parts of today's modern law, such as establishing a state-designated agency responsible for planning programs.

However, the act still limited coverage to cerebral palsy, epilepsy, and mental retardation (Hightower-Vandamm 1979). Although it mentioned "other neurological conditions" it did not clearly define them for adequate coverage. It was not until the current law was enacted in 1975 and amended several times afterwards that the definitions for disabilities were expanded. With the modern law, the term "mental retardation" was replaced with "developmental disabilities." Behind each of the amendments since 1975 is the advocacy of coalitions to help people with various conditions. For example, the National Association for Retarded Citizens (The Arc), a group strongly associated with the DDA, has advocated for better conditions for people with developmental disabilities in institutional and educational environments (National Council on Disabilities 1997).

By 1975 the climate was right for enactment of the current law, as other federal acts helping people with disabilities were being enacted at the same time. These other public policies included the RA and the EHA. The 1960s and 1970s were an important and creative time period for the disability rights movement. The intent of the DDA was to promote independent living, productivity, and community integration as well as to provide protection and advocacy for persons with developmental disabilities (Graney 2000; Rothstein 1992).

The current Developmental Disabilities Act is divided into several titles. Title I has four parts, each of which is interpreted differently by the individual states. These parts include: (1) state councils on developmental disabilities, (2) protection and advocacy systems, (3) university affiliated programs (UAPs), and (4) projects of national significance. States have some discretion under the law to design their own systems for the councils, protection and advocacy agencies, and university-affiliated programs. As a result, these programs have different forms in the various states (Gordon 2000). The state councils help advocate for people with developmental disabilities (Graney 2000). State councils have four purposes: consumer **empowerment,** systems change, obtaining recourses for people with developmental disabilities and their family members, and promoting community inclusion (NADDC 2000). The protection and advocacy agencies mediate and handle legal situations for people with developmental disabilities. The university-affiliated programs provide interdisciplinary education and training for professionals and conduct applied research. In addition, the UAPs provide training and technological assistance for people with disabilities, their families, and others. The projects of national significance involve research, evaluation, and demonstration projects (Graney 2000).

Title II of the DDA provides support to families with children who have disabilities. Examples of family support are respite care and subsidies to families (Title II, section 202). Title III is a limited scholarship program for staff assisting individuals with developmental disabilities.

Barriers and Concerns with the DDA

The largest controversy surrounding the DDA is the perception of some advocates that the act seems to offer better support to people with developmental disabilities living in the community than in institutions. People who favor institutional settings are concerned that the DDA and the programs it supports are focused almost exclusively on community-based placement. These advocates for institutions feel that some people with developmental disabilities are safer and better served in institutions. They are concerned that as the DDA pushes for greater community inclusion, the institutional choice could be eliminated (Gordon 2000; Kelley 2000).

The DDA and Therapy

The Developmental Disabilities Act was meant to manage the arrangement of services and advocacy efforts on behalf of those with developmental disabilities and not to provide direct services (Graney 2000). Therefore, most therapists are not directly involved with the act and it does not directly reimburse therapy services. The DDA has much the same philosophical intent as therapy services, namely, helping people achieve maximal independence and potential (Gordon 2000). Nevertheless, over the years the American Occupational Therapy Association has taken an active role in lobbying for the different amendments (Boyd et al. 1996). Therapists working in university-affiliated programs are directly affected by the DDA.

Work-Related Policy Acts

The Rehabilitation Act (RA)

Maintaining or promoting the ability of people to work is a strong value that has consistently been part of American society (see Chapter 1). Therefore it is not surprising that health-related public policy, even at the beginning of the twentieth century, was related to this value. Both the workers' compensation law and the Rehabilitation Act (RA) have roots at the beginning of the twentieth century (see Chapter 6 for more about workers' compensation). Review Table 5–5 for a listing of key public policies related to work throughout the twentieth century. Some of these laws remain in force and still have an impact on today's health-care environment (e.g., workers' compensation insurance).

Therapists, however, may not be as familiar with the RA, which also helps clients with work-related concerns. Refer to Table 5–6 for an overview of the history of this law.

The Rehabilitation Act was rooted in the Smith-Fess Act of 1920. The Smith-Fess Act provided federal funds for people who had become disabled in industrial settings and funded services for persons with physical disabilities (Dunn 2000; Reed 1996). Coincidentally, the Smith-Fess Act was instituted around the time that the disciplines of physical therapy and occupational therapy were founded. Occupational therapy was affected by this law during this period. The Smith-Fess Act originally limited occupational therapy practice to a medical, not educational service, and therefore would not reimburse for services titled "occupational therapy" (Reed 1996). The Smith-Fess Act also did not include physical rehabilitation in the

Table 5–5.   Key Public Policy Related to Work

1916 National Defense Act Ch. 134, 39 Stat. 166	Assisted people with instruction and study of occupations. Did not have a specific focus on disabilities but was a model for later legislation.
1900–1910 Workers Compensation Laws	Not a federal act, but passed by most states between 1900 and 1910. Helped people who were injured on the job.
1917 Smith Hughes Act (Vocational Education Act of 1917) Ch. 114, 39 Stat. 929	Created the federal board for vocational education.
1918 Smith-Sears Act Ch. 107, 40 Stat. 617	Soldiers' and Sailors' Vocational Rehabilitation Act. Later expanded the role of the vocational board to include vocational and medical rehabilitation for injured war veterans.
1920: PL 66236, Smith Fess Act (Vocational Rehabilitation Act) Ch. 219, 41 Stat. 735	Provided counseling and guidance, vocational training, and job placement. Limited support services were available for prosthetics and transportation. Is the root of the Vocational Rehabilitation Act. This act was amended several times until the modern act in 1973.
1935: PL 74271, Social Security Act Ch. 531, 49 Stat. 620	Provided continuous funds for vocational rehabilitation training programs for civilians. Part of this act includes unemployment compensation and old-age insurance. Also provided medical and therapeutic services for children with disabilities.
1973-PL 93-112, 87 Stat. 355 Rehabilitation Act of 1973	Modern rehabilitation act. Has sections including affirmative action in employment (section 503) and nondiscrimination in facilities (section 504).
1984-PL 98–524, 98 Stat. 2435 Carl D. Perkins Vocational Education Act	Provided state funding for vocational programming. Act continues to be amended.
1990-PL 101-336, 104 Stat. 324 Americans with Disabilities Act of 1990 (ADA)	Civil rights act, which among other areas provides protection in employment.
1999: H.R. 3433 Ticket to Work and Work Incentives Improvement Act	Allows people with disabilities to keep their federal health insurance benefits of 1999 (Medicare and Medicaid) if they become employed. Helps people with disabilities be employable to reduce dependence on benefits and assistance.

Dunn, personal communication (2000); Reed, The beginning of occupational therapy (1992); Johansson, Disability advocates say more could be done (2000); Rothstein, *Disability and the Law* (1992).

Table 5–6.   History of the Rehabilitation Act (RA)

1920 Smith Fess Act (Vocational Rehabilitation Act) Ch. 219, 41 Stat. 735	Precursor to modern act. Provided counseling and guidance, vocational training, and job placement. Limited support services were available for prothetics and transportation. Is the root of the vocational rehabilitation act. This act was amended several times until the modern act in 1973.
1943 Barden-LaFollette Act (Voc-ational Rehabilitation Act) Ch. 190, 57 Stat. 374	Precursor to modern act. Amendment to PL 66236. Added more diagnoses, including psychiatric diagnoses. Began covering rehabilitation services. Established an Office of Vocational Rehabilitation.
1954-Ch. 655, PL 83-565, 68 Stat. 652 Hill-Burton Act (Vocational Rehabilitation Act Amendments of 1954)	Precursor to modern act. Intent was to expand building of hospitals. These amendments addressed many areas, including expanding rehabilitation facilities, making facilities more assessable, and financing therapy education. Funded research and program development. Provided funding for occupational therapy, physical therapy, and other services.
1965- PL 89-333, 79 Stat. 1282 Vocational Rehabilitation Act Amendments of 1965	Precursor to modern act. Replaced the Office of Vocational Rehabilitation with the Vocational Rehabilitation Administration. Provided construction money to rehabilitation facilities and increased the scope of diagnoses coverage to the more severely disabled by the Vocational Rehabilitation Act. Considered for the first time the impact of social disability. Established the National Commission on Architectural Barriers, which studied architectural design.
1973-PL 93–112, 87 Stat. 355: Rehabilitation Act of 1973	Is the modern-day act. Included more severe disabilities. Expanded to include personal and vocational needs.
1974	Attempted to change focus from only considering employability.
1978-PL 95-602, 92 Stat. 2955 Amendments to the Rehabilitation Act of 1973, Rehabilitation Comprehensive Services, and Developmental Disabilities Amendments of 1978	Included 504 and 505 regulations. Added independent living with Title VII. Created the National Institute of Handicapped Research. Added a Protection and Advocacy for Individual Rights program.
1984: PL 98-524, 98 Stat. 2435 Carl D. Perkins Vocational Act	Authorized more funding for state vocational education and programs.

(*continued*)

1986: PL 99-357, 100 Stat. 761Carl D. Perkins Vocational Education Act Amendment	Dealt with state allocation of funds. Addressed technology.
1992 Amendments (PL 102-569, 106 Stat. 4334)	Mandated state vocational rehabilitation agencies to provide for individual choices of services and service providers, focused on careers, not jobs, and made the assumption that people with disabilities are employable.
1998-Amendments (PL 105-220, 112 Stat. 936)	Reorganized the way employment services were provided. Made vocational rehabilitation programs part of state workforce investment systems. Enhanced section 508: Strengthened federal government's existing obligation to ensure that technology is available to people with disabilities. Added complaint procedure and reporting requirements.

Bristo, *Achieving Independence* (1996); Dunn, personal communication (2000); Reed, History of federal legislation for peoples with disabilities (1992); Rothstein, *Disability and the Law* (1992); Jacobs, (1996); *http://www.access-board.gov/sec508/Section*

scope of covered services (Dunn 2000). Persons with psychiatric diagnoses who were seen by occupational therapists were also not covered. These restrictions impeded the early growth of occupational therapy.

In 1943, the Smith-Fess Act was amended to permit reimbursement for occupational therapy services. The resulting new law, known as the Barden-LaFollette Act, expanded coverage beyond physical disabilities to include funding for both physical and mental restoration services. Although the Barden-LaFollette Act did not specify rehabilitation services, occupational therapy was covered under the expansion of services (Dunn 2000; Jacob 1996). Work-related activities continued to be part of occupational therapy practice, and in the 1950s a major debate at the national occupational therapy convention over the usage of work evaluations in therapy results in some therapists leaving occupational therapy to join the new field of **vocational rehabilitation** (Marshall 1985).

Between 1943 and 1973, when the modern act was instituted, the Rehabilitation Act was amended several times. These amendments increased services for people with disabilities (PL 78–113) and increased rehabilitation facilities by providing grant money (PL 83–565). With the amendments in 1965, which coincided with changing American values about social disability, the social impact of disabilities was considered for the first time (Reed 1992). The 1965 amendments changed the eligibility criteria to include "behavioral disorders" as a disability and removed the idea that a handicap to employment could only be caused by or result from physical and mental disabilities. However, as psychological assessments at the time were culturally insensitive, most minorities, public offenders, and impoverished people receiving testing ended up with a diagnosis of behavioral disorder. Although these populations had employment needs based on social concerns, they did not necessarily have real mental and or physical disabilities. Also, to deal with the institutionalized mentally retarded (MR) population, the 1965 amendments created an 18-month period of "extended evaluation" during which vocational rehabilitation (VR) agencies attempted to enhance the employability of the institutionalized individuals (Dunn 2000). The 1965 amendments also focused on the social rehabilitation of the most severely disabled in the institutions (Reed 1992).

In 1973, the modern act (PL 93-112) was instituted. With the modern act, the definition of disabilities was extended to include more severe disabilities, and rehabilitation services were included for all people with disabilities (Bristo 1997). The changed definition of disabilities was a response to the concern of people with physical disabilities that vocational rehabilitation programs were no longer servicing them and instead were prioritizing those diagnosed with behavioral disorders. Thus, with limited funding, priorities were set on the most severely disabled with physical disabilities (Dunn 2000). Sheltered workshops were seen as an adequate substitution of work for the most severely disabled. The modern act included a broader focus by emphasizing **independent living** (instituted by amendments in 1978). In addition, individual, written rehabilitation plans for qualified people were instituted (Reed 1992). This act has subsequently been amended to include independent living programs (PL 95-602), more funds for vocational education and programming (PL 88-210), increased consumer control and access to technology for people with disabilities (PL 102-569, 106), and even more consumer control with the 1998 amendments (PL 105–220). These amendments have redefined who is considered to be disabled (Rothstein 1992).

An underlying theme of these amendment changes over the years has been the demedicalization of vocational rehabilitation programs and the development of an independent-living philosophy, the "new paradigm of disability" (Berland and Seelman 2000; Dunn 2000). This philosophy, discussed at the beginning of the chapter (and in Chapter 1), involves looking at disability as a dynamic interaction between the individual's impairment, functional status, and personal and social qualities with "natural, built, cultural, and social environments" (Berland and Seelman 2000, 5). Disability is perceived on a continuum from disablement to enablement (Berland and Seelman 2000).

The Rehabilitation Act set a precedent for the subsequent Americans with Disabilities Act, including sections 501, 503, and 504. Section 501 established "a federal interagency committee on employees who are individuals with disabilities" (Tucker 1994, 48). A key part of section 501 is the requirement that federal agencies must have an affirmative action plan for employment of people with disabilities. Section 503 requires nondiscrimination on the basis of disability and puts an affirmative action plan in place for federal agencies that contract for $10,000 or more. Section 504 prohibits discrimination in employment, education, architectural accessibility, and health, welfare, and social services for recipients of federal financial assistance (Tucker 1994). Section 504 was landmark legislation, for it was the first civil rights declaration for people with disabilities (Bristo 1997; Tucker 1994). With the elevation of this law to a civil rights act, people with disabilities were allowed a legal means to advocate for their rights. Because of the controversies over this regulation, people in the disabilities movement had increased public visibility (Bristo 1997).

Barriers and Concerns with the Rehabilitation Act

Although the intent of the Rehabilitation Act was positive, it has always been controversial. When the modern act was instituted it was not properly enforced. It was only after public concern and a lawsuit that regulations were implemented under section 504 (Rothstein 1992). A recent concern has dealt with the usage of funds appropriated by the RA. In some cases, funding abuses have occurred, with vocational rehabilitation programs being charged for rehabilitation instead of the Medicaid program. These abuses led to a modification in the 1998 amendments. The 1998 amendments also specify that any rehabilitation intervention should be expected to eliminate or reduce the impediment to employment and not be just for the condition (Dunn 2000).

In spite of policies related to work, people with disabilities, particularly minorities and women, have higher rates of unemployment or underemployment than the general population. Access to health insurance remains a prime concern, especially for those who are disabled and employed in part-time work. Finally, vocational rehabilitation programs have not changed the nationwide employment rate for people with disabilities (Bristo 1996).

The Rehabilitation Act and Therapy

The Rehabilitation Act helps people with disabilities by providing many beneficial services. Section 103 of the act (Workforce Investment Act of 1998, 105-220, § 404) lists many services including but not limited to training programs and centers, vocational rehabilitation services, prosthetic and orthotic services, diagnosis and treatment for mental and emotional disorders, and transportation services. Section 103 also mentions visual services and reading services for people who are blind and interpreter services for people who are deaf. In addition, Section 103 lists technical and consultation services assistance for individuals seeking self-employment, establishing a small business, or who need assistance on the job. The RA also provides consultative and technical assistance to educational programs to help students with disabilities transition to post-school activities and employment (refer to Section 103 of the RA for a full listing of the available services covered by the act).

Neither physical therapy nor occupational therapy has been strongly involved with the modern act. However, therapy can become involved to help people improve function and become more independent with self-care in order to engage in employment (Dunn 2000). Vocational rehabilitation specialists primarily work with people who have disabilities and need these services. The 1998 amendments more clearly defined the Rehabilitation Act as an employment program, which results in even less involvement from therapists. It specifies that therapy can become involved only if therapy services cannot be funded by another source (Dunn 2000). Thus, if Medicaid (see Chapter 9) covers rehabilitation services for a person, the RA would not reimburse for rehabilitation. In addition, the Rehabilitation Act is a state-federal program, with states responsible for delivery of services according to a state plan, and state agency programs vary widely in focus (Dunn 2000). Therapists wishing to provide services funded by this law will need to be familiar with community-based models vs. medical-based models and should communicate with their state agencies.

Finally, newer legislation, such as the Ticket to Work and Work Incentives Improvement Act of 1999, may open up more opportunities for therapists to work with disabled persons in order to facilitate their return to employment. With this new legislation, clients can receive services beyond the traditional vocational rehabilitation programs (Johansson 2000). However, the therapists would only be paid after the patient gets and maintains gainful employment and is earning more than $700 per month (Dunn 2000).

The Americans with Disabilities Act (ADA)

The most broadly reforming civil rights act, helping disabled people of all ages, is the Americans with Disabilities Act (ADA) of 1990. The ADA is a federal antidiscrimination law guaranteeing equal opportunity and not just equal treatment for those with disabilities (Wells 2000). Previous acts, such as the Civil Rights Act of 1964, the RA, and the EHA, established the climate for the development of the ADA (Bristo 1997; Wells 2000). The Civil Rights Act of 1964 was the first federal act to consider discrimination in public places and tie the promise of nondiscrimination to the receipt of federal funds (Wells 2000). The ADA expanded some of the premises of the RA, especially section 504 (Rothstein 1992). The perspective of inclusion under the EHA helped influence public opinion about the ADA (Bristo 1997).

The Americans with Disabilities Act was revolutionary in many ways. One was its use of language. The act changed the verbiage of public policy from "handicapped" people to people "who have disabilities" (Rothstein 1992). This "people first" language reflected a change in societal values toward empowerment and respect for people with disabilities. Another unique aspect was the focus on the abilities and aptitudes of people with disabilities, with emphasis on societal inclusion (Bowman 1992). Thus, the ADA considered work along with other related societal areas to help keep people with disabilities working and included in the larger fabric of society. For example, it dealt with the dilemma of people who might be able to work at a job but not successfully access the transportation system to get there or not be able to get to the actual job-site location in a facility. The act made public areas accessible even for disabled persons who were not working. Therefore the inclusion of public transportation and architectural accessibility in the ADA reflects the law's broad perspective.

As stated, a primary purpose of the ADA is to help people with disabilities be employed and have the same advantages as others who are not disabled (Goren 1999). To qualify as having a disability the person must have "the physical or mental impairment that substantially limits one or more major life activities, a history or record of such an impairment, or a person is perceived by others as having such an impairment" (*www.peublo.gsa* 2000).

The law has four titles. Title I deals with employment and requires employers that have 15 or more employees to provide equal employment opportunities to qualified individuals with disabilities. This title also mentions protection against discrimination in hiring, promotion, and pay. It provides restrictions on questions about disabilities before the job is offered. In addition, Title I requires that employers make "reasonable accommodations" to allow the person to work, unless there is "undue hardship." Title II covers state and local governments. It requires that people with disabilities be provided with equal opportunity to benefit from such services as public education, employment, transportation, health care, social services, courts, voting, and town meetings. Title II also requires that governments follow architectural standards in the construction and renovation of buildings. In addition, Title II requires reasonable modification of policies and procedures to avoid discrimination against those who have disabilities. Another part of Title II is the provision of coverage for public transportation so that there is no discrimination against people with disabilities in using the services. Title III covers public accommodations—businesses such as retail stores, hotels, and restaurants. Public accommodations must comply with standards and requirements in terms of architecture and access. Title IV covers telephone accessibility for people with hearing and speech disabilities. It requires telephone companies to enable people with hearing and speech disabilities to use special adaptive phones, such as TDDs (AOTA 1993;*www.peublo.gsa* 2000).

Barriers and Concerns with the ADA

The ADA has resulted in very positive results throughout the United States, but there is still room for improvement. The very fact that there have been so many employment discrimination suits filed with the Equal Opportunity Commission exemplifies that there remains much discrimination toward people with disabilities (Bristo 1997). In particular, there is discrimination toward minorities with disabilities. As Bristo (1999, 1) states, "But for a large segment of the population with disabilities, particularly those from diverse racial, cultural, and ethnic communities, a shameful wall of exclusion continues to hinder their ability to participate fully in all aspects of American society. Whether the exclusion stems from one's disability, one's race, one's language, one's culture, one's ethnicity, or a combination of these, the sting of rejection is just as painful." In particular Native Americans do not benefit from the ADA and other disability policies because they were not established in collaboration with tribal governments (Bristo 1997). Public hearings held by the National Council on Disability (Bristo 1999) identified the following barriers for minority people with disabilities: (1) employment, public accommodations, transportation, and culturally competent service delivery, (2) citizenship, and (3) accurate demographic data.

Therapy and the ADA

In different ways, the Americans with Disabilities Act has an impact on therapists and involves therapy with the law (AOTA 2000). From a manager's perspective, it influences hiring decisions. Direct questions concerning a disability cannot be asked of a person during an interview. The manager should be interested in whether the qualified person can perform the "essential functions" of a job in the therapy department. As discussed, the ADA requires employers to make "reasonable accommodations" to allow the qualified person to work as long as these accommodations do not entail "undue hardship." Therefore, managers of therapy departments may be involved in the process of implementing reasonable accommodations.

A unique way for therapists to get involved with the ADA is as consultants (Hanebrink and Brown-Parent 2000). Therapists have the skills to be ADA consultants. However, it is important that they have a strong knowledge base about the law in order to implement it in practice. Redick, McLean, and Brown (2000) studied occupational therapy practitioners (N = 152 qualified participants) to ascertain their knowledge of Title III of the ADA and its application to clients who use wheelchairs to access public accommodations. The study concluded that the occupational therapists were not knowledgeable about ADA and were inactive in respect to implementing Title III, even though they recognized that occupational therapy had a role under the ADA. This shows that it is important to become more knowledgeable about applications of the ADA. Hanebrink and Brown-Parent (2000) suggest that therapists can increase their knowledge base by participating on local private and government committees for people with disabilities, and attending continuing education courses. Simply networking with people involved in implementing the act may be very beneficial.

With a knowledge base about the Americans with Disabilities Act, therapists can consult about legislation and architectural codes, assist local government agencies, and provide suggestions for reasonable accommodations (AOTA 2000). Consulting with human resource departments may involve doing job site analysis and writing job descriptions (Wells 2000). In addition, therapists should address ergonomic adaptations (Stockdell and Crawford 1992) and adaptive equipment needs, and perhaps provide expert-witness testimony (Hanebrink and Brown-Parent 2000). Therapists may also choose to conduct research for intervention strategies and related programs (Bowman 1992). Suggested areas for consultation include government agencies, public transportation and communication bodies, businesses, the individuals who have a disabilities (Hanebrink and Brown-Parent, 2000). Furthermore, therapists may consider working as a team with architects, engineers, and others to help meet the requirements of the ADA (Wells 2000).

Working to implement the ADA can be difficult in many areas because the act is so broad. For example, many of the adaptations can help elders remain part of society. Especially as society ages, worksite adaptations may help elders who chose to remain working (McGinty, Bachelder, and Hilton 1994). Or adaptations can be made to help children and adolescents with disabilities remain in appropriate environments (Kalscheur 1992). Some suggested areas for interventions to meet ADA requirements with youth are in play, sports, education, gathering places, and entertainment environments (Kalscheur 1992). Therapists may also help qualified disabled students in higher education (Bowman and Marzouk 1992). Furthermore, occupational therapist with a strong background in mental health may become involved with making reasonable accommodations for those with mental health diagnoses. With mental health interventions, the focus may be on the psychosocial aspects of employment, such as communication skills, time management, multitasking, concentration, and self-efficacy (Crist and Stoffel 1992).

Technology and Persons with Disabling Conditions

The Assistive Technology Act of 1998

The Assistive Technology Act (ATA) became law in 1998. It promotes the usage of technology to improve function, independence, and quality of life for persons with disabilities. The ATA reflects the rapidly changing and increasingly sophisticated development of technology for people with disabilities. It developed after World War II when advancing technology for health care became a societal value (Lenker 2000). As Bristo (2000, 1) states, "for people with disabilities . . . technology changes the most ordinary of life activities from impossible to possible."

The intent of the original act was "systems change" to be initiated by state technology-assistance programs. The focus was on advocacy for and modeling of changes in systems that would increase access to and funding of assistive technology. Amendments in 1994 increased the focus on advocacy as a strategy for systems change. The 1998 act shifted the focus to system capacity building. This shift, while not removing a responsibility to conduct systems-change activities, appears to allow for activities that would enhance or expand the delivery of assistive technology services (as well as development of new assistive technology and alternative financing systems) (Schultz 2000). Refer to Table 5–7 for a brief history of the Assistive Technology Act and its related amendments.

The ATA defines technology as "any item, piece of equipment, product system, whether acquired commercially, modified, or customized, used to increase, maintain, or improve the functional capabilities of individuals with disabilities" (Assistive Technology Act, as cited by Bristo 2000, 2). Title I defines state obligations to educate about technology, improve access to technology, provide technical assistance and services, including developments of laws and policies, and provide outreach to the statewide community. This title authorizes grant money for states to carry out these functions (Reyes-Akinbileje 1999). Title II deals with national activities, such as coordination of federal research and providing small business in-

Table 5–7.   History of the Assistance Technology Act

Section G of the Education of the Handicapped Act	Precursor to modern act. Addressed access to existing technology but did not address development of technology.
Section 508 of the Rehabilitation Act Amendments of 1986 (P.L. 99-506, 100 Stat. 1807).	Precursor to modern act. Addressed access to existing technology but did not address development of technology.
The Technology-Related Assistance for Individuals with Disabilities Act of 1988 (The Tech Act) (P.L. 100-407, 102 Stat. 1044)	Focus on advocating for and modeling of changes in systems that would increase access to and funding of assistive technology. Addressed lack of information about technology, lack of training, lack of accessibility of technology. Established grant money for state technological assistance programs. Focused on providing funds for technological development.
Technology-Related Assistance for Individuals with Disabilities Amendments of 1994 (P.L. 103-218, 108 Stat. 50).	Increased focus on advocacy as a strategy for systems change. Expanded program authorizations. Continued authoriza tion of grant money for state technological assistance programs, some of which remained unfunded.
Assistive Technology Act of 1998 (P.L. 105-394, 112 Stat. 3627).	Shifted focus to system capacity building to address assistive technology needs of individuals with disabilites. Mandated state activities include public awareness, interagency coordination, technical assistance and training, and outreach. Title III created opportunties for microloan program to individuals for purchase of assistive technology devices or services. Repealed 1988 Act.

Schultz, personal communication (2000); Reed, *The beginnings of occupational therapy* (1992); Reyes-Akinbileje, CRS Report for Congress (1999).

centives. Title III authorizes funding for assistive technology and considers alternative financial areas (Reyes-Akinbileje 1999; RESNA 2000). In addition, a Protection and Advocacy Technology (PAAT) program was created with amendments to this act. This program provides legal advocacy for assistive technology obtainment (RESNA 2000).

Concerns and Barriers with the Assistive Technology Act

Even though the ATA is available to help U.S. citizens, there remain barriers to obtaining assistive technology. A recent report to the president from the National Council on Disability identified several barriers, with recommendations to reduce their effect (Bristo 2000). A prime barrier is the need to improve awareness of the available assistive technology and access to expertise about the technology. One recommendation addressing this concern suggests that therapists and other personnel should have training about assistive technology. Another interesting recommendation from this report calls for broadening the descriptors for assistive technology within the Medicare and Medicaid programs. It mentions that the current definitions for durable medical equipment came from the original laws enacted in the 1960s. During that time the philosophical approach toward medical care was for curing and palliative care, "with little consideration for the individual's functional status (Bristo 2000, 9)." Thus, equipment that would enhance a person's safety and independence, such as shower chairs or reachers, is not covered by current laws.

Therapists and the ATA

The purpose of this law is more for education than for provision and funding of technology. However, utilization of resources provided by this act helps therapists understand current assistive technology, especially because technology is such a rapidly developing area. Therapists may refer their clients to centers established by this law in order to familiarize them with the most current technology available. In addition, this act may help therapy clients through funded research for the development of new technology. On a state level, therapists may become involved with educational programs about assistive technology.

Working with Disability Policies

As therapy moves into community-based practice it will be beneficial to become aware of these disability policies. Even if therapists do not receive direct reimbursement from some of these acts, they can help many of the patients they serve by becoming familiar with programs so that they can advise clients.

Therapists can learn how to access and work with these policies through networking and advocacy skills. Therapists must recognize that disability policies are laws that can be changed by legislative systems on both the federal and state level. As with any law, revision involves issue identification, the design of policy, involvement of public support, and legislative decision-making (McGregor 2001). The histories of the different policies presented in this chapter show that these laws have gone through many changes over time. Some of the amendments have improved therapy access and coverage, such as the amendments to the IDEA. Other amendments have tightened therapy coverage, such as the amendments to the RA. Prior to each amendment therapists should advocate for their concerns on the state and national level (refer to Chapter 15 for a discussion of advocacy and for hints on how to become involved in the legislative process).

It is also beneficial for therapists to understand the philosophy and priorities of the state agencies that institute these policies. Each state program institutes policies a little differently. It takes networking to find out a given state's priorities about disability policies. Networking will also help locate special-interest groups that may influence these policies. State agencies often have grant funding for research which therapists might choose to access. Furthermore, therapists must understand that the federal laws are superseded by any state statutes that provide greater protection for people with disabilities (Wells 2000).

In addition, it is important to be aware that for any federal law with state mandates there is a constant tension between federal and state control, especially related to funding issues. Johansson (2000, 1) recently reflected that there has been "a 'shift' in developing policy and programs from the federal government to the states. This offers opportunities for innovation, but it also introduces 'new tensions and complexities' into the process of securing benefits." Thus, funding controversies are an economic certainty (Reed, 1992).

Therapists must also be aware of trends in public policy related to disability. For example, all of these acts profess the philosophy of inclusion or integration into the "least restrictive environment" in society and enhancement of function. All of these laws have similar definitions of disability, with the exception of the IDEA (Turner 1996), and specific requirements for which a person must qualify (Rothstein 1992). With amendments some policies may adapt parts of other policies. For example, several policies have adapted protection and advocacy boards. Trends will change and as, discussed at the beginning of the chapter, views about disability will also change.

Finally, as has been suggested throughout this chapter, even though there are federal laws available to help people with disabilities, there remain many barriers, controversies, and room for improvement with all of these acts. Several plausible explanations exist for these problems. First, the history of legislation for people with disabilities has not been a planned effort but rather a piecemeal attempt to deal with concerns (Bowman 1992). Thus many of the discussed policies overlap in some areas and over the years have become more similar. Second, public policy can be very incremental and may involve multiple levels of federal and state bureaucracy (McGregor 2001). It is the bureaucrats who actually institute the policies, and interpretations can vary. As Bristo (1997, 25) states, "The customer with disabilities seeking services faces a maze of programs, requirements and bureaucratic obstacles." Furthermore, decisions regarding service provision continue to be made by bureaucrats rather than by people with disabilities, thus promoting dependence (Bristo 1997). Third, because public policies are federal laws, compromises are made during the debates in the House and Senate (Reed 1992). These compromises often deal with the practical funding aspects of these policies. Fourth, the written language and regulations of the acts may also include limitations (Nosek 1992). For example, the terminology "readily achievable" is not clearly defined in the ADA. Fifth, even though these policies are in effect, people in society may not understand the issues related to the provision of services for disabilities (Wells 2000). For example, people who are minorities and have a disability may encounter dual discrimination and have trouble obtaining services (Wells 2000). Even congressional members may present a barrier because of lack of understanding and support of disability policies (Bristo 1996). Last, the real power of all these laws is how they are actually implemented in reality and not on paper (Nosek 1992). For even with all these policies, people with disabilities are older, more impoverished, and less educated than those without disabilities (Bristo 1996). Thus, the ultimate analysis of all these policies is how they really help the disabled members of our society.

Conclusion

Numerous public policies have been enacted in the last 35 years to address social disability by reducing social barriers and empowering persons with disabling conditions. We have discussed the history, purpose, and effectiveness of many of these policies. Social disability that affects children and youth, persons with disabling conditions who work, and restrictions on access to assistive technology have been reduced by these government actions. Together, these policies have created a more inclusive society.

CHAPTER REVIEW QUESTIONS

1. Define "inclusion," "mainstreaming," "barriers," and "empowerment."
2. Review the history and purpose of the following disablement-related laws:
   a. Individuals with Disabilities Education Act
   b. Developmental Disabilities Act
   c. Rehabilitation Act
   d. Americans with Disabilities Act
   e. Assistive Technology Act
   Who is eligible for services? What types of services are provided? How are physical and occupational therapists involved in delivering services to eligible populations?

CHAPTER DISCUSSION QUESTIONS:

1. Reflect on the paradigm switch in the twentieth century regarding views about disability. What were the different values influencing disability prior to the 1960s and after the 1960s?
2. Briefly describe the focus of each policy. What are some of the similarities and differences between the different disability policies?

3. Discuss why it is beneficial for therapists to know about policies (such as the DDA and the ATA) for which they do not provide direct services.

INTERNET RESOURCES

http://www.adata.org/ ADA Technical Assistance Program: Enhances public consciousness, technical assistance, training, materials and referrals throughout the country.

Http://fedlaw.gsa.gov/ Contains the full texts of the federal disability laws.

http://www.igc.apc.org/ Provides information on DDA programs.

http://naric.com/ Provides information on each state's assistive technology program.

http://www.igc.apc.org/ Developmental disabilities council information.

REFERENCES

American Occupational Therapy Association. 1992*a*. Occupational therapy services in work practice. *Am J Occup Ther* 46: 1086–88.

———. 1993*b*. The role of occupational therapy in the independent living movement. *Am J Occup Ther* 47: 1079–80.

———. 1995. Occupational therapy: A profession in support of full inclusion. *Am J Occup Ther* 50: 855.

———. 2000. Occupational therapy: and the Americans with Disabilities Act (ADA). *Am J Occup Ther* 54: 622–25.

American Physical Therapy Association. 2000. *House of delegates policies*, 1–55. (WWW document). URL *http://www.apta.org*

Bachelder, J. M. and C. List-Hilton. 1994. Implications of the Americans with Disabilities Act of 1990 for elderly people. *Am J Occup Ther* 48: 73–81.

Berland, B. J. and K. D. Seelman. 2000. Overview of NIDRR's long range plan. Chapter 1: Introduction and Background. (WWW document). URL *http://www.ncddr .org/rpp/lrp_ov.html*

Bowman, O. J. 1992. Americans have a shared vision: Occupational therapists can create the future reality. *Am J Occup Ther* 46(5): 391–96.

——— and D. K. Marzouk. 1992a. Implementing the Americans with Disabilities Act of 1990 in higher education. *Am J Occup Ther* 46(6): 521–33.

——— and ———. 1992b. Using the Americans with Disabilities Act of 1990 to empower university students with disabilities. *Am J Occup Ther* 46(5): 450–56.

Boyd, K., C. DeMarco, K. Figetakis, S. Robinson, S. Sullivan, J. Young, C. Custard, M. DiCarlo, M. Laners, K. Serfas, and K. Vigil. 1996. Developmental Disabilities Act. Unpublished manuscript, Creighton University, Omaha, Nebraska.

Bristo, M. 1996. *Achieving Independence: The Challenge for the 21st Century*. Washington DC: National Council on Disabilities.

———. 1997. *Equality of Opportunity: The Making of the Americans with Disabilities Act*. Washington DC: National Council on Disability.

———. 1999. *Lift Every Voice: Modernizing Disability Policies and Programs to Serve a Diverse Nation.* Washington DC: National Council on Disabilities.

Crest, P. A. and V. C. Stifle. 1992. The Americans with Disabilities Act of 1990 and employees with mental impairments: Personal efficacy and the environment. *Am J Occup Ther* 46(5): 434–43.

Dunn, D. 2000. Personal communication, November.

DeJong, G. and B. O'Day. 2000. Contrast of Paradigms: "Old" paradigms vs "new" paradigms. (WWW document). URL *www.ncddr.org*

Gordon, M. 2000. Personal communication, November.

Goren, W. D. 1999. *Understanding the Americans with Disabilities Act: An overview for lawyers.* Chicago: General Practice, Solo and Small Firm Section, American Bar Association, ABA Publishing Co.

Graney, P. J. 2000. RS20194: Developmental Disabilities Act: 106th Congress legislation. Washington DC: Domestic Policy Division. Congressional Research Service, Library of Congress.

Hanebrink, S. and B. Parent-Brown. 2000. ADA consulting opportunities. *OT Practice* 5(17): 12–16.

Hightower-Vandamm, M. D. 1979. Nationally speaking: Developmental Disabilities Act: An historical perspective, part 1. *Am J Occup Ther* 355–59.

Jacobs, K. 1996. Work assessments and programming. In *Willard and Spackman's occupational therapy,* eds. H. L. Hopkins and H. D. Smith 226–48, 8th ed. Philadelphia: J. B. Lippincott.

Johansson, C. 2000a. Disability advocates say more could be done. (WWW document). URL *http://www.aota.org*

———. 2000b. Work incentives bill signed. (WWW document). URL *http://www.aota.org*

Kalscheur, J. A. 1992. Benefits of the Americans with Disabilities Act of 1990 for children and adolescents with disabilities. *Am J Occup Ther* 46(5): 419–27.

Kelley, M. 2000. Personal communication, November.

Lenker, J. A. 2000. Certification in assistive technology. *OT Practice* 5(16): 12–16.

Marshall, E. M. 1985. Looking back. *Am J Occup Ther* 39(5): 297–300.

McClain, J. 1996. Personal communication, January.

McGregor, D. 2001. Health policy. In *Delivering Halth Care in America: A Systems Approach,* eds. L. Shi and D. A. Singh. Gaithersburg, MD: Aspen.

Mellard, E. 2000. Impact of federal policy on services for children and families in early intervention programs and public schools. In *Best practice occupational therapy,* ed. W. Dunn. Thorofare, NJ: Slack.

Muchlenhaupt, M. 2000. OT services under IDEA 97: Decision-making challenges. *OT Practice* 5(24): 10–16.

NADDC. 2000. National Association of Developmental Disabilities Council. URL *http://www.igc.apc.org*

National Information Center for Children and Youth with Disabilities (NICHCY). January 2000. *NICHY News Digest 21 (2nd ed.),* 1–35. Accessed at *http://www.nichcy.org/pubs/newsdig/nd2ltxt.htm* on Dec. 5, 2000.

Nosek, M. A. 1992. The Americans with Disabilities Act of 1990: Will it work? *Am J Occup Ther* 46(5): 466–67.

Perinchief, J. 1996. Service management. In *Willard and Spackman's occupational therapy*, eds. H. L. Hopkins and H. D. Smith, 375–93, Philadelphia: J. B. Lippincott.

Redick, A. G., L. Mclean, and C. Brown. 2000. Consumer empowerment through occupational therapy: The Americans with Disabilities Act Title III. *Am J Occup Ther* 54(2): 207–213.

RESNA. 2000. Rehabilitation Engineering and Assistive Technology Society of North America Internet site: RESNA Government Affairs. (WWW document). URL *http://www.resna.org*

Reed, K. L. 1992. History of federal legislation for peoples with disabilities. *Am J Occup Ther* 46(5): 397–409.

———. 1996. The beginnings of occupational therapy. In *Willard and Spackman's occupational therapy*, eds. H. L. Hopkins and H. D. Smith, 26–39, Philadelphia: J. B. Lippincott.

Reyes-Akinbileje, B. 1999. CRS Report for Congress: Technology assistance for people with disabilities: Summary of P.L. 100–407 and P.L. 103–218. Washington DC: Congressional Research Service, Library of Congress.

Rothstein, L. F. 1992. *Disability and the law*. Colorado Springs CO: McGraw-Hill.

Schultz, M. 2000. Personal communication, December.

Stockdell, M. and M. S. Crawford. An industrial model for assisting employers to comply with the Americans with Disabilities Act of 1990. *Am J Occup Ther* 46(5): 427–33.

Tomlin, G. 2000. The history of P & A programs. (WWW document). URL *http://boots.law.ua.edu/*

Tucker, B. P. 1994. *Federal disability law*. St. Paul, MN: West Publishing Co.

Wells, S. A. 2000. The Americans with Disabilities Act of 1990: Equalizing opportunities. *OT Practice* 5(6): CE1–8.

www.peublo.gsa 2000

Workforce Investment Act of 1998, Pub. L. No. 105–220, § 404, 112 Stat. 936, 1148–49 (codified as amended at 29 U.S.C. § 723 Supp. IV 1998).

6

Fundamentals of Insurance

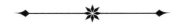

CHAPTER OBJECTIVES

At the conclusion of this chapter, the reader will be able to:

1. Discuss the social purpose and organization of health care insurance.
2. Define and relate the basic features of an insurance contract.
3. Describe insurance contracts using three methods of classification.
   a. By Sponsorship
      1. Private Insurance
      2. Self-Insurance
      3. Direct Contracting
   b. By Method of Cost Sharing
      1. Indemnity
      2. Service Benefit Plans
   c. By Covered Events/Services
      1. Long-Term Care Insurance
      2. Workers Compensation
      3. Casualty Insurance
4. Discuss the rationale for regulation of health care insurance markets.

KEY WORDS: Actuarial Analysis, Assignment of Benefits, Beneficiary, Community
Rating, Cost Limits, Moral Hazard, Premium, Risk, Underwriting

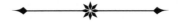

Introduction

Insurance is a financial mechanism that shares and disperses the risk of financial loss due to the occurrence of an adverse event within a population. Insurance performs an important social function by improving the financial stability of individuals and organizations. Individuals and organizations pay a fee (premium) to create a pool of resources that will provide income or service benefits to holders (beneficiaries) of an insurance contract (policy). A beneficiary who experiences an adverse event covered by the contract is eligible to receive benefits. Since insurance funds the majority of therapy services, physical therapists and occupational therapists need to understand the form and structure of insurance in order to meet contractual obligations for the reimbursement of their care.

In this chapter, we will introduce the social function of insurance, the basics of an insurance contract, a classification system of insurance contracts, and how insurance is regulated. Chapter 7 is devoted to the most common form of health care insurance today: managed care. Chapters 8 and 9 will discuss the largest social insurance programs in the world: Medicare and Medicaid. We begin the chapter with an explanation of the social purpose and organization of health care insurance.

Why Have Health Care Insurance?

Purpose of Insurance

Insurance performs an important social purpose in protecting individuals and organizations against unforeseen and severe financial loss. For many employees, health care insurance is an important part of a work-related benefit package. In 1994, about 60 percent of national income loss due to short-term illness was replaced by employee benefit plans, such as health care insurance, disability insurance, sick leave, and worker's compensation (Kerns, 1997). Without insurance, many ill or injured persons would be forced into liquidation of assets and bankruptcy to pay for the costs of medical illness and disability.

Risk and Insurance

The basic purpose of insurance is to share and disperse the negative consequences of an adverse event. Health care insurance prevents any one individual or group of individuals from suffering serious financial hardship or poor health due to an illness or injury. To prevent this from occurring, individuals come together to form a **risk** pool which collects a fee (**premium**) from each member (**beneficiary**) which can be disbursed to individuals who actually incur an event covered by the contract. The purchase of insurance does not guarantee that one will receive benefits equal to the amount of money contributed to the pool. In fact, if all the beneficiaries received benefits equal to or greater than the amount they contributed, the risk pool would be financially bankrupt. Implicit to the concept of insurance is the sharing of risk. Insurance exists to provide "peace of mind" in that the individual will receive benefits in case of the occurrence of the adverse event. Those without insurance are placed at risk of significant loss of financial resources and/or health.

Organization and Administration of Health Care Insurance

The organization and administration of an insurance program is performed by private companies and by the government. Private insurance companies are regulated by state governments that, at a minimum, require insurance plans to maintain adequate financial reserves to cover the needs of the risk pool. The United States, unlike most industrialized countries, does not provide universal medical care coverage for its citizens. As a consequence, health care insurance in the United States is a dualistic mix of public and private insurers (see Chapter 1). This results in both the freedom of individuals to purchase an insurance contract as well as the reality that a large segment of the population is without any health care insurance coverage at all (see Chapter 2).

Actuarial Adjustment and Insurance

In order for insurance to be a stable source of funding for therapy and medical care, the collected premiums must cover the benefits to pool members, the administrative expenses of the insurance plan, and, in the case of private insurers, generate a profit. The premium fee is determined by a process called **actuarial analysis**. Actuarial analysis commonly considers demographic factors (e.g., age, gender, medical history), past medical care utilization rates, and known cost data to make statistical decisions about future utilization and costs. An actuarial adjustment determines the premium fee based on the information included in the actuarial analysis. For example, people over the age of 65 would pay a greater amount for medical care insurance than individuals in their early twenties. Actuarial adjustment provides for equity in cost sharing based on likely need for benefits. If performed improperly, actuarial methods can result in excessive profits or losses for the insurer and can affect the availability and affordability of health care insurance to the public.

Moral Hazard and Insurance

Moral hazard is an insurance problem which can be caused by both the beneficiary and the insurer. Moral hazard is financially irresponsible behavior regarding insurance. Individuals create moral hazard by choosing not to purchase health care insurance when they have the capability to do so or by utilizing unnecessary medical care services covered by the insurance. People who choose not to purchase health care insurance shift the costs of their unpaid medical care to people who pay into the risk pool. People who overutilize services raise the costs of health care for all insured individuals.

Insurance companies commit moral hazard through the process of actuarial analysis or actuarial adjustment. Favorable selection results from an actuarial process that preferentially identifies people with anticipated low health care costs. This will result in lower beneficiary premiums and higher insurer profits. Favorable selection also creates a pool of individuals with higher health care costs who may not be able to obtain affordable insurance. Individuals in this pool are affected by adverse selection.

By the mid-1990s, the problems of rising insurance costs and moral hazard made it increasingly difficult for people to obtain or maintain health care insurance. To address the problem caused by insurance moral hazard, some states attempted to mandate a form of actuarial adjustment called **community rating.** Community rating requires insurance companies to set a premium fee not based on individual experience but on the experience of everyone in a given city, county, or other geographic area. Individuals with high costs and low costs are included in the geographic region. Community rating has been less than successful. Premium rate increases to cover all persons, both the healthy and the sick, resulted in many people disenrolling from the insurance plans. In effect, community rating caused adverse selection.

Basics of an Insurance Contract

A medical care insurance contract with a beneficiary defines eligibility for benefits, what events and services are covered by the plan, what the cost limits of the insurance plan are, and how coordination of benefits will occur (see Table 6–1). Insurance contracts with providers define the mechanisms and circumstances of payment for services (see Table 6–2). It is important to understand that an insurance contract does not pay for all of the services that can be requested by a beneficiary or delivered by a provider. For example, most insurance contracts exclude payment for luxury or experimental services. Insurance contracts do not tell providers what to do. Insurance contracts inform the beneficiary and the provider about what services are covered and how much of the cost of care will be paid for by the insurance company. Insurance contracts only provide benefits to eligible beneficiaries for covered events and covered services.

Eligibility

Eligibility is established based upon criteria set by the sponsor of the insurance plan. The United States lacks a comprehensive single source for health care insurance which is open for enrollment by all Americans. Instead, the United States has a mix of programs that determine eligibility based on the motivation of the sponsor and the willingness of the beneficiary to participate. For example, employment-based coverage is offered only to employees of a given business or members of a

Table 6–1. Basic Features of an Insurance Contract

A. Eligibility
  1. Established by the sponsor of the plan.
B. Covered Events
  1. Medical problem diagnosed by a credentialed physician.
  2. Contract is responsible for event precipitating the illness or injury (e.g., worker's compensation insurance is responsible for work-related illness or injury).
  3. Excludes illness or injury caused by war, riot, or self-inflicted.
C. Covered Services
  1. Stated in contract
    a. Reasonable and necessary
    b. Acceptable medical practice
  2. Excludes experimental and certain elective procedures (e.g., cosmetic surgery).
C. Beneficiary Cost Limits
  1. Plan limits: lifetime, overall limit, annual, out-of-pocket limit.
  2. First-dollar coverage: deductible or co-payment.
  3. Co-insurance: shared percentage-based reimbursement between insurer and beneficiary up to out-of-pocket limit.
  4. Limits on utilization: pre-authorization, day-dollar-visit limits, provider selection, documentation or expectation for improvement.
D. Coordination Of Benefits
  1. Primary and secondary insurance: "Birthday" rule for children.

given labor union. Eligibility can be further restricted by previous or anticipated utilization of health care services. The process of **underwriting** determines whether an individual's personal characteristics (e.g., age, medical history), qualify the person to purchase the insurance. Strict application of underwriting rules resulted in problems with insurance portability in the mid-1990s. We will discuss this issue later. An insurance contract defines who is eligible to join the risk pool and contribute premiums.

Covered Events

Covered events are usually medical illnesses or injuries that have been diagnosed by a credentialed physician. The credentialing process is an insurance procedure that verifies that the provider has met minimum qualifications for the relevant area of practice. Typically, an insurance contract will not list events that are covered but rather events that are excluded from coverage under the contract. Events due to war, civil disturbance, or self- inflicted injuries are usually not covered. Some insurance contracts exclude preventive health services. It is important to note that the type of insurance must match the covered event. For example, if a person is injured on the job, insurance will be provided by worker's compensation insurance, not an employer-sponsored group health insurance plan.

Covered Services

Once insurance eligibility is established and a covered event has occurred, a beneficiary or provider is eligible to receive benefits for covered services from the plan. Benefits may be financial remuneration for expenses incurred due to a covered event or, more commonly, the services themselves. Services typically include physician care, hospital stays, outpatient care, rehabilitation therapy, behavioral health care, short-term nursing facility stays, and prescription drug benefits. At a minimum, services need to be "reasonable and necessary" to treat the covered event. In general, services should contribute to the recovery of the patient and meet locally acceptable standards of patient care. "Reasonable and necessary" and "acceptable" are determined by an internal review process (utilization review) performed by the insurer.

Cost Limits

Finally, an insurance contract will establish rules that limit the cost of services to the insurance plan. For the beneficiary, this occurs through plan limits, "first dollar coverage" limits, co-insurance, and limits on utilization of care. Insurance contracts between the insurance plan and providers will limit costs to the plan by means of fee schedules, case rates, and capitation. These limits define how the insurance plan will pay for professional services.

Beneficiary Cost Limits

Insurance contracts will establish two types of plan limits: an overall plan limit and an out-of-pocket limit. The overall plan limit is the maximum dollar amount the plan will pay over the lifetime of a covered member. An out-of-pocket limit is the maximum amount a beneficiary is responsible to pay during a plan year.

Second, an insurance contract will define when plan coverage begins. It is typically calculated on an annual basis by plan year. This first-dollar-coverage limit will vary by type of health care insurance plan. For example, a deductible is the amount of money to be paid out of pocket by the beneficiary before any reimbursement by the insurance company. In this form of insurance cost limit, the beneficiary is responsible for all covered costs during the plan year up to a set amount of money (e.g., $250). Another example of a first-dollar-coverage limit is a **co-payment.** A co-payment is a flat fee (e.g., $10) paid by the beneficiary each time a health care service is utilized. This form of first-dollar-coverage limit is common to the health maintenance organization (HMO) form of managed care.

A third form of cost limit in insurance contracts is co-insurance. It is used in indemnity plans and some forms of managed care to share a percentage of costs between the beneficiary and the insurance plan until the out-of-pocket limit is reached. For example, a "70–30" co-insurance means that the insurance plan is responsible for 70 percent of the costs and the beneficiary for 30 percent after the deductible is paid and before the out-of-pocket limit is reached. Once the out-of-pocket limit is reached, the insurance contract will typically pay all remaining costs for the plan year up to the overall plan limit.

A fourth form of cost limit in insurance contracts is limits on the utilization of covered services. Physical therapy and occupational therapy services typically require pre-authorization by physician referral and, in some cases, by the insurer. Therapy services may have day, dollar, or visit limits for the plan year. An insurance contract may limit beneficiary selection of providers to a contracted panel. A typical standard for reimbursement of occupational therapy and physical therapy services in all insurance contracts is the expectation and documentation of improvement in function or health status in order to justify the continuation of services.

Provider Cost Limits

The various types of provider cost limits are summarized in Table 6–2. A fee schedule is a predetermined list of procedure payments that are negotiated between the provider and the insurance plan. A fee schedule is used in many types of insurance contracts, including managed care, service benefit plans, and social insurance. Case rates are all-procedure-inclusive payments that take three forms: per diem (daily), per visit, and per episode. A per diem rate is a flat payment for a day of services. A per visit rate sets reimbursement for each therapy visit. A per episode rate is a negotiated fee for an entire episode of care. Capitation is a form of reimbursement that pays the provider for each member of a health care insurance plan. Capitation will be fully discussed in Chapter 7.

Table 6–2.   Provider Cost Limits in Health Care Insurance Contracts

A. Fee Schedules
   1. Negotiated list of payment rates by health care procedure.
B. Case Rates
   1. Per diem
      a. All-procedure-inclusive daily payment rate.
   2. Per visit
      a. All-procedure-inclusive payment rate for each visit.
   3. Per episode
      a. All-procedure-inclusive rate for a treatment episode.
C. Capitation
   1. Payment to provider based on members in health plan.

Coordination of Benefits

Some individuals will be covered by more than one insurance contract. This is a common situation in marriages where both spouses have employment-based insurance for themselves and their dependents. In such cases, a coordination of benefits occurs. The policy held by the insured person seeking services is considered to be the primary insurance, and the other coverage is considered to be secondary insurance. For children with dual parental coverage, the birthday rule is commonly used. The insured parent whose birthday is the earliest in the calendar year is considered to be the primary insurer.

Types of Insurance

Health care insurance is offered to the public through different insurance product types. One way to classify health care insurance is to determine its sponsorship (e.g., commercial insurance, social insurance, self- insurance, direct contracting). The method of cost-sharing between the insurance plan, provider, and beneficiary is another method to classify insurance. For example, indemnity insurance, service benefit plans, and managed care are different types of health care insurance. Finally, the type of covered services can classify type of insurance (e.g., health care insurance, workers compensation, long-term care insurance).

In this next section, we will introduce several of these types of insurance. The next three chapters of the book will explore the managed care and social insurance forms of health care insurance in more detail. For now, we will consider these types of health care insurance:

- By sponsorship
  - private insurance
  - self-insurance
  - direct contracting
- By method of cost sharing
  - indemnity insurance
  - service benefit plans
- By covered events/services
  - long-term-care insurance
  - worker's compensation
  - casualty insurance

It is important to understand that this classification system for health care insurance does not create mutually exclusive categories of insurance. For example, a private insurance company may sponsor an indemnity, long-term-care insurance product. This classification system will help you understand the variety of insurance products that affect the practice of physical therapy and occupational therapy. Since there are many types of health care insurance available in the market, the therapist needs to understand the specific features of each product in order to understand the eligibility, covered events, covered services, and cost limitations for the patient's episode of care.

Sponsorship

Private Insurance

Private insurance is most commonly provided as a benefit of employment. Health care insurance sponsored by for-profit insurance companies is commonly termed commercial insurance. Individuals may purchase commercial insurance on their own or through a group plan. Group health care insurance is also sponsored by non-profit organizations (e.g., labor unions, the Blue Cross insurance plans).

Self-Insurance

Nearly one-half (47%) of the holders of employment-based insurance are covered by employers who self-insure (Park 1999). Self-insurance means that a company or organization chooses not to participate in a risk pool organized by an insurance company (commercial insurance)and instead establishes its own separate insurance fund internally to pay for covered events and benefits. Sponsors usually contract with a health insurance company to administer the plan. Many self-insured companies and organizations supplement this method of insurance by purchasing "stop-loss" coverage to cap their liability for claims that are higher than anticipated.

Self-insurance is most common in businesses or labor unions with at least 100 members (Garfinkel 1995; Park 1999) . This method of insurance enables large organizations to manage health care insurance costs by predicting and dispersing risk in a known risk pool while simultaneously avoiding expensive marketing and administrative costs. Self-insured health care insurance plans are exempt from state regulation (ERISA exemption). As a result, this form of insurance is popular with multi-state organizations that would be affected by individual state mandates and regulations.

Direct Contracting

In the late 1990s, two new forms of financing for medical care services emerged that are in competition with health care insurance: buyer-sponsored organizations and provider-service organizations. Both of these types of contract mechanisms bypass the traditional insurance company actuarial function and incorporate this process into the operations of either employer purchasers or large provider organizations. In this way, direct contracting occurs between employer purchasers of health care and health care providers. Few in number, these forms of "insurance" are risky for their organizers, and the financial performance of these endeavors on a national scale has been both positive and negative.

The increasing interest and sophistication of large employers in purchasing medical care insurance products has caused some of them to form cooperatives and directly contract with providers to obtain care for their employees. This type of contracting group is called a buyer-sponsored organization. A Minneapolis and St. Paul, Minnesota coalition of large employers has formed the Buyers Health Care Action Group to competitively bid and contract for employee health coverage with area health care providers (Christianson et al. 1999). Provider-sponsored organizations are structures established by health care providers to market a package of benefits directly to employers and other purchasers of health care. This new method of obtaining health care has applications for physical therapists and occupational therapists (Cohn 1999).

Method of Cost Sharing

Indemnity Insurance

The first health care insurance products were called indemnity insurance plans. Indemnity insurance reimburses a beneficiary for covered health care expenses. The provider is paid by the beneficiary, who is subsequently reimbursed by the insurance company. Indemnity insurance plans utilize plan limits, a deductible form of first-dollar coverage, and co-insurance to limit costs. "Managed" indemnity plans also include limits on the utilization of services. This insurance structure is paperwork-intensive, and providers often need to wait a long time for payment. To address the problem of delayed payments, the **assignment of benefits** clause was created to permit direct payment to the provider by the insurance company. Assignment of benefits is routinely obtained from the patient on admission to a physical therapy or occupational therapy practice.

Indemnity insurance is also associated with open choice, fee-for-service reimbursement structures. Beneficiaries have the right to choose any provider who will accept their insurance plan (open choice). In this structure, patients and insurers pay the provider for the reasonable and necessary charges of care on a per procedure basis. Indemnity insurance products provide financial incentives that provide maximum beneficiary choice of provider, broaden the range of services delivered, and increase the cost of health care.

Service Benefit Plans

Service benefit plans developed as a modified form of indemnity insurance. Service benefit plans originated several features common to today's health care insurance plans. First, service benefit plans established panels of providers to deliver services. A provider panel is a list of physical therapists, occupational therapists, physicians, hospitals, and other providers who contract with an insurance company to provide care. Second, service benefit plans utilize assignment of benefits and pay providers directly from the insurance company. Third, service benefit plans utilize a fee schedule to pay for provider services. A fee schedule establishes the payment rates for contracted services.

Covered Events/Services

Long-Term-Care Insurance

The increased risk of expensive long-term care and the limitations of private health care and social insurance plans in sponsoring this coverage have spawned the development of long-term-care insurance. In 1994, one-fifth of the country's population over age 65 (7.1 million people) experienced disablement (Urban Institute 1999). For the severely impaired, the average cost of a nursing home stay for a year was $46,000 in 1995 (Urban Institute 1999). To protect against this risk, about 5 million Americans have purchased long-term-care insurance policies at an annual cost of $2,000 per year for an individual age 65 (National Association of Insurance Commissioners 1999). Most long-term-care insurance is sold in the individual insurance market, but employment-based long-term-care insurance is increasing. Unlike the post-acute care benefits in medical care or social insurance plans, eligibility for long-term-care insurance benefits is not limited to the aftermath of an episode of acute medical illness.

Long-term-care insurance provides benefits to people with physical illness, cognitive impairments, and other chronic diseases that result in impairments and functional limitations. Eligibility for benefits is based on the loss of function in activities of daily living (ADL) or the onset of a significant cognitive impairment. Six ADLs are commonly examined to determine eligibility: bathing, continence, dressing, eating, toileting, and transferring. An inability to perform at least two of these tasks without assistance will usually initiate benefits (NAIC 1999).

Long-term-care insurance benefits cover services at home, or in skilled nursing facilities, assisted living facilities, and adult day care centers. Services include personal assistance and professional care (e.g., occupational therapy, physical therapy). Typically, cost limits on benefits are established as a per diem rate. Case management to determine eligibility and coordinate benefits is used in long-term-care insurance plans (NAIC 1999).

Worker's Compensation

Worker's compensation insurance originated in the early part of the twentieth century. It was precipitated by the increasing incidence of industrial workplace injuries, lost worker wages, worker disabilities, and workplace litigation. The purpose of worker's compensation insurance is to protect workers, free employers from excessive litigation, and decrease the incidence of occupational injuries. The prevalence of musculoskeletal injury in this population makes worker's compensation insurance a program of importance to physical therapists and occupational therapists. Back pain is the most common worker's compensation claim (Guo et al. 1999).

Worker's compensation insurance is an example of no-fault insurance. Employers are liable for damages due to workplace-related illness and injury regardless of the circumstances surrounding the event. The source or severity of the injury, however, can be disputed (Hirsch 1997). Worker's compensation laws establish statutorily determined benefits for workers and also protect employers from suits over expenses related to workplace injuries. Worker's compensation laws are state-specific within broad guidelines established in federal law. Some states require employers to participate in state-operated programs. Other states permit employers to purchase worker's compensation insurance in the private market. Employers pay the full premium for worker's compensation insurance. About 95 percent of the American workforce is covered by worker's compensation insurance (Himmelstein et al. 1999).

Worker's compensation insurance consists of three benefit programs: health care insurance, disability income replacement, and vocational rehabilitation. To be eligible for worker's compensation, an individual must be injured or acquire an illness while performing employment activities or functions (Calfee 1998). The benefits may be temporary or permanent depending on the injury or illness. About 70 percent of claims are temporary in nature, but the most expensive claims are due to permanent disability (Hirsch 1997). The medical benefits start immediately after the injury and are unlimited. Medical benefits are provided until "maximal medical improvement" or a return to employment has occurred (Durbin 1997).

Outpatient services are the dominant mode of medical care delivery in worker's compensation programs (Himmelstein et al. 1999). Medical benefits are paid without deductible or co-insurance to the injured employee. Choice of physician and provider is a source of contention in worker's compensation law (Himmelstein et al. 1999). Since eligibility for benefits is based on a determination that an injury or illness is work-related, the choice of provider to make the determination is important. Some states allow open choice of provider by the injured employee. Other states permit the employer to select the physician to determine eligibility for benefits.

The Occupational Health and Safety Act of 1970 established income replacement cash benefits and vocational rehabilitation benefits as part of a minimum worker's compensation benefit package. This program accounts for 60 percent of the costs of the worker's compensation program (Himmelstein et al. 1999). Durbin (1997) has reviewed the process that determines the amount of income replacement for a worker's compensation claim. Disability is classified using five categories:

- fatal
- permanent total
- permanent partial
- temporary total
- temporary partial

Disability benefits are paid as an income replacement payment (typically 66 percent of pre-injury income) while the worker is not employable. Temporary benefits are paid after a three- to seven-day waiting period until maximal medical improvement is reached or the worker has a medical release to return to work (Hirsch 1997). Permanent benefits are provided after maximal medical improvement has been attained.

A physical impairment rating and a schedule of benefits are used to determine permanent disability. Certain types of injuries are non scheduled (e.g., injury to the visceral organs, trunk, or neck and head, claims of psychological disability). Scheduled injuries include the limbs, eyes, and ears. Each of these body parts is assigned a statutory length of time in weeks of disablement based on a schedule. Impairment of function is rated using the *American Medical Association Guide to the Evaluation of Permanent Impairment.* This percentage rating is multiplied by the schedule of weeks for benefits to determine the degree of permanent disability. This figure is multiplied by the pre-injury wage to determine the total disability award.

Worker's compensation insurance costs have been rapidly rising in the last 15 years. In response to this trend, 24 states had authorized or mandated worker's compensation managed care programs by the mid-1990s (Dembe et al. 1997). Fraud and abuse in the worker's compensation system is commonly alleged (Hirsch 1997; Durbin 1997). Several types of moral hazard have been described in the worker's compensation program (Hirsch 1997; Durbin 1997). First, the generous benefit packages in worker's compensation plans provide incentives for employees to file false claims or to exaggerate symptoms. Second, the high costs of the program have incentivized employers to aggressively manage these costs and jeopardize the medical care of persons with legitimate injury or illness. Third, the presence of insurance tends to make employers more safety conscious and employees less safety conscious. Fourth, the fee-for-service reimbursement mechanism of some worker's compensation plans incentivizes providers to overtreat conditions.

Recent trends in worker's compensation include the use of managed care and self-insurance programs to restrain the growth in costs. Disability case management and utilization review are now in widespread use for worker's compensation insurance. Contracted provider networks that limit open choice of providers are also used. A newer trend is for the development of integrated primary, secondary, and tertiary care networks in worker's compensation plans that can provide 24-hour coverage.

Casualty Insurance

Automobile or homeowner's insurance will include a medical care benefit. A person must have been injured in an automobile accident or home accident to be eligible for covered benefits. Depending on the state, determination of fault in the accident situation will establish responsibility of claims. In these cases, a legal judgement is sometimes necessary to determine who will pay for therapy services. Casualty insurance is most commonly provided using a fee-for-service reimbursement structure, although managed care principles are sometimes used to reimburse providers. A recent report in *Physical Therapy Reimbursement News* stated that managed care automobile plans have appeared in seven states. These products utilize case management, utilization reviews, contracted-provider networks, and discounted fee mechanisms to control costs.

Regulation of Insurance

Insurance is only useful if it provides contracted benefits when needed at an affordable cost. The failure of insurance to meet these obligations has prompted the intervention of government into the insurance marketplace. States have primary responsibility to regulate insurance. The ability of states to regulate medical care insurance is affected by federal legislation. In this section, we will explore the role of the state and federal governments in regulating the insurance marketplace.

Insurance Regulation

Each state has an insurance department that licenses and regulates the activities of insurance companies doing business in the state. Klein (1995) has defined two primary areas of state insurance regulation: maintaining solvency requirements and market regulation. Insurance companies are required to be licensed in their state of incorporation and in the states where they sell insurance products. Solvency requirements mandate that insurance companies maintain capital reserves and financial strategies to cover their anticipated losses. This lessens the possibility of an insurance company facing bankruptcy due to a simultaneous increase in claims and inadequate financial reserves. Some states regulate the premiums charged by insurers, and all states monitor the marketing and eligibility determination (underwriting) practices of insurance companies.

Insurance departments also investigate consumer complaints regarding insurance. The rise of managed care and changes in health care insurance have resulted in the enactment of laws restricting insurance practices in some states. Examples of these laws include the prohibition of "gag clauses" on providers and of insurance limits on maternal stays after childbirth. The ability of states to regulate health care insurance, however, is significantly limited by federal law, specifically, the Employee Retirement Income Security Act.

Employee Retirement Income Security Act of 1974

The Employee Retirement Income Security Act of 1974 (ERISA) is a federal statute enacted to standardize regulation of pension and employee benefit plans. The law establishes minimal reporting requirements on pensions and prohibits state regulation of health care self-insurance plans. ERISA prevents state regulators from establishing consumer advocacy, minimal solvency, or benefit requirements in this popular form of employment-based insurance (Polzer and Butler 1997). In addition, it protects managed care organizations from lawsuits about decisions made by the plan unless the provider is employed by the plan (Mariner 1996). As a result, providers bear the brunt of malpractice lawsuits even when insurance coverage decisions are made by managed care plans (Griffin and Adelman 1998).

Continuation Issues

The high cost of medical care insurance has made it increasingly difficult for some people to obtain coverage. This is especially true for those who lose employment-based coverage due to a change in life status or employment. The Consolidated Budget Reconciliation Act of 1985 (COBRA) was enacted to deal with the problem of loss of health care insurance due to change in life status or employment. The Health Insurance Portability and Accountability Act of 1996 limits the ability of insurance companies to deny coverage based on pre-existing conditions.

COBRA mandates that individuals who lose employment-based health care insurance for reasons other than gross misconduct are eligible to continue coverage for 18 months at full cost to themselves. This law provides that insurance must be also offered to the spouse and dependents of employees who had family-type coverage. In the event of an employee death, a divorce, or a child no longer maintaining eligible-dependent status, the spouse or dependents can purchase coverage for up to three years. Coverage is terminated on the first occurrence of one of the following events: end of the mandated period, the employer discontinues health care insurance for all employees, or the premiums are not paid. COBRA has been criticized for being too expensive for both the employee (Retsinas 1998) and the employer (Fronstin 1998). Fronstin (1998) reports that 10 percent of an employer's workforce is usually eligible for COBRA continuation coverage. Only about one in four eligible employees accept COBRA continuation coverage. These tend to be persons who have higher incomes and higher medical care expenses.

In the mid-1990s, people with employment-based coverage found their employment opportunities limited by stringent restrictions on eligibility for health care insurance. New hires were either not offered health care insurance if they had certain pre-existing medical conditions or had to wait for long periods before coverage would begin for these problems. As a result, people became less willing to change jobs. This portability problem was called "job lock." It was remedied by the Health Insurance Portability and Accountability Act of 1996 (HIPAA). This law established limits on an insurance company's ability to restrict eligibility for health care insurance. It allows an insurance company to establish one 12-month waiting period for pre-existing conditions (Health Insurance Association of America 2000). This is modified by the date of diagnosis of the condition and previous nondisrupted medical care insurance coverage prior to the new employment situation. Like COBRA, HIPAA does not regulate premium costs. As a result, individuals with high health care costs may still not be able to obtain affordable health insurance.

Conclusion

In this chapter we have discussed the structure and forms of insurance that reimburse for health care services, including occupational therapy and physical therapy. Health care insurance prevents financial disaster for those who are ill or disabled and provides a source of funding for health care providers. It does not cover all the costs of health care; some services are excluded, and many services require financial participation by the beneficiary and place limits on reimbursement to the provider. Insurance contracts define eligibility, covered events, covered services, and the sharing of the costs of health care insurance. Health care insurance is sponsored by many types of organizations, has different forms of cost sharing, and at times provides covered benefits only for certain events (e.g., worker's compensation insurance). Primary oversight of the health care insurance industry is performed by state government. Several federal laws have been enacted that affect access to health care insurance.

CHAPTER REVIEW QUESTIONS

1. Define the purpose of health care insurance.
2. Define and discuss the concept of risk in health care insurance.
3. What are actuarial analysis and actuarial adjustment?
4. Define moral hazard, favorable selection, and adverse selection.
5. Define the basics of an insurance contract:
   a. Eligibility
   b. Covered events
   c. Covered services
   d. Cost limits for the beneficiary and the provider
   e. Coordination of benefits
6. Compare and contrast health care insurance contracts:
   a. By sponsorship
   b. By method of cost sharing
   c. By covered events and services
7. Define the role of state and federal government in regulating health care insurance.

DISCUSSION/CASE QUESTIONS

1. Mary is a 22-year-old single woman who has just accepted an entry-level position as a telemarketer. She is provided with a pool of benefit dollars from which she can purchase a variety of benefits, including vacation, retirement plan, and health care insurance. Consider and discuss the effects of a decision to purchase or decline to purchase health care insurance on Mary and the community.

2. Mr. Smith is receiving therapy services in your outpatient clinic. He has a service benefit plan with a $200 annual deductible, $500 out-of-pocket maximum, 75–25 co-insurance, and a $1 million overall plan limit. To date, he has utilized $100 worth of covered plan benefits. Therapy charges are $500. What is the out-of-pocket cost of therapy services to Mr. Smith?
3. Consider this statement: "Insurance contracts do not tell providers what to do. Insurance contracts inform the beneficiary and provider about what services and how much of the cost of care will be paid for by the insurance company." Define and discuss the implications of this statement for the practice of occupational therapy and physical therapy.

REFERENCES

Calfee, B. E. 1997. Workers compensation litigation review. Part I. *AAOHN J* 45(11): 609–11.

———. 1998. Workers compensation litigation review. Part II. *AAOHN J* 46(1): 45–46.

Christianson, J., R. Feldman, J. P. Weiner, and P. Drury. 1999. Early experience with a new model of employer group purchasing in Minnesota. *Health Affairs* 18(6): 100–14.

Cohn, R. 1999. Direct contracting: Is it for you? *PT Magazine* 7(5): 22–24.

Dembe, A. E., J. E. Himmelstein, B. A. Stevens, and M. P. Beachler. 1997. Improving worker's compensation health care. *Health Affairs* 16(4): 253–57.

Durbin, D. 1997. Workplace injuries and the role of insurance: Claims costs, outcomes and incentives. *Clin Orthop* 336: 18–32.

Garfinkel, S. A. 1995. Self-insuring employee health benefits. *Med Care Res Rev* 52(4): 475–91.

Griffin, F. D. and S. H. Adelman. 1998. ERISA and medical professional liability. *Bull Am Coll Surg* 83(7): 16–21.

Guo, H. R., S. Tanaka, W. E. Halperin, and L. L. Cameron. 1999. Back pain prevalence in US industry and estimates of lost workdays. *Am J Pub Health* 89(7): 1029–35.

Health Insurance Association of America. Guide to Health Insurance. Accessed at *http://www.hiaa.org/cons/guidehi.html#law* on March 3, 2000.

Himmelstein, J., J. L. Buchanan, A. E. Dembe, and B. Stevens. 1999. Health services research in workers compensation medical care: Policy issues and research opportunities. *Health Serv Res* 34(1 pt. 2): 427–37.

Hirsch, B. T. 1997. Incentive effects of worker's compensation. *Clin Orthop* 336: 33–41.

Kerns, W. L. 1997. Cash benefits for short term sickness, 1970–1994. *Soc Sec Bull* 60(1): 49–53.

Klein, R. W. Insurance regulation in transition: Structural change and regulatory response in the insurance industry. Accessed at *http://www.naic.org/1misc/about naic/about/regutra3.htm* on March 3, 2000.

Mariner, W. K. 1996. Liability for managed care decisions: The Employee Retirement Income and Security Act (ERISA) and the uneven playing field. *Am J Pub Health* 86(6): 863–69.

National Association of Insurance Commissioners. 1999. *A shoppers guide to long-term care insurance.* Kansas City MO.: NAIC

Managed Auto Insurance and Physical Therapy. 1998. *Phys Ther Reimbursement News* 6(3): 1, 9.

Park, C. H. 1999. State variation in self-funding of employer-sponsored health insurance. *Abstr Book Assoc Health S* 14: 362.

Polzer, K. and P. A. Butler. 1997. Employee health plan restrictions under ERISA: Employee Retirement Income Security Act. *Health Affairs* 16(5): 93–102.

Urban Institute. Long term care for the elderly: Ten basic questions answered. Accessed at *http://222.urban.org/news/factsheets/elderlyFS.html* on March 3, 1999.

7

Managed Care

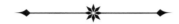

CHAPTER OBJECTIVES

At the conclusion of this chapter, the reader will be able to:

1. Discuss the goals of managed care.
2. Define and describe the main principles employed by managed care organizations.
   a. limited access to the entire universe of providers
   b. payment mechanisms that reward efficiency
   c. enhanced quality-improvement monitoring
3. Describe the primary features of managed care products (plans).
   a. managed indemnity
   b. preferred provider organization
   c. health maintenance organization
   d. point-of-service plan
3. Define and discuss different provider-network models that contract with managed care organizations.
   a. staff model
   b. group model
   c. network model
   d. independent practice association
4. Discuss the advantages and disadvantages of managed care for physical therapists and occupational therapists.
5. Discuss successful strategies therapists have used to adapt to the age of managed care.

KEY WORDS: Benchmarking, Bundled, Case Management, Credentialing, Gate-keeper, Leverage, Panel, Penetration

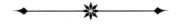

Introduction

Many forces, (e.g., employer awareness of the cost of care, the disincentives that make fee-for-service inefficient) have come together to change the medical delivery system that was once based on solo providers receiving fee-for-service payments. This change includes a move toward an "integrated" delivery system that is often referred to as managed care.

In the preceding chapter (Chapter 6), we introduced the basic purpose and characteristics of several types of health care insurance. In Chapters 8 and 9, we will discuss social insurance: the primary form of government-sponsored health insurance. This chapter addresses one of the most important developments with regard to the organization and payment of health care services in recent decades: managed care. The principles of managed care affect both the private and government-sponsored health insurance systems. We will begin by defining managed care, looking historically at how managed care became such an important player in the delivery of health care services. We will then discuss the basic principles of how managed care operates and how providers have responded to these changes. We will conclude by discussing how managed care policies affect physical and occupational therapists.

Because of years of being sheltered from the rising costs of health care and due to the availability of the latest and greatest medical technology, many working Americans used the health care system without much restriction or awareness of costs. Likewise, hospitals and physicians did not feel constrained to contain costs or hold back on providing services. As concerns rose with regard to rising health care costs in the 1970s, the federal government and employers looked for new ways to reduce health care expenditures. One of their ideas was the use of provider prepayment in order to encourage cost-conscious, efficient, effective care (Sultz and Young 1999). Though the concept of prepayment for services had been adopted by various employers to care for their employees, it was not until the passage of the Health Maintenance Organization (HMO) Act in 1973 that managed care and the concept of prepayment were thrust into the forefront of health insurance policy. Employer concerns about the costs of health care expedited the growth of managed care plans beginning in the late 1980s. The growth of managed care was also propelled by the ERISA exemption that prevented states from regulating employer-sponsored, self-insured health insurance plans (Noble and Brennan 1999; see Chapter 6).

It is important to note the difference between managed care and HMOs. Whereas HMOs are organizations that serve beneficiaries for a fixed fee and provide both financing and delivery of health care services, managed care is a broader concept referring to the principles that payment and the provision of service are interdependently linked. All HMOs represent some form of managed care, while most insurance companies apply at least some managed care principles in different forms of their insurance products (see the section on managed care products later in this chapter).

Defining Managed Care

In 1994, David Mechanic commented that the term "managed care" is used so "promiscuously" that it has limited meaning. While many people use the term, they may all have different ideas about what it really means. Thus, the term may describe one type of system for some people, but a totally different system to someone else. A minimal definition of managed care is "a system that integrates the financing and delivery of health services" (Barton 1999). Because of the widespread disparity in the definitions of "managed care," it has become an umbrella term to describe the many different organizational structures that try to accomplish the goal of linking the delivery and financing of health care services.

Though managed care has many definitions, all managed care organizations (MCOs) have some certain features in common (Kongstvedt 1999). Recall that in traditional indemnity insurance, the provider is paid a "reasonable and necessary" fee after delivering a service, without restriction on the number or type of services provided. The insurer acts as a processor of claims and makes no determination on the appropriateness of the care that was provided. Managed care health insurance plans expand the role of the insurer using three principles: limited access to the universe of providers, payment mechanisms that reward efficiency and enhance quality-control procedures. The insurer's role in managed care organizations is expanded from claims processing to determining on some level, the appropriateness of the care and the access by the beneficiary to plan benefits.

How widely and strictly these principles are utilized varies between managed care products. In general, managed care plans that are more restrictive and uniform in their benefits packages (e.g., HMOs) are less expensive than other forms of managed care and traditional indemnity insurance. Other types of managed care organizations (e.g., PPO and POS plans) provide some but not all features of managed care. Open access to care is improved, but these plans are more expensive. Thus, a variety of insurance options at different prices are available to consumers in the marketplace. Before we discuss the specific types of managed care products, let us explore each of these managed care principles in more detail.

Managed Care Principles

The three managed care principles are presented in Table 7–1. A short description and application of each principle is included in the table. We will consider each principle separately.

Limited Access to the Universe of Providers

Managed care organizations typically establish a **panel** of health care providers (i.e., a group of physicians, therapists, hospitals, etc.) that are contracted with or employed by the managed care organization to deliver care to plan beneficiaries.

Table 7–1.   **Managed Care Principles**

Principle	Description	Application
Limited access to providers	Controlled number of providers	Open/closed panels
		Credentialing
	Controlled patient access	Gatekeeper
Payment rewards efficiency	Discounts	Discounted fee-for-service
	Bundling	Case-based payment
	Capitation	Per member per month
Quality improvement	Data collection	Utilization review
	Peer review	Clinical pathways
		Benchmarking
		Case management

The panel should be geographically distributed and be inclusive of all necessary services in order to serve the population of patients covered by the plan. A panel may be short of the universe of providers in the area. This is important because this situation sets up a competitive situation in marketplaces with heavy managed care **penetration,** where the MCO has **leverage** in order to force providers to accept lower rates in order to maintain a patient base.

Provider panels may be either open panels or closed panels. An open panel allows any provider who agrees to the terms of the contract to join and be a part of the panel. A closed panel only allows a finite number of providers to participate in the panel even if there are others who qualify and desire to be part of the panel. When HMOs organize their provider panels, the providers often go through a **credentialing** process that reviews their education, clinical experience, and professional behavior. Regardless of how a panel of providers is put together or how big the panel may be, the extent to which patients view the provider panel as sufficient is highly subjective and depends greatly on whether or not "their" provider is on the list. This situation has led to many consumer complaints about closed-panel managed care plans. Later in this chapter, we will discuss how providers organize themselves in response to the insurer's initiative to create panels (see the discussion of managed care provider structures).

Most MCOs also limit or refuse benefits to members if they receive care from noncontracted providers. In some managed care models, authorization is done through primary care physicians who act as **gatekeepers.** Patients who want to visit a specialist, such as a physical or occupational therapist, must first go to their primary care provider and obtain a referral. The purpose for using some form of authorization is to reduce the number of "unnecessary" visits to more expensive specialists and thus save money. A less strict pre-authorization policy may allow patients to visit any physician directly without getting a referral from the primary care physician, but requires them to get authorization for the more expensive procedures, such as hospital admissions. While all managed care products utilize a provider panel, authorization schemes vary.

Payment Mechanisms That Reward Efficiency

As stated at the beginning of the chapter, traditional indemnity insurance provides few incentives for patients or providers to be efficient users of health care. The financial risk of health care is borne by the insurer; hence, the importance of actuarial analysis. Also, payment is made retrospectively, that is, after the intervention has occurred. In a managed care environment, providers are reimbursed for their services through a variety of mechanisms that either "bundle" individual services and procedures into one fee category or create new payment mechanisms altogether (i.e., discounted fee-for-service, case-based payment, capitation) (see Chapters 3 and 6). Some of these payment models utilize retrospective reimbursement (e.g., discounted fee-for-service), and other schemes utilize prospective payment systems (e.g., case-based payment, capitation). For further discussion of retrospective and prospective payment systems, see Chapter 8. With these incentives, the provider assumes either some or all the financial "risk" associated with patient care. Sharing of financial risk between the provider and the insurer is a very important concept in managed care. No longer are providers not at risk of losing money for the decisions they make in providing care and allocating financial resources. Let us consider how this works.

In a discounted fee schedule environment, providers accept a contract that is less than the full charge for certain services. In return for accepting this discounted fee, the provider is assured of a set of patients from those who subscribe to the contracted health plan and is paid per procedure, but at a lower rate than "reasonable and necessary." Most of the financial risk in this system is still borne by the insurer. The insurer must anticipate usage rates for plan benefits and collect enough premium dollars to pay providers. The insurer has little control over the amount of services that are utilized.

Under a **bundled** payment system, the insurer begins to limit financial risk. This is done by paying one fee to the provider for a set of patient services. It may be as simple as an insurer collating several procedures on a fee schedule that are commonly performed together to create one new fee category (while typically discounting or eliminating certain fees). Or, as in the case of Medicare, the insurer may deny payment for certain procedures that are billed at the same time as another procedure. Bundling can also occur when payment is made for an entire visit or day or episode of care, inclusive of all individual procedures and services. These payment mechanisms are all examples of case-based payment, which was introduced in Chapter 2. All of these payment mechanisms share financial risk between the insurer and provider. The more procedures, visits, or days of treatment provided, the greater the cost of delivering services. In the traditional indemnity and discounted fee-for-service systems, these costs are passed on to the insurer.

Bundled and case-based payment mechanisms separate reimbursement from procedure incidence. Instead of being paid more money for more procedures, providers receive fixed fees. The type and incidence of individual procedures is left to the provider, who assumes the financial risk of the cost of this care. Therefore, an incentive is created for the provider to control costs of care within the reimbursement amount provided by the insurer.

Capitation completely separates payment from treatment incidence. Capitation prospectively pays the provider a predetermined sum for each covered member of the plan on a regular basis (usually monthly). The provider is paid even if the plan member does not access covered services during that month. Conversely, the provider is not paid extra for the cost of delivering services that exceed the capitation payment. Capitation payment systems transfer financial risk almost entirely to the provider. If the provider's expenses are greater than the capitation payment for the plan members for the month, then the provider loses money. However, if the provider can care for that population for less than the capitation reimbursement amount, then profits are realized. Thus, the incentive is to engage in coordinated preventive care and keep patients healthy while avoiding expensive or extensive health care services. These incentives are so powerful that in some cases, the withholding of necessary services has been alleged against providers and MCOs using capitated payment models.

A number of ethical concerns about the effect of managed care reimbursement structures have been raised. One concern is that HMOs have little incentive to provide high-quality treatment, because success attracts costlier patients (Nayyar et al. 1998). Furthermore, physicians receive financial incentives, such as capitation or financial bonuses, to not refer patients to specialists (Spragins 1995). There have been occasions of physicians being dismissed from MCOs for over-referring patients and exceeding spending guidelines (Nayyar et al. 1998). Unchecked, these incentives sometimes create the moral hazard of favorable selection—marketing a low-cost but profitable managed care plan to healthy people while avoiding persons who are less healthy. Finally, it needs to be recognized that managed care is a dynamic system. MCOs have been forced in recent years to respond to consumer as well as provider concerns about some of their practices. For example, a majority of HMOs permit direct access to hospital and specialist physician services with pre-authorization by a HMO staff member (Freudenheim 2001). Other managed care practices have resulted in government intervention and, as a result, 41 states allow appeal to independent reviewers about decisions that deny access to health care (Freudenheim 2001).

Enhanced Quality Improvement Monitoring

Managed care plans intend to integrate the financial and delivery mechanisms of health care. As we have discussed, they do this by controlling access to health care services and by creating payment mechanisms that encourage efficiency. True integration of the financing and delivery of health care services requires policy related to quality as well as access and cost. Since quality is clearly in the purview of providers, this has been the most difficult policy principle for MCOs to implement.

To affect the quality of health care, MCOs perform utilization review, critical pathways, benchmarking, and case-management functions. Utilization review and critical pathways were discussed in Chapter 4 (see also Reynolds 1996). MCOs use these procedures to track the care of plan members. **Benchmarking** is an ongoing process of evaluating practice and outcomes against the evidence (i.e., industry standards, expert opinion, scientific literature). The report cards discussed in Chapter 4 are an application of benchmarking. Case management is used to coordinate care that is provided to managed care plan members. We will have more to say about working with case managers at the conclusion of this chapter.

In summary, managed care organizations use three principles: controlled access, cost incentives for efficiency, and quality-improvement mechanisms in order to integrate the financing and delivery of health care. A number of managed care products have been developed that incorporate the principles just discussed. The following section examines some of these managed care products.

Managed Care Products

Several types of managed care products exist that vary in their organizational structure and how they reimburse providers. These managed care plans range from those that are less aggregated (discounted fee-for-service) to those that are more aggregated (i.e., bundle payments either by episode of illness, per day/visit, or per member). This section briefly discusses the following managed care products: managed indemnity, preferred provider organizations, health maintenance organizations, and point-of-service plans. The primary features of these products are described in Table 7–2.

Managed indemnity

Managed indemnity, the least aggregated form of managed care, is a fee-for-service reimbursement strategy that adds a pre-authorization component along with utilization review. Thus, it is just one step removed from the fee-for-service systems of the past. The beneficiary in this system is required to obtain pre-authorization for inpatient stays and other services. Failure to do so could result in no reimbursement. On a more positive note, beneficiaries in this system have maximum choice in selecting their health care provider.

Preferred provider organizations

A preferred provider organization (PPO) is a contracted relationship between a panel of providers and the purchaser of health care services (i.e., the managed care organization). The contract is usually an agreed discounted fee-for-service for

Table 7–2.   Managed Care Products

Product	Characteristics
Managed indemnity	Open panel
	Discounted fee-for-service
	Pre-authorization
	Utilization review
Preferred provider organization	Open or closed panel
	Discounted fee-for-service and case-based payment
	Pre-authorization/utilization review
Health maintenance organization	Closed panel
	Discounted fee-for-service, case-based payment or capitation
	Gatekeeper authorization
Point of service plan	Contains both HMO and PPO plans
	Rules based on which option patient chooses

a set of specific services provided to beneficiaries. The plan uses pre-approval, utilization review, and discounted reimbursement to control costs. Health care providers benefit from an increased pool of patients, low financial investment, and more autonomy than in other managed care products. Beneficiaries have a choice of providers within the panel. Limited or no reimbursement is available for providers who are not contracted panel members.

Health Maintenance Organizations

A health maintenance organization (HMO) is a highly aggregated form of managed care. HMOs typically utilize gatekeeper physicians, pre-approval, and utilization review to control plan costs.

Beneficiaries can access plan benefits only upon referral from their primary care physician and only from panel providers. There is no reimbursement for providers not on the HMO panel. Provider payment can take various forms, including discounted fee-for-service, case-based, and capitation. Capitation is most common in the HMO form of managed care.

Point of Service (POS)

A hybrid managed care plan is the point of service (POS) plan. POS products contain both an HMO and PPO form of managed care. In this plan, beneficiaries are able to choose their provider at the time services are needed. Benefits are typically paid at a higher percentage for persons choosing their primary care providers (HMO product) rather than other providers in the panel (PPO product). Thus, patients have more flexibility to choose the provider they think is most appropriate for the current condition.

Managed Care Provider Structures

In order to establish managed care organizations, insurers or other entities must develop relationships and contracts with the provider community. These relationships can take various forms that result in the provider panels discussed in the preceding section. In broad terms, MCOs adopt four general model types that describe how provider contracts are established; specifically, a staff model, a group model, a network model, and an independent practice association (IPA) model (see Table 7–3). The more integrated models are characterized by a tightly structured organization that allows them to have more control of the delivery and cost of health care service. These models typically limit patient choices when it comes to how care is obtained. Those models that have relatively less integration are less structured and offer more choice to their patients. They also describe how providers choose to organize themselves in order to contract with MCOs.

Staff model

In a staff model, individual providers are employed by the HMO and receive a base salary for their services. Some HMOs may also pay incentives based on performance. The largest example of a staff model HMO is Kaiser of California, which salaries its physicians, and even owns many of its network hospitals. Other staff model HMOs may not own the hospitals, but salary providers and contract with hospitals. Beneficiaries in a staff model HMO receive coverage for a comprehensive set of conditions for a fixed price per month, but must be treated within the HMO. This is a highly integrated form of managed care.

Table 7–3. Managed Care Provider Structures

Staff model	Providers are salaried employees of the MCO. MCO may own many of the institutional providers (e.g., hospitals).
Group model	MCO contracts with a multispecialty provider group for services.
Network model	MCO contracts with several provider groups for services.
Independent practice association (IPA)	Organization of independent or small group practices that contract with a MCO.

Group model

Group model HMOs contract with provider group practices to deliver health care services. The HMO contracts with just one multispecialty group to provide health care services. Some of these models have exclusive relationships with their provider group practice, referred to as a captive group, in which the provider group only serves patients from one HMO. In a nonexclusive relationship, also known as an independent group, the provider group practice may have contracts to provide service to multiple HMOs. The provider group may be paid by various mechanisms, including fee-for-service or capitation.

Network model

The network model HMO is similar to the group model, but it contracts with multiple provider group practices, including both primary care groups. This model may offer greater geographical coverage than the group model. Compared to the staff and group models, the network model is significantly less integrated.

Independent practice associations

Independent practice associations (IPAs) are organizations that contract with individual providers or small provider group practices for the purposes of managed care contracting. The HMO then contracts with the IPA to provide health care services to the patients that belong to the HMO. Providers in this model are able to keep their individual or group practices. Thus, they see patients from multiple HMOs as well as patients who do not participate in an HMO.

Effect of Managed Care on Physical Therapy and Occupational Therapy

Managed care has had an impact on all areas of health care, including physical and occupational therapy practice. It has not been easy for some therapists who had been out in the field before managed care to adjust to the restrictions of managed care policies. This section addresses the practical realities of the enactment of managed care policy into therapy practice. It will include a discussion of typical benefits and concerns about managed care and skills for adapting to change.

MCOs: Benefits and Concerns for Therapists

In the therapy literature, there is not a clear consensus about whether managed care is beneficial or problematic (Poole 1996; Wynn 1999). Table 7–4 lists key benefits and concerns about MCOs that have been voiced by therapists.

Table 7–4.   Benefits and Concerns About Managed Care

Benefit	Concern
Patients take more responsibility for therapy secondary to fewer visits	Fewer patient visits with less therapy time
More outcomes research and use of outcomes in clinical practice	Less reimbursement
More streamlined services	Loss of autonomy
Stronger emphasis on preventive care	Increased administrative demands
Increased interdisciplinary team interdependence and better communication	Increased productivity demands
Improved care from pre-set treatment protocols, such as clinical pathways	Holistic approach to patient care is incompatible with business emphasis
Improved care from educating other health professionals about the latest treatments	Consumers may have less choice of therapists
Increased problem-based learning in therapy education	Bureaucratic demands may result in delayed treatment
Greater emphasis in therapy education on the health care environment and business principles	Patients with chronic conditions may not have adequate coverage

Source: Brayman 1996; Wynn 1999; Coffey et al. 1992; Spragins 1995; Vanleit 1996; and Varela-Burstein et al. 1997.

Managed Care Benefits

Managed care results in patients taking more responsibility for their care, as visits are fewer than in traditional forms of health insurance. With managed care there are more outcome measures and research, more streamlined coordinated services, stronger emphasis on preventive care, and increased health care team interdependence with better communication (Brayman 1996; Wynn 1999). Treatment can be effective with pre-set treatment protocols, such as clinical practice guidelines (Coffrey et al. 1992). In some MCOs, physicians are educated about the most current treatments, which may ultimately help therapy outcomes (Spragins 1998).

Professional educators maintain that managed care results in increased problem-based learning, more emphasis on clinical research, more education about working in the current health care environment, and increased interest in the business aspects of therapy (Wynn 1999). Developing outcome measures and research has been very beneficial for therapists. Although therapists struggle with time constraints and the best methodology for doing clinical research, they recognize the importance of scientific research to validate the therapy fields (Foto 1996; Miller 1999; Wynn 1999).

Managed Care Concerns

Therapists express concerns about having fewer visits with patients and less treatment time, lower reimbursement, loss of autonomy in patient care, and greater administrative and productivity demands (Vanleit 1996; Varela-Burstein, Voight, and Pantel 1997; Wynn 1999). Therapists are also concerned about adequate coverage for patients with chronic conditions, because the managed care environment seems more supportive of acute treatable conditions (Wynn 1999). In addition, in a business-minded system, it is difficult to provide true holistic health care (Lohman and Brown 1997). Further concerns are that consumers have less choice of health care professionals, including therapy practitioners. This may result in patients being referred to generalist therapists who contract with a plan rather than specialist therapists (e.g., a certified hand therapists). Moreover, because of the bureaucracy of MCOs, there often is a lapse of time from referral to treatment, which may adversely affect therapy results (Fisher 1997; Miller 1999).

Adapting to the Changes Brought about by Managed Care

The changes wrought by managed care have revolutionized the delivery of therapy services in the United States. They have caused confusion and new opportunities for therapists across the nation. We conclude this chapter with a discussion of successful strategies that have been adopted by occupational therapists and physical therapists to manage the changes initiated by managed care.

According to Kauffmann (1996, 193), "the occupational therapy manager and practitioner have experienced more changes in the past 10 years than in any other decade in the history of the profession." Managed care is now in its more mature stages of development (Nugent 1996), and depending on the area of the United States, therapists may be very used to working in the managed care environment. However, in some areas of the country, managed care continues to slowly integrate into therapy practice. Therapists have learned to adapt to managed care changes over time. Education about managed care and a good understanding of one's own organization helps with this adaptation. Finally, as Daniel states (as quoted in Wynn 1999, 38), "In terms of overall career satisfaction there are two types of therapists in the profession. There are therapists who are survivors who see change as challenges and they are more able to adapt and there are therapists who have a less adaptive nature. These are the therapists who perhaps have less satisfaction with managed care."

Importance of Good Communication

Good communication skills have emerged as crucial therapist competencies during the era of managed care. Several of the strategies we will discuss are summarized in Table 7–5. It is important to develop rapport with key people in the

Table 7–5.   Good Communication Skills

1. Develop and strengthen rapport with key players (e.g., case managers, utilization review coordinators, gatekeepers).
2. Communicate the outcomes of your treatment to key players.
3. Be aware of the goals of the managed care organization.
4. Educate the managed care organization about the benefits of therapy.
5. Understand the needs and values of all of your customers.
6. Advocate for your patients and profession.

managed care system, such as case managers, utilization review coordinators, and primary care gatekeepers. Regular communication helps increase awareness of therapy outcomes. Communication and demonstrating treatment effectiveness will enhance respect for therapy in the managed care arena. Furthermore, effective communication will keep therapists aware of the MCO's goals, such as achieving quality care in a cost-effective, timely manner. Doing in-house **case management** by collecting and communicating outcome data to the MCO about length of stay (LOS), functional status at discharge as compared to entry, costs of providing care, and patient satisfaction enhances the respect of the MCO for the provider (Foto 1996). Since some case managers have nonmedical backgrounds, and even those from medical backgrounds may not have an in-depth understanding of rehabilitation, good communication can make a big difference in patient ability to access and benefit from therapy services.

Therapists need to carefully analyze their customers and what they value. In the managed care environment, the key customers are MCOs, primary care physicians, patient employers, and patients. Each may have a different perspective on what is expected from the therapist. MCOs usually value the most economical, streamlined, quality care (Foto 1997). Therefore, a therapy clinic that offers diversified care will have an edge in getting contracts over one that specializes in one type of care. Additionally, belonging to a therapy network helps market to a MCO (Lansey 1996). Producing outcomes that are functional and sustainable will also enhance marketing efforts (Foto 1996). Practitioners from therapy clinics should also market to get coverage from several MCOs so that if they lose a contract they will still have adequate coverage.

Finally, patients are the main customers therapists regularly see. Patients value caring health care, clear and courteous communication, and an overall satisfactory experience from therapy (Foto 1997). One way to demonstrate care so as to improve patient satisfaction is to advocate for the patient. Advocacy is done by preauthorizing an adequate treatment amount, and by communicating about the treatment plan. Advocacy also means being assertive about the patient's rights if there are problems with the MCO. All MCOs offer appeal processes, which can be accessed if there is a perception of unfair treatment coverage or some other problem. If the appeals process is accessed it is important to have clear objective documentation. In addition, providing effective treatment through careful planning in the time restricted managed care world is an important marketing tool for both the patient and the managed care provider (Miller, 1999).

Case Managers and Managed Care

The key health care professionals in the managed care environment are the case managers. Case managers coordinate, in a holistic manner, all aspects of a patient's care. Case management is defined as "a collaborative process that assesses, plans, implements, coordinates, monitors, and evaluates the options and services to meet an individual's health needs, using communication and available resources to promote quality, and cost effective outcomes" (Commission for Case Management Certification 1996, preface). Although nurses dominate the case-management field, occupational and physical therapists are assuming case-management roles. In the professional literature in both fields, there have recently been numerous articles addressing the role of therapists in case management (Fosnought 1996; American Occupational Therapy Association 1991; Fischer 1996; Lohman 1998, 1999).

Therapists have much to offer to case management thanks to their background in rehabilitation practice (Fosnought 1996). However, working in a medical model may be difficult, because therapists often do not have the same depth of medical-management knowledge as nurses (Lohman 1998). Lohman (1999) reflects that occupational therapists can assume case-management roles in all settings, including medical settings, by learning the medical aspects of care from a functional perspective. One can also break into case management by demonstrating the ability to case manage, making sure that the formal institutional policies include therapists becoming certified as case managers (Lohman 1998, 1999). A new case-management role that therapists can assume is internal case manager. This person coordinates admissions and service delivery within an institution (Fosnought 1996).

Whether or not therapists assume case-management roles, they will work with case managers in the managed care environment. Therefore, it is beneficial to learn how to best work with case managers. One suggestion, as discussed earlier, is to think like a case manager when monitoring internal cases. Therapists who consider the perspective of the case manager will look at discharge planning from the initiation of therapy. It also helps to maintain good communication with the case manager from the initiation of treatment. Having regular communication and contact keeps communication open. Another suggestion is to demonstrate the value of therapy by providing effective treatment resulting in patient satisfaction and cost savings (Fosnought 1996; Foto 1997). Additionally therapists can educate case managers from other disciplines about the rehabilitation aspects of patient care (Lohman 1998).

Conclusion

This chapter defines and describes the philosophy and organization of managed care. Managed care changes the traditional role of the insurer from actuarial analyst and claims processor to one that includes access/cost control and quality management. These functions are performed by limiting the size of the provider pool, implementing payment schemes that reward efficiency, and measuring provider performance and, in some cases, patient health status. Providers respond to the emergence of managed care by organizing themselves into groups of practitioners and institutions that can provide the geographic coverage necessary for population-based contracts. Managed care has changed the practice of physical therapy and occupational therapy. These changes have caused confusion as well as new opportunities. Case management has emerged as a new opportunity for therapists to explore as a career option and also to understand as an important player in the implementation of managed care.

CHAPTER REVIEW QUESTIONS

1. Define managed care.
2. Identify and describe the three principles used by managed care organizations to influence the delivery of health care.
3. Compare and contrast the four types of managed care products.
4. Compare and contrast the four types of managed care provider structures.
5. Discuss the advantages and disadvantages of managed care as it affects physical therapy and occupational therapy.
6. Identify successful adaptations for working in managed care systems.
   a. communication skills
   b. case management

CHAPTER DISCUSSION QUESTIONS

1. You have been working as a manager in a department that has contracted for the past two years with Happy MCO. Although its rates are on the low side, you have been able to meet budget. This year, when you renegotiate the contract with Happy HMO, it will request even lower rates. You know that with the lower rate your department will not be able to meet budget. What will you do?
2. You are starting a clinic in an area that is highly infiltrated by MCOs. Other therapy clinics currently have all the contracts. Provide a minimum of three suggestions as to how you might get a contract that is financially feasible for your clinic.
3. You are following a patient who had a cerebral vascular accident (CVA) one month ago. The MCO has discharged the patient and will not authorize any additional time. What will you do?

REFERENCES

American Occupational Therapy Association. 1991. Statement: The occupational therapist as case manager. *Ameri J Occup Ther* 45: 1065–66.

Barton, P. L. 1999. *Understanding the U.S. Health Services Systems.* Chicago: Health Administration Press.

Brayman, S. J. 1996. Managing the occupational environment of managed care. *Amer J Occup Ther* 50: 442–46 .

Coffey R. J., J. S. Richards, C. S. Remmert, S. S. LeRoy, R. R. Schoville, and P. J. Baldwin. 1992. Introduction to critical paths. *Quality Management in Health Care* 1: 45–53.

Commission for Case Mangement Certification. 1996. CCM Certification Guide. Rolling Meadows IL: By the author.

Fisher, T. 1996. Roles and functions of a case manager. *J Amer Occup Ther Assoc* 50: 452–54.

Fosnought, M. 1996. PT is as case managers: An evolving role. *PT: Magazine of Physical Therapy* 4: 46–53.

Foto, M. 1996. Excelling in a managed care environment. *OT Practice,* 20–22. (January)

———. 1997. Preparing occupational therapists for the year 2000: The impact of managed-care on education and training. *Amer J Occup Ther* 51: 88–90.

Freudenheim M. 2001. A changing world is forcing changes on managed care. *New York Times,* July 2, A1, A13.

Ginzberg, E. and M. Ostow. 1997. Managed care: A look back and a look ahead. *N Engl J Med* (14): 1018–20.

Kassirer, J. P. 1997. Is managed care here to stay? *N Engl J Med* 336 (14): 1013–14.

Kauffman, S. H. 1996. Management of rapid change. In *The Occupational Therapy Manager,* Bethesda MD: American Occupational Therapy Association.

Kongstvedt, P. R. 1999. Managed health care. In *Health Care Administration: Planning, Implementing, and Managing Organizational Delivery Systems,* L. F. Wolper, 3rd ed., 522–44. Gaithersburg MD: Aspen.

Lansey, D. 1996. Reimbursement: Keeping track of managed care. *PT: Magazine of Physical Therapy* 4(12): 22–23.

Lohman, H. 1998. Occupational therapists as case managers. *Occupational Therapy in Health Care* 11: 65–76.

———. 1999. What will it take for more occupational therapists to become case managers? Implications for education, practice, and policy. *Ameri J Occup Ther* 53: 111–13.

Lohman, H. and K. Brown. 1997. Ethical issues related to managed care: An in depth discussion of an occupational therapy case study. *Occupational Therapy in Health Care* 10(4): 1–12.

Mechanic D. 1994. Managed care: Rhetoric and realities. *Inquiry* 31(2): 124–28.

Miller, R. E. 1999. Hands in the new millennium: Therapist commentary. *J Hand Ther* 12: 182–83.

——— and H. S. Luft. 1994. Managed care plan performance since 1980. *JAMA* 271(19): 1512–19.

Nugent, J. 1996. Reimbursement: Planning for managed-care. *PT Magazine* 4: 32–34 (March).

Peloquin S. M. 1996. The issue is—Now that we have managed care, shall we inspire it? *Amer J Occup Ther* 50: 455–60.

Poole, D. L. 1996. Editorial: Keeping managed care in balance. *Health and Social Work* 21: 163–65.

Reynolds, J. P. 1996. LOS: SOS? *PT Magazine,* 38–47. (February).

Spragins, E. E. 1995. Beware your HMO. *Newsweek,* 54–55. (October 23).

Stahl, C. 1995. Who's doing the managing in managed-care? *Advance for occupational therapists,* 14–15.

Sultz, H. A. and K. M. Young. 1999. *Health Care USA: Understanding its Organization and Delivery.* Gaithersburg MD: Aspen.

Vanleit, B. 1996. Managed mental health care: Reflections in a time of turmoil. *Amer J Occup Ther* 50: 428–34.

Varela-Burstein, E. A., E. A. Voight, and E. S. Pantel. 1997. The impact of managed care on the practice of occupational therapy by hand therapists. *Occupational Therapy in Health Care* 10(4): 33–52.

Wynn, K. E. 1999. The pearls and perils of managed care. *PT: Magazine of Physical Therapy* 1: 34–44.

8

Medicare

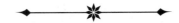

CHAPTER OBJECTIVES

At the conclusion of this chapter, the reader will be able to:

1. Explain the history of the Medicare program.
2. Describe the organization and scope of the Medicare program.
3. Relate the eligibility criteria and benefits in the Medicare Part A program.
   a. Hospital inpatient program
   b. Skilled nursing facility
   c. Hospice
   d. Home health care
4. Discuss the mechanisms of provider reimbursement under Medicare Part A.
   a. Cost-based reimbursement
   b. Prospective payment
      1. Hospitals: Diagnosis-Related Groups
      2. Skilled nursing facilities: Resource Utilization Groups
      3. Inpatient rehabilitation facilities: Case Mix Groups
      4. Home health agencies: Home Health Resource Groups
5. Relate the eligibility criteria and benefits in the Medicare Part B program.
   a. Outpatient hospital programs
   b. Comprehensive Outpatient Rehabilitation Facilities (CORFs)
   c. Physical Therapist in Private Practice/Occupational Therapist in Private Practice
6. Discuss the structure of fee schedules as a method of provider reimbursement in the Medicare Part B program.

7. Relate the eligibility criteria and benefits in the Medicare Part C program.
8. Describe the quality-control procedures employed in the Medicare program.
   a. Recognize fraud and abuse in Medicare.
9. Define the structure and interaction of private health insurance plans with Medicare.
10. Relate the proposals for reform of the Medicare program.

KEY WORDS: Benefit Period, Carrier, Case Mix Adjustment, Certification, Consolidated Billing, Cost-Based Reimbursement, Cost Shifting, Defined Contribution Plan, Defined Benefit Plan, Entitlement, Fee Schedule, Intermediary, Medically Necessary, Medicare Assignment, Medigap, Peer Review Organization, Prospective Payment, Social Insurance, Vested

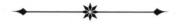

Introduction

Medicare is the most influential insurance program affecting the United States health care system. This is for two reasons. First, Medicare is the largest single payer of health care services in the United States. Second, it is organized and managed by the federal government, which has enormous statutory and regulatory authority over many activities performed by health care providers, including occupational therapists and physical therapists. It is important, then, for therapists and all health care providers to understand this program. Changes in the program affect the daily delivery of health care in the United States.

We will open this chapter by briefly reviewing the history of how Medicare came to be such a large and influential program. Second, we will introduce how Medicare is organized and administered. Third, we will explore the major components, or "parts," of Medicare that provide services to many Americans. During this discussion, we will pay close attention to the methods by which providers, including therapists, are paid for services. These payment systems have powerful effects on the organization of the health care delivery system. Fourth, we will review the organization of quality-control programs in Medicare with special attention to fraud and abuse detection. Fifth, we will examine efforts to reform Medicare, including proposals to increase private insurance participation in the delivery of Medicare services.

History of Medicare

The origin of Medicare needs to be considered in the context of the movement to provide universal national health insurance to all Americans (Ball 1995; Friedman 1995). Prior to 1965, Americans who needed institutional health care services had two broad choices: pay privately or receive services in public health care facilities (Blaisdell 1992). This two-tiered system had developed in the first half of the century as medical care began to rely increasingly on technology (Blaisdell 1994). Medical care was not delivered primarily in the patient's home by a private physician. Hospitals became institutions where a person could receive the latest technology applied to the treatment of disease and illness. At the same time, social movements began to call for improved access to medical care for people with limited financial resources. Beginning in the late nineteenth century and into the twentieth century, many European countries began to institute universal health insurance for their citizens. American efforts at universal coverage (still incomplete) can be traced back to 1912 and have continued to the current date (Friedman 1995).

Medicare has been identified as an interim step in the development of universal health insurance for all Americans. By the early 1960s, one in two elderly Americans lacked health care insurance to pay for hospital care (Davis and Burner 1995). Elderly Americans were known to have an increased need for hospital services, and they had fewer resources to pay for this care. Legislative attempts to enact an insurance program for older Americans commenced in 1957, and after the landslide election of Lyndon Johnson as President in 1964, proponents of public health insurance for older Americans had firm control of the Congress and the executive branch. Medicare was vigorously opposed by organized medicine, which had defeated all previous attempts at federal health insurance. In July 1965, however, Medicare was passed by Congress, and shortly thereafter, it was signed into law by President Johnson.

Hospital insurance for elderly Americans was enacted as part of a package of benefits. This package is sometimes referred to as a "three-level cake" (Friedman 1995). Hospital insurance (HI), or Part A Medicare, provided coverage for inpatient hospital stays and short-term residential care for rehabilitation in other facilities. Supplementary Medical Insurance (SMI), or Part B Medicare, was intended to provide coverage for professional services (e.g., physicians, occupational therapists, physical therapists). Medicaid, the third tier of the cake, was enacted as an extension of the 1960 Kerr-Mills legislation that provided funds to states to care for the poor. We will discuss Medicaid in Chapter 9.

Medicare and Medicaid have been effective in increasing access to health care services for people who are older, people with a disability, people with low incomes (Medicaid), and people with end-stage renal disease (Medicare). Enactment of comprehensive national health insurance has not yet occurred. Rothman (1993) identified four reasons for this situation. First, private health insurers have been aggressive and successful in meeting most needs of middle-class Americans.

Second, many components of the health care delivery system remain suspicious and opposed to more government involvement in health care. Third, the principle of charitable health care as a means to provide services for people who lack care remains alive in America. Finally, the existing programs (i.e., Medicare and Medicaid), appear to be adequate in meeting the needs of vulnerable Americans.

Almost since its inception, concerns have arisen about the cost of the Medicare program (Russell and Burke 1978). In its first year, Medicare cost less than $2 billion. It was funded by a 0.35 percent payroll tax on the first $6,600 of a worker's earnings (Davis and Burner 1995). Today, Medicare pays out over $200 billion in reimbursement for health care services. A 2.9 percent payroll tax on all earnings pays for Medicare, and there are concerns about the long-term financial viability of the program.

There are several reasons for the explosive growth of Medicare. First, many providers, including physical therapists and occupational therapists, had access to major new sources of funding intended to expand access to their services. In addition, the federal government expanded health science educational programs and supported the development of new occupations and fields. Medicare created special financial support for graduate medical education in academic medical centers. As new treatments emerged, born out of expanded biomedical research in academic medical centers, Medicare funded their widespread application to the general population. As a result of its successes in expanding access to care for people in need of services, the costs of the program grew rapidly.

In this chapter, we are going to discuss several methods that have been devised by the Center for Medicare and Medicaid Services to cope with the problem of program costs. The Medicare program became a leader in developing alternative payment methods for services, and these have a powerful influence on health care providers. Initially, Medicare followed the regular payment methods used by private insurers. Hospitals were paid based on the costs of caring for persons who received services. Providers, including therapists, were paid "usual and customary" charges for their services, using prevailing regional rates and fees. The growth of the program and rise in costs necessitated the development and implementation of new "prospective" payment systems for Medicare charges. **Prospective payment** means that the insurer identifies what it will pay prior to the delivery of care. The previous "retrospective" payment methods paid providers based on what care was delivered after the care was given (see Chapters 6 and 7). Beginning in 1983 with hospitals, and continuing up to 2002 with inpatient rehabilitation facilities, the Medicare program has instituted a variety of prospective payment systems (e.g., Diagnosis-Related Groups, Resource Utilization Groups) and the fee schedule.

The Medicare program has changed the health care system in many ways since 1965. Friedman (1995) identifies an oversupply of hospitals, the birth of the for-profit hospital industry, the development of payment inequities and **cost shifting** between private and public payers, the need to generate and use data to understand a very large health care system, and the formation of quality oversight bodies as some of the legacies of the Medicare program. Blaisdell (1994) notes that public hospitals have shrunk in size since Medicare's inception because private providers have gained access to public funds to care for persons who are indigent. Medicare was also an influential force in ending discrimination against the ability of minority Americans to access hospitals (Reynolds 1997). Medicare is a very important and influential program. In this next section, we will introduce the Medicare program by reviewing how it is organized and the size of its various components.

Scope and Organization of Medicare

Medicare is the largest payer of health care services in the United States. In 1998, the Medicare program spent $216.6 billion on health care for 38.8 million beneficiaries. These payments accounted for 19 percent of all health care spending in the United States that year (Levit et al. 2000). Table 8–1 describes the overall characteristics of the Medicare program. Medicare provides health insurance to about one in six Americans. It is the dominant form of insurance for persons over age 65 (aged) and persons with long-term disabilities. Two in three dollars of Medicare expenditures are paid out of the Hospital Insurance Trust Fund (Part A) to hospitals, home health agencies, and skilled nursing facility providers. Medicare oper-

Table 8–1.   Characteristics of the Medicare Program

A. Enrollment: 39,100,000 (1998)
    1. By Gender   2. By Eligibility Category
      a. Males: 16,497,000   a. Aged: 33,608,000
      b. Females: 21,598,000   b. Disabled: 4,846,000
B. Expenditures: $208 billion (1997)
    1. Part A/Hospital Insurance: $136 billion
    2. Part B/Supplementary Medical Insurance: $71.1 billion
C. Utilization Rates (1997)
    1. Hospital discharges: 11.8 million
    2. Persons served in skilled nursing facilities: 1.4 million
D. Providers Receiving Medicare Payments (1997)
    1. Hospitals: 6,293
    2. Skilled nursing facilities: 14,860
    3. Home health agencies: 10,807
    4. Outpatient physical therapy clinics: 2,758
    5. Comprehensive outpatient rehabilitation facilities: 531
    6. Physicians: 807,674
E. Program Administrative Costs: 1.2 percent (Part A) to 2.0 percent (Part B)

Source: Health Care Financing Administration. HCFA Data and Statistics. Accessed at *www.hcfa.gov/stats/stats.htm* on October 23, 2000.

ates in all states and territories and affects all providers. It operates at a low 1–2 percent administrative cost.

As mentioned in the first section, Medicare was designed as part of a "three-tiered cake" of benefits. Part A Medicare, the hospital insurance benefit, provides for hospital, short-stay skilled nursing facility, and home health care for eligible beneficiaries. Part B Medicare, or Supplementary Medical Insurance, provides coverage for outpatient hospital, office visits to therapists and physicians, and durable medical equipment needs. The third tier was originally the Medicaid program, which provides insurance coverage for people who meet certain categorical or income eligibility criteria. We will discuss Medicaid in Chapter 9. In 1997, Congress created a new third component, Medicare Part C, that includes all of the managed care options in the Medicare program.

Medicare is a good example of a federal **entitlement** program. In an entitlement program, eligible persons have a guarantee to services identified in the law. Once in place, entitlement benefits are difficult to change (see the discussion of public vs. private policy in Chapter 1). Medicare (and Medicaid) is also an example of **social insurance.** Social insurance means that economic resources are transferred from one group to another group to meet a defined social need, in this case health care. Taxes are paid by working Americans to provide health care benefits to nonworking Americans: the elderly and the permanently disabled. Unlike private health care insurance, those who pay the premiums (in this case, taxes) are not eligible for program benefits.

Medicare policy, (e.g., eligibility and program benefits), is established by congressional legislation. Changes in the policy structure of Medicare require changes in the statute and cannot be made administratively. Failure to provide benefits to eligible beneficiaries can be enforced in the courts. As an entitlement program, Medicare differs from Medicaid in one important aspect. Everyone who meets the eligibility requirements, regardless of income, can participate in Medicare. In contrast, Medicaid is a means-tested program that limits benefits to people who often have not made regular contributions to the program (e.g., low-income persons, children). The popularity of Medicare as the "third rail" of American politics can be tied to its structure as a "pay as you go" program with guaranteed benefits to those who have made regular contributions to the program.

Medicare procedures (e.g., eligibility, reimbursement), are developed and implemented by the Center for Medicare and Medicaid Services (CMS), an agency formerly known as the Health Care Financing Administration (HCFA). This agency is part of the Department of Health and Human Services. Claims processing and review is performed by private organizations, usually insurance companies, that each service a defined region of the country. These claims review organizations are called intermediaries and carriers. **Intermediaries** process and review claims for Part A Medicare (e.g., hospital physical or occupational therapy). **Carriers** process and review claims for Part B Medicare (e.g., physical therapists and occupational therapists in private practice).

We are now ready to explore the Medicare program in detail. For each part, we will introduce the eligibility criteria, benefits package, and mechanisms of reimbursement. The first two components of our presentation address program areas experienced primarily by the beneficiary. Reimbursement mechanisms affect the provider in profound ways by establishing market incentives, cost controls, and documentation requirements. To help us understand the benefits and payment structure of the Medicare program, we will introduce and follow a patient case: Mrs. Miller, a 76-year-old Medicare beneficiary who needs a total hip replacement.

Case Example: Mrs. Smith is a 76-year-old widow who has health insurance coverage through Parts A and B of Medicare. She worked for 15 years as a bookkeeper and made regular payroll contributions into the Hospital Insurance trust fund. She is vested in the Medicare program.

Part A: Hospital Insurance

Eligibility

Eligibility for Medicare Part A benefits is based on a record of payroll or premium contributions, age, marital status, and the presence of permanent disability. Most individuals qualify based on age (currently age 65; gradually being raised to age 67) and a record of payroll contributions into the program for 40 quarters (10 years). After paying into the program for 10 years, an individual is **vested** and eligible for benefits after reaching the minimum eligibility age. Spouses of vested Medicare beneficiaries are also eligible for Medicare at age 65. No monthly premium is required of vested beneficiaries or their spouses.

Persons who are not vested in the program can receive Medicare benefits after reaching age 65 and agreeing to pay a monthly premium. Individuals younger than age 65 are eligible for Medicare benefits if they have been declared permanently disabled by the Social Security Administration for 24 months or have end-stage renal disease.

Benefits

Table 8–2 outlines the four basic benefits included in Medicare Part A: inpatient hospital care, short-term skilled nursing facility care, home health care, and hospice. These benefits include room and board (hospital and skilled nursing facility) and **medically necessary,** professional services provided by the institution. Medically necessary services, including physical therapy and occupational therapy, must meet program requirements (see the discussion of skilled care below) and be authorized by a provider with physician status (e.g., a medical or osteopathic physician). Although vested beneficiaries do not pay a monthly premium, the most commonly used Part A benefits are not free. Beneficiary out-of-pocket costs include a deductible (hospital care) and daily co-insurance fee (after 60 days of hospital care and 20 days of skilled nursing facility care).

Table 8–2.   2001 Medicare Part A Benefits/Beneficiary Costs

A. Monthly Premiums: $0 for vested individuals
       $165 for persons with 30–39 quarters of payroll
        contributions
       $300 for persons with < 30 quarters of payroll contributions
B. Hospital Inpatient Coverage
 1. Deductible: $792
 2. Ninety days of "medically necessary" care per benefit period.
  a. Co-insurance
 1. First 60 days: $0
 2. Day 61–90: $198 per day
 3. Sixty lifetime reserve days
  a. Co-insurance: $396 per day
C. Skilled Nursing Facility Coverage
 1. Deductible: $0
 2. One hundred days of post-hospital care
  a. Co-insurance
   1. First 20 days: $0
   2. Day 21 to 100: $99 per day

Source: Medicare Premium Amounts for 2001. Accessed at
www.medicare.gov/Basics/Amounts2001.asp on October 24, 2000.

Case Example: Mrs. Miller has been experiencing pain and limited mobility in her left hip for many years. It has reached the point where she has elected to receive a total hip replacement to relieve the pain and disablement. She understands that Medicare will pay for most of her hospital and post-hospital care.

Benefit Period

The Part A deductible and co-insurance is calculated using a **benefit period.** Unlike most forms of private health insurance, Medicare does not determine out-of-pocket expenses based on an annual period. Instead, a single episode of Part A benefits is determined from the time of admission to the hospital until the patient is out of a hospital or skilled nursing facility for 60 days. All Part A benefits during this period are covered by one deductible and co-insurance fee (including the case of a readmission). Conversely, a beneficiary who needs two episodes of Part A benefits in the same year that are more than 60 days apart owes two deductibles and the appropriate co-insurance fee for each episode of care.

 In our hypothetical example, consider the implications of the benefit period on the potential cost of care to be paid by Mrs. Miller. Mrs. Miller enters the hospital for a total hip replacement. She pays the initial $796 in charges as her deductible. Scenarios A and B in Case I illustrate the effect of the benefit period in calculating Medicare Part A benefits. Both scenarios describe another hospital admission for a complication related to her total hip replacement. In scenario A, Mrs. Miller owes nothing for the care because it occurred within 60 days of the discharge from the skilled nursing facility (i.e., the same benefit period). In scenario B, Mrs. Miller is required to pay another deductible expense for the care because it occurred after the first benefit period expired. Even though this problem may have occurred within the same calendar year, Mrs. Miller needs to pay an additional $796 deductible for this hospital stay.

Case Example: Mrs. Miller receives five days of hospital care for the total hip replacement, including physical therapy and occupational therapy. Since she uses only five days of inpatient hospital care, she owes no co-insurance for these days.

Case Example 8–1 Medicare Part A Benefit Period

Mrs. Miller is admitted to the hospital for a total hip replacement. She spends six days in the hospital and another 20 days in a skilled nursing facility receiving nursing care, physical therapy, and occupational therapy services.

Out-of-Pocket Cost to Mrs. Miller

Deductible: $796
Co-Insurance: $0
Total: $796

A. Ten days after returning home, Mrs. Miller develops hip pain due to a dislocation and re-enters the hospital for a five-day inpatient stay. She returns home after being dicharged from the hospital.

Out-of-Pocket Cost to Mrs. Miller

Deductible: $0
Co-Insurance: $0
Total: $0

OR

B. Three months after returning home, Mrs. Miller develops hip pain due to a dislocation and re-enters the hospital for a five-day inpatient stay. She returns home after being discharged from the hospital.

Out-of-Pocket Cost to Mrs. Miller

Deductible: $796
Co-Insurance: $0
Total: $796

The total cost to her for this stay is the $796 deductible. She is then transferred to a skilled nursing facility for further recuperation.

Skilled Nursing Facility Benefit

The skilled nursing facility (SNF) benefit under Medicare Part A provides short-term nursing and skilled rehabilitation services (up to 100 days) in a Medicare-certified unit per benefit period that is related to the recovery from an acute hospital stay. Medicare does not pay for long-term institutionalization, nor can beneficiaries access the SNF directly without a hospital stay. Medicare-certified skilled nursing facility units are located both in free-standing nursing homes and in hospitals. Hospital units are commonly referred to as sub-acute, swing bed, transitional care, or restorative care units (see Chapter 11). Although they are physically within an acute care hospital, these units are licensed as skilled nursing facility beds, and Medicare patients receiving unit services are covered by the SNF benefit. Prior to admission to a SNF unit, a patient must have had at least a three-day stay in a hospital during the preceding 30 days and be certified for admission to the SNF by a physician.

Need for rehabilitation is a major criterion that qualifies an individual for a Medicare-funded stay in a skilled nursing facility. The intent of the benefit is to continue the process of recovery after an acute illness and hospital stay. The advent of prospective payment systems for hospitals in 1983 fostered the growth and need for the skilled nursing facility benefit. This change was one factor that fueled the increased demand for occupational therapists and physical therapists in the late 1980s and 1990s. General exercise and routine assistance with activities of daily living and ambulation are not covered by the Medicare SNF benefit. These "restorative therapy" services are provided by nonprofessional nursing personnel.

Skilled rehabilitation services are covered under the SNF benefit. The guidelines in the *Medicare Skilled Nursing Facility Manual* for the determination of skilled physical therapy and occupational therapy services are listed in Tables 8–3 and 8–4. Table 8–5 provides examples listed in the Medicare regulations of skilled and nonskilled services. It is important for occupational therapists and physical therapists to understand the rules defining skilled and nonskilled services. Billing Medicare for the provision of a nonskilled service is considered to be fraud. Maintenance therapy is excluded from coverage as a skilled benefit, but the development (not the execution) of a maintenance therapy program by a therapist is covered. The professional activities of patient examination, observation, assessment, evaluation, and education, as well as the planning and supervision of a treatment program, are central to the determination of whether a service is skilled.

Each Medicare beneficiary who receives services in a skilled nursing facility is assessed and reassessed using a standardized examination set called the *Resident Assessment Instrument,* or RAI. The Resident Assessment Instrument was mandated by congressional action in the late 1980s in an effort to reform and improve care received by Americans residing in nursing homes. The RAI consists of two parts: the Minimum Data Set for Nursing Home Resident Assessment and Care Screening

Table 8–3.   Medicare Definition of Skilled Physical Therapy

1. The services must be directly and specifically related to an active written treatment plan designed by the physician after any needed consultation with a qualified physical therapist.
2. The services must be of a level of complexity and sophistication, or the condition of the patient must be of a nature that requires the judgment, knowledge, and skills of a qualified physical therapist.
3. The services must be provided with the expectation, based on the assessment made by the physician of the patient's restoration potential, that the condition of the patient will improve materially in a reasonable and generally predictable period of time, or the services must be necessary for the establishment of a safe and effective maintenance program.
4. The services must be considered, under accepted standards of medical practice, to be specific and effective treatment for the patient's condition.
5. The services must be reasonable and necessary for the treatment of the patient's condition; this includes the requirement that the amount, frequency, and duration of the services must be reasonable.

Source: Health Care Financing Administration, *Skilled Nursing Facility Manual* chapter 2. Coverage of Services. 214.3 C Skilled Physical Therapy. Accessed at *www.hcfa.gov/pubforms /12%5Fsnf/sn201.htm# 1 19* on November 2, 2000.

(MDS) and Resident Assessment Protocols (RAPS). The MDS is administered at admission, at routine post-admission intervals, and when a significant change in patient status occurs during a skilled nursing facility stay. A list of the major sections of the MDS can be found in Table 8–7. The MDS provides a comprehensive description of the status and problems being experienced by the nursing home resident. Identified problems or changes in patient function trigger a process called Resident Assessment Protocols (RAPS). RAPS are a structured process for the care team to identify, analyze, address, and follow up on patient problems.

Case Example: Mrs. Miller enters the skilled nursing facility. Within the first three days, the staff completes an assessment of Mrs. Miller's status using the MDS. She stays in the skilled nursing facility for 20 days, receives necessary rehabilitation care, and then is discharged to her home. A home health agency is contacted to follow up on Mrs. Miller's continued recovery at home.

Home Health Care Benefit

Patients qualify for the home health care benefit based on home confinement and the need for skilled nursing and/or rehabilitation services, including physical therapy and occupational therapy. Home health care therapy is provided in the patient's residence, which need not be an institutional setting. Physician certification of home confinement is necessary. In general, patients may not leave the

Table 8–4. Medicare Definition Of Skilled Occupational Therapy

1. The evaluation, and reevaluation as required, of a patient's level of function by administering diagnostic and prognostic tests.
2. The selection and teaching of task-oriented therapeutic activities designed to restore physical function (e.g., use of wood-working activities on an inclined table to restore shoulder, elbow, and wrist range of motion lost as a result of burns).
3. The planning, implementing, and supervising of individualized therapeutic activity programs as part of an overall "active treatment" program for a patient with a diagnosed psychiatric illness (e.g., the use of sewing activities which require following a pattern to reduce confusion and restore reality orientation in a schizophrenic patient).
4. The planning and implementing of therapeutic tasks and activities to restore sensory-integrative function (e.g., providing motor and tactile activities to increase sensory input and improve response for a stroke patient with functional loss resulting in a distorted body image).
5. The designing, fabricating, and fitting of orthotic and self-help devices (e.g., making a hand splint for a patient with rheumatoid arthritis to maintain the hand in a functional position, constructing a device that would enable an individual to hold a utensil and feed himself independently).
6. Vocational and prevocational assessment and training.

Source: Health Care Financing Administration. *Skilled Nursing Facility Manual,* chapter 2, Coverage of Services. 230.3 C. Occupational Therapy. Accessed at *www.hcfa.gov/ pubforms/12%5Fsnf/sn201.htm# 1 19* on November 2, 2000.

home except for necessary medical treatments (e.g., radiation therapy) or occasional, community outings (e.g., attending a church service). Home health care services are ordered by a physician, who is required to recertify the continued need for skilled care every 62 days. The criteria for a skilled therapy service are the same as the criteria in the skilled nursing facility benefit.

Patients may qualify for Medicare reimbursement of home health care as a Part A benefit or a Part B benefit (Health Care Financing Administration 1998). Those who are enrolled in both Part A and Part B Medicare are entitled to 100 visits of home health care if they meet the general eligibility criteria and have had a three-day hospital stay within the prior 14 days. If they exceed the 100-visit limit, they are able to continue necessary home health care though Part B Medicare financing.

Everyone receiving home care services is evaluated using a tool called the Outcome and Assessment Information Set, or OASIS (Health Care Financing Administration 2000). OASIS has been implemented since the Balanced Budget Act of 1997 to describe the care needs of persons receiving home health care and to serve as the primary data set used to determine home health prospective payment. There are several forms of the OASIS survey: start of care and resumption of care, follow up, transfer to inpatient facility, and discharge. OASIS *collects information* in a checklist format

Table 8–5.   Selected Examples of Medicare Definitions of Skilled vs. Nonskilled Rehabilitation Services

A. Physical Therapy

Skilled	*Nonskilled*
1. Assessment	1. Maintenance exercise or gait activities
2. Therapeutic exercise	2. Hot packs, infrared, paraffin baths
3. Gait training	3. Routine care of braces
4. Ultrasound, diathermy	

B. Occupational Therapy

Skilled	*Nonskilled*
1. Evaluation	1. Maintenance activities
2. Task-oriented therapy activities	2. Temporary loss or reduction in function
3. Upper limb prosthetic training	3. Patient activity programs
4. Functional training	4. Motivation problems unrelated to psychiatric illness.

Source: Health Care Financing Administration, *Skilled Nursing Facility Manual,* chapter 2, Coverage of Services. 214.3 A Direct Skilled Rehabilitation Services to Patients: Skilled Physical Therapy. 230.3 C. Occupational Therapy. Accessed at *www.hcfa.gov/pubforms/ 12%5Fsnf/sn201.htm# 1 19* on November 2, 2000.

about patient demographics, history, diagnosis, living arrangements, social support, patient attributes (e.g., sensation and integument), activities of daily living performance, medications, equipment and therapy need. OASIS is to be completed within five days of the start of a home health care episode, between day 55 and 60 of a continuing episode, and within two days of the completion of a home health care episode. Data are reported to the Center for Medicare and Medicaid Services through state contacts on a monthly basis.

Case Example: Upon admission to the home health agency, Mrs. Miller is evaluated using the OASIS instrument and her care needs are identified. The nurse, physical therapist, and occupational therapist each see Mrs. Miller two to three times per week for a month to help her successfully transition to living at home. At the end of the month, Mrs. Miller is discharged from home health care. She is functional with her adaptive equipment in moving about her home and performing her activities of daily living.

Hospice Benefit

Hospice services are provided to Medicare beneficiaries who select this treatment option and have been diagnosed with a terminal illness. Core hospice services identified by Medicare for coverage are nursing, social services, medicine, and counseling. Physical therapy and occupational therapy are among the optional hospice benefits.

Part A: Payment Structures

From the time Medicare was established until 1983, Part A providers were paid based on the costs they incurred when caring for Medicare beneficiaries. The intent was to reimburse providers a fee for each service received by a beneficiary based on "reasonable and necessary" charges in their region. This method of payment, common to private insurance plans at the time, was known as **cost-based reimbursement.** Under the cost-based reimbursement mechanism, Part A providers were paid a preliminary amount for care provision during the year, and final reimbursement amounts were determined at the end of the year after reconciliation between a cost report and the periodic interim payment. Every provider was required to produce a detailed cost report to Medicare on the direct and indirect costs of caring for beneficiaries for the year. At the end of the year, providers and the government reconciled the difference between the interim payment and final costs for the year. This retrospective system of payment provided few incentives for providers to be efficient when delivering services. As long as costs could be documented and were allowed by Medicare, providers had every incentive to provide as much care as possible and expect government payment.

Beginning with hospitals in 1983 and, since 1997, continuing with skilled nursing facilities, home health agencies, and rehabilitation hospitals, Medicare has been phasing out cost-based reimbursement as a payment mechanism in favor of various forms of prospective payment. Cost reports are still required as an accounting report, but payment is determined based on sets of predetermined criteria. Prospective payment identifies payment amounts up-front based on sets of patient characteristics, service needs, and facility characteristics determined at the time of admission to, during, or discharge from a Part A service. These mechanisms are all examples of case-based payment systems. Instead of being paid for each individual service (e.g., nursing, physical therapy) and procedure (e.g., ADL training) based on individual facility costs, providers are paid an all-inclusive rate for a day or multiple days (an episode) of care. This payment is a lump sum for all Medicare services with few exceptions. As we will see, prospective payment is determined using a sophisticated process of classifying patients or procedures and determining average, adjusted, national costs of the services. Provider behavior incentives in prospective payment systems are the opposite of cost-based reimbursement systems. Acceptance of a case rate incentivizes the provider to keep the cost of care (number or intensity of services) lower than the fixed case rate amount. In effect, providers are placed on a predetermined budget with which to deliver care. We discussed the incentives of these systems in detail in Chapter 7.

Hospital Prospective Payment

In 1983, the federal government initiated prospective payment for inpatient hospital stays by classifying patients into groups that could predict resource utilization. This system of patient classification is called **case mix adjustment**. Several patient characteristics are used to determine which group a patient should be assigned to: diagnosis, surgery, patient age, patient sex, and discharge destination. Using these criteria, the Center for Medicare and Medicaid Services has established 511 Diagnosis-Related Groups, or DRGs, in order to classify patients at discharge from the hospital into payment groups (Medicare Program Rule 1998). Reimbursement amounts for each group are established based on cost report and billing information collected by CMS. DRG payments are intended to be inclusive of all direct and indirect hospital costs. Hospitals can receive other payments for patients who justifiably exceed day or cost limits and if the hospital treats a "disproportionate share" of low-income Medicare beneficiaries. The DRG methodology has been adopted internationally (Chaix-Couturier et al. 2000; Forgione and D'Annunzio 1999).

Table 8–6 provides an example and information about a Diagnosis-Related Group: DRG 210. This DRG is a surgical DRG for a hospital stay for a hip or femur surgery. As can be seen by the provider charges and Medicare reimbursement data, providers billed Medicare $2.3 billion in 1998 for care provided to beneficiaries for this procedure. Medicare DRG payments covered about half of the covered Medicare charges ($1.1 billion) for this DRG. The discrepancy between covered charges and actual Medicare reimbursement increases the pressure on hospitals to be more efficient. For example, Clancy et al. (1998) reported that the DRG payment amount for care of a Medicare beneficiary with hip fracture resulted in a net loss of $1,000 per patient to the hospitals in their sample. For many years, hospitals would **cost shift** Medicare underpayments to private insurance companies. This was successful until the early 1990s. With the advent of managed care, many private

Table 8–6. Diagnosis-Related Groups: Example

Diagnosis Related Group:	210
Description:	Hip and Femur Procedures
Type:	Surgical
Total Charges (1998):	$2,322,932,212
Covered Charges:	$2,306,768,066
Medicare Reimbursement:	$1,078,891,513
Total Days:	912,731
Number of Discharges:	134,991
Average Total Days:	6.8

Sources: Medicare Provider Analysis and Review, DRG Description Profile (1998). Accessed at *www.hcfa.gov/stats/medpar/drg98dsc.xls* on November 3, 2000. Medicare Provider Analysis and Review, Short Stay Hospital Profile (1998). Accessed at *www.hcfa.gov/stats/medpar/ss98d&s.xls* on November 3, 2000.

insurers imposed their own form of payment constraints and were not open to paying a disproportionately higher amount of medical care expenses in the system. The result has been a significant reorganization of the health care system.

The effect of hospital prospective payments on the health care system was dramatic. When implemented, the DRG cost-control mechanism resulted in a sharp reduction in inpatient hospital utilization (Whetsell 1999; Takemura and Beck 1999; Menke et al. 1999). Patients spent fewer days in the hospital and received fewer services than in the previous cost-based reimbursement environment. The effect of the DRG system on occupational therapists and physical therapists, however, was positive. Patients needed rehabilitation services to move out of inpatient hospitals. Cost-based reimbursement was maintained in skilled nursing facilities, inpatient rehabilitation facilities, outpatient hospital rehabilitation, and home health care. As a result, the demand for rehabilitation expanded in all of these settings in order to meet the needs of an increasing number of patients who were being discharged from hospitals to these levels of care at ever earlier periods. More care that was originally provided in hospitals was transferred to skilled nursing facilities and home health agencies. The demand for therapists increased.

The reorganization of care from inpatient hospital care to sub-acute or SNF care has caused CMS and Congress to act to limit the ability of providers to unfairly profit from an early patient discharge from the hospital to an SNF or home health care. In 1997, Congress established a "transfer rule" that reduces the DRG payment to the acute hospital for patients who are discharged more than one day earlier than the average for the 10 DRGS with the highest rate of acute hospital transfers to post-acute care (Gilman et al. 2000).

Case Example: Mrs. Miller received seven days of room, board, and professional services for her total hip replacement procedure. We can estimate that the hospital received a payment of about $8,000 for this care ($1,078,891,513 total Medicare reimbursement divided by 134,991 discharges). Since Mrs. Miller stayed in the hospital about the average length of time for DRG 210, the hospital will receive the full DRG payment and is not limited to a lower payment due to the transfer rule. As long as the cost of delivering this care was less than $8,000 the hospital earned a profit. Hospital costs greater than $8,000 resulted in a financial loss to the hospital. As a result, hospital administrators and utilization-review nurses closely monitor all Medicare Part A admissions to ensure efficient and effective care.

Skilled Nursing Facility Prospective Payment

In 1989, the Medicare program paid out $2.8 billion to skilled nursing facilities for the SNF benefit. By 1997, this amount had increased to $12.2 billion (Office of the Inspector General 1999). Concerned about rising program costs and the growing national debt, Congress enacted a reformed payment system for the Medicare post-acute care benefit in 1997. The Balanced Budget Act of 1997 authorized the implementation of a national prospective payment system for Medicare Part A skilled nursing facility care that replaced the facility-specific, cost-based reimbursement system that existed prior to 1997. This system is currently being phased in for the payment of Medicare Part A services and, in many states, for Medicaid-covered long-term care services.

SNF prospective payment is based on the classification of persons residing in nursing homes into Resource Utilization Groups (Medicare Program Rule 1998). The intent is to identify the service needs of persons in skilled nursing facilities and to pay an all-inclusive per diem payment to providers for this care.

The determination of the RUGS class for a person is based on the results of the MDS assessment, the medical diagnosis, documented therapist contact time, nursing restorative interventions, and certain behavioral observations. MDS assessment is regularly completed by SNF staff for a 5-day, 14-day, 30-day, 60-day and 90-day report on patient status (see Table 8–7). The Resource Utilization Group classification system has seven categories: rehabilitation therapies, extensive care, special care, clinically complex, impaired cognition, behavioral, and physical. These groups were developed from extensive field testing in several states during three clinical demonstrations in the 1990s.

The Rehabilitation category is of most interest to occupational and physical therapists working in skilled nursing facilities. Table 8–8 describes the Rehabilitation subcategories of the RUGS-III classification system. Patients are classified into one of five rehabilitation subcategories (ultra high, very high, high, medium, and low) based on the number of therapy disciplines involved in the care and the

Table 8–7. Minimum Data Set for Nursing Home Resident Assessment and Care Screening: Major Data Sections

A. Identification and Background Information
B. Cognitive patterns
C. Communication/hearing patterns
D. Vision patterns
E. Mood and behavior patterns
F. Psychosocial well-being
G. Physical functioning and structural problems
H. Continence in last 14 days
I. Disease diagnoses
J. Health conditions
K. Oral/nutritional status
L. Oral/dental status
M. Skin condition
N. Activity pursuit patterns
O. Medications
P. Special treatments and procedures
Q. Discharge potential and overall status

Source: Health Care Financing Administration, September 2000 Update to the MDS Form. Accessed at *http://www.hcfa.gov/medicaid/mds20/mds0900b.pdf* on November 8, 2000.

Table 8–8.   Resource Utilization Groups: Rehabilitation Subcategories

Ultra-High
  At least 720 minutes of therapy per week
  At least two disciplines involved, one at least five days per week
  ADL Index Score 16–18   RUGS Group RUC
  ADL Index Score 9–15   RUGS Group RUB
  ADL Index Score 4–8   RUGS Group RUA
Very High
  At least 500 minutes of therapy per week
  At least one discipline with patient five days per week
  ADL Index Score 16–18   RUGS Group RVC
  ADL Index Score 9–15   RUGS Group RVB
  ADL Index Score 4–8   RUGS Group RVA
High
  At least 325 minutes of therapy per week
  One discipline five days per week
  ADL Index Score 13–18   RUGS Group RHC
  ADL Index Score 8–12   RUGS Group RHB
  ADL Index Score 4–7   RUGS Group RHA
Medium
  At least 150 minutes of therapy per week
  Five days of therapy across three disciplines
  ADL Index Score 15–18   RUGS Group RMC
  ADL Index Score 8–14   RUGS Group RMB
  ADL Index Score 4–7   RUGS Group RMA
Low
  45 minutes of therapy per week over at least three days
  Nursing rehabilitation six days per week, two activities
  ADL Index Score 14–18   RUGS Group RLB
  ADL Index Score 4–13   RUGS Group RLA

Source: Health Care Financing Administration, Medicare Program: Prospective Payment System and Consolidated Billing for Skilled Nursing Facilities; Final Rule Federal Register 63(91): 26262. May 12, 1998.

amount of time spent in therapy each week. Once classified into a subcategory, patients are classified into a resource utilization group based on the ADL Index Score of the MDS.

Prospective payment for skilled nursing facility care is based on the calculation of a per diem amount based on a federal standard base rate that is adjusted by a conversion factor based on Resource Utilization Group classification and a cost of living factor for local wage conditions. An example of the payment calculation for RUGS- III group RUC is provided in Table 8–9. Using historical cost report and project demonstration data, CMS determines two (urban and rural) base rates for

Table 8–9.   SNF Prospective Payment: Federal Per Diem Rate Calculations for RMB

Unadjusted Federal Per Diem Rate

Nursing case mix: $109.48   Therapy case mix: $82.67

Therapy non-case mix: $10.91   Non-case mix: $55.88

RMB Conversion

Nursing case mix (1.09): $119.33

Therapy case mix (0.77): $ 63.66

Non-case mix: $55.88

Total per diem rate: $238.87

Wage Conditions Adjustment

Total labor-related component: $181.27

    Adjusted for Omaha: $171.68 (x 0.9471)

    Adjusted for San Francisco: $257.04 (x 1.4180)

Total non-labor-related component: $57.60

Total per diem rate in Omaha: $229.28

Total per diem rate in San Francisco: $314.64

Source: Health Care Financing Administration. Medicare Program: Prospective Payment System and Consolidated Billing for Skilled Nursing Facilities; Final Rule Federal Register 63(91): 26252–26316. May 12, 1998.

various components of skilled nursing facility care: nursing case mix, therapy case mix, therapy non-case mix, and non-case mix. For the Rehabilitation subcategories, nursing case mix, therapy case mix and the therapy non-case mix rates are used. The nursing and therapy case mix component rates are multiplied by a factor that accounts for resource intensity needs as determined by the RUGS class. Adding each of these components identifies the total per diem rate: $384.21.

This RUGS-adjusted national rate is then adjusted for local wage conditions. The labor-related and non-labor-related components for each Resource Utilization Group payment are determined. The labor-related component of the RUGS adjusted rate is multiplied by a factor based on local health care worker wage conditions. The intent is to reflect that the cost of providing services differs, based on the cost of labor, between areas of the country. In this example, the wage conversion factor lowers payment rates to SNF providers in Omaha vs. providers with similar patients in San Francisco. This reflects local differences in the costs of providing care to patients in these different local economies.

CMS has been phasing in this prospective payment system since 1998. Starting in 2001, facility-based, cost-based payments were no longer made to skilled nursing facilities. Federal examination of therapy services has reaffirmed the value of the SNF therapy benefit for most Medicare beneficiaries (Office of the Inspector General 1999). Most nursing home administrators support this payment system, although they have reported a need to more closely examine the medical condition of the patient before accepting admission. SNF prospective payment has not adversely affected access to the SNF benefit (Office of the Inspector General 1999). SNF prospective payment has incentivized physical therapists and occupational therapists to move away from discipline-specific examinations and interventions. Innovations like the MDS and RUGS require therapists to expand teamwork and closely count minutes of therapy intervention.

Case Example: Mrs. Miller was evaluated using the MDS. Based on these results she was classified into a Medium Rehabilitation subcategory: RGM. While she was classified as RGM, her nursing home was paid $238.87 per day (using the national per diem rate). As she improved and this was documented by MDS, Mrs. Miller was reclassified in less expensive RUGS and the per diem payments were reduced. The amount of services Mrs. Miller needed before she was discharged declined. For this 20-day stay, we can estimate that the nursing home was paid about $4,500.

The physical therapist and occupational therapist paid close attention to the level of care Mrs. Miller received. The documentation reflects that Mrs. Miller required a skilled service, received regular evaluations, and made progress during her therapy episode, and that the therapists counted therapy minutes to be included in the RUGS determination.

Inpatient Rehabilitation Facility Prospective Payment

In November 2000, HCFA released a proposed rule for the prospective payment of inpatient rehabilitation services for Medicare beneficiaries to be implemented in April 2001 (Medicare Program Rule 2000). Growth in inpatient rehabilitation program costs paralleled the growth in skilled nursing facility costs. Between 1990 and 1996, program costs increased 18 percent per year from $1.8 billion to $4.3 billion.

Originally, the foundational data system for this payment model was intended to be a modification of the MDS called the Minimum Data Set—Post Acute Care, or MDS-PAC. In the spring of 2001, CMS changed its position in favor of a new case mix adjustment system to be based on the Functional Independence Measure (Stineman, et al. 1994). Each patient will now be evaluated with a standardized "patient assessment instrument" upon admission and discharge from the inpatient rehabilitation facility (CMS 2001). Using the results of this evaluation, the patient will be assigned to one of 100 Case Mix Groups (CMGs) for payment purposes (CMS 2001).

Home Health Agency Prospective Payment

Home health agency prospective payment was implemented on October 1, 2000 (Medicare Program Rule 2000). In this prospective payment system, home health agencies are paid using a 60-day episode of care. This payment is intended to cover all home health services (including physical therapy and occupational therapy) received by the beneficiary during this period of care. Durable medical equipment is excluded from this payment mechanism and is paid using a fee schedule (see Part B reimbursement). Using historical claims and cost report data, CMS determines a "standardized prospective payment rate." In 2001, this rate was $2,115.30 per episode of care. Similar to the SNF prospective payment formula, this rate is adjusted for individual patient needs and the geographic costs of care delivery.

The effect of individual patient needs on provider reimbursement is based on the determination of a home health resource group (HHRG) classification. Data for HHRG classification are generated from the OASIS completed at admission and a record of the number of therapy hours received by the beneficiary. These data determine three domains used to classify the patient into one of 80 HHRGs. These domains are clinical severity factors, functional severity factors, and services utilization factors (see Table 8–10). Points are awarded for patient status in each of these criteria, and the total in each domain scores the domain as minimum, low, moderate, high, or max. The combination of three domains with five different scores creates 80 Home Health Resource Groups (HHRGs).

Each HHRG is assigned a case mix weight factor that reflects the intensity of services or health problems experienced by the beneficiary. This case mix factor is used in combination with a local wage condition factor to determine the prospective payment rate. Table 8–11 provides an example for HHRG C0F0S0 (clinical domain—minimal, functional domain—minimal, service domain—minimal) that is assigned a case mix value of 0.5265. This value is multiplied by the standard

Table 8–10.   Home Health Prospective Payment: HHRG Case Mix Classification Criteria

Clinical Severity	*Functional Status*	*Service Utilization*
Primary home care diagnosis	Dressing	No discharge last 14 days
IV/infusion/parenteral/ enteral therapies	Bathing	IP rehab/ SNF discharge past 14 days
Vision	Toileting	10 or more therapy visits
Pain	Transfers	
Wound/lesion	Locomotion	
Multiple pressure sores		
Most problematic pressure ulcer stage		
Stasis ulcer status		
Dyspnea		
Urinary incontinence		
Bowel incontinence		
Bowel ostomy		
Behavioral problems		

Source: Health Care Financing Administration, 42 CFR Parts 409, 410, 411, 413, 424 and 484. Medicare Program; Prospective Payment System for Home Health Care Agencies; Final Rule. Table VII Federal Register; 65(128): 41194.

Table 8–11. Home Health Prospective Payment: Federal per Episode Rate Calculation for C0F0S0

Standardized prospective payment rate:	$2,115.30	
Case mix adjustment for C0F0S0:	0.5265	
Case mix adjusted rate:	$1,113.71	
Wage conditions adjustment		
Labor component (x 0.7768)		$865.13
Adjusted for Omaha (x 1.0456)		$904.58
Adjusted for San Francisco (x 1.4002)		$1,211.36
Non-labor-related component:		$248.58
Total per episode rate in Omaha:		$1,153.16
Total per episode rate in San Francisco:		$1,459.94

prospective payment rate to determine the effect of patient characteristics and service needs on provider reimbursement ($2,115.30 x 0.5265 = $1,113.71). Similar to the provider reimbursement system in skilled nursing facilities, the case mix adjusted rate is then modified based on local wage conditions. In 2001, the government determined that the labor portion of the prospective payment rate was 78 percent (0.77668) of the total rate. This proportion of the prospective payment rate requires adjustment for local wage conditions (0.7768 x $1,113.71 = $865.12). Wage indices differ across the country (Omaha: 1.0456; San Francisco: 1.4002). In either case, the labor proportion of the payment rate is multiplied by the local factor to determine a wage-adjusted rate. This is added to the nonwage portion of the prospective payment rate to determine the final per home health care episode prospective payment rate ($1,153.16 in Omaha; 1,459.94 in San Francisco). Similar to the results of the SNF prospective payment system, providers in more expensive areas of the United States are reimbursed at higher rates to care for the same case-mix adjusted patient as providers in less expensive areas of the country.

As a result of the implementation of home health prospective payment, there are fewer home health agencies across the country but nearly all Medicare beneficiaries are receiving necessary services (Office of the Inspector General 2000). There has not been an increase in hospital admissions or emergency room visits as a result of this new payment system (Office of the Inspector General 2000).

Case Example: The home health agency received a payment of $1,113.71 for Mrs. Miller's home health care. The therapist documentation demonstrated that Mrs. Miller required and received skilled therapy visits during her home recuperation. Overall, Mrs. Miller's care cost $14,409.71. All of this cost, except for the $796 Medicare deductible, was paid by the Medicare Part A trust fund to each of her providers based on a separate prospective payment system.

Part A: Medicare Reform and Prospective Payment

The development and implementation of prospective payment systems in the Medicare program has reformed the program and halted the rapid rate of growth in post-acute program expenditures. In 1999, Part A program costs for skilled nursing facility care declined 15 percent, and home health program costs declined 35 percent with the introduction of prospective payment (Board of Trustees 2000). These program savings can be attributed to the change from facility-based, cost-based reimbursement to a case rate payment structure based on national cost averages, case mix adjustment for patient characteristics and service needs, and legislative mandates to reduce program expenditures. Cost efficiencies are created by standardizing the data used to make payment decisions. Federal budget surpluses are increasing the pressure on policymakers to increase Part A Medicare funding. Demographic change, political realities, and legislative action will continue to define the Part A program in this next decade.

Part B: Supplementary Medical Insurance (SMI)

Eligibility

Persons who are eligible for premium-free Medicare Part A (vested persons over age 65, spouses of vested beneficiaries, persons with permanent disabilities, and persons younger than age 65 with end-stage renal disease) are automatically eligible for Part B Medicare. Other American citizens or permanent residents over age 65 may also enroll in Part B Medicare (Health Care Financing Administration 1999).

Part B Medicare is an optional benefit package. Many people enroll in Medicare Part B when they become eligible for Medicare Part A. A person who declines Medicare Part B is eligible to enroll at a later date during special enrollment periods at a higher cost. About 25 percent of Medicare Part B program costs is paid by enrollees. The monthly premium in 2002 is $54.00. This is usually deducted automatically from Social Security checks. There is a $100 annual Part B deductible and a 20 percent co-insurance rate.

Benefits

Medicare Part B pays for most of the costs of health-related professional services, outpatient care, home health care, durable medical equipment, prosthetics, and orthotics (Health Care Financing Administration 2000). Each beneficiary is responsible for a $100 annual Part B deductible before receiving program benefits. Medicare Part B pays for therapy services in outpatient hospital, rehabilitation agency, comprehensive outpatient rehabilitation facilities, and private practice settings.

Patients receive these benefits when a medically supervised, skilled rehabilitation service is provided (see Table 8–12). Medicare Part B will pay for therapy services provided in outpatient departments, homes, and other inpatient environments (e.g., skilled nursing facilities). Until 1997, many Medicare beneficiaries in skilled nursing facilities received physical and occupational therapy services from therapists who were independent contractors or worked for agencies that billed Medicare Part B directly for their services. The Balanced Budget Act of 1997 required **consolidated billing** of all Part A and Part B Medicare services by the skilled nursing facility (Health Care Financing Administration 1998).

Provider Types

Medicare Part B regulations define different types of therapy providers. At one time, this typology had important implications for the way therapists were paid for their services. Since the Balanced Budget Act of 1997, all Medicare Part B provider types are reimbursed using a fee schedule. We will discuss the fee schedule payment mechanism shortly.

Outpatient Hospital Programs

Hospital outpatient programs (e.g., radiology, rehabilitation, laboratory services) provide a wide range of medically necessary, skilled services to community-dwelling Medicare beneficiaries. Until 1997, these programs were reimbursed using a cost-based mechanism. Beginning in January 1999, Medicare initiated a fee schedule

---

Table 8–12.   Conditions For Coverage of Outpatient Physical Therapy and Occupational Therapy Services

A. Definition of Outpatient Physical Therapy and Occupational Therapy
   1. Provided to patients in homes, outpatient facilities, or other inpatient environments
   2. Persons who have exhausted their Part A benefits
B. Physician Certification and Recertification
   1. Occurs at admission to therapy services and every 30 days thereafter.
C. A written plan has been established for the patient's episode of care.
   1. Created by the physical therapist, occupational therapist, or physician.
   2. Type, amount, duration, and frequency of therapy activities are outlined.
     a. Is a reasonable and necessary intervention.
     b. Skilled intervention
   3. Patient diagnosis is identified.
   4. Measurable therapy goals are identified.
   5. Plan of care must be kept on file.

Source: Health Care Financing Administration, Outpatient Physical Therapy, Comprehensive Outpatient Rehabilitation Facility and Community Mental Health Center Manual. Chapter 2–Coverage of Services. Section 270. Accessed at *http://www.hcfa.gov/ pub-forms/09 opt/op202.htm# 1 126* on November 10, 2000.

for outpatient rehabilitation services. A prospective payment system for other outpatient hospital programs was implemented in 2001.

Comprehensive Outpatient Rehabilitation Facility

A comprehensive outpatient rehabilitation facility (CORF) is a Medicare Part B type provider that consists of at least the following services: physician care, physical therapy, and social services (Medicare Program Manual 2000). In addition, occupational therapy, speech/ language therapy, respiratory therapy, nursing, prosthetics, and orthotics services can be offered through a CORF.

Physical Therapists and Occupational Therapists in Private Practice

Physical therapists in private practice (PTPP) and occupational therapists in private practice (OTPP) are two other recognized Medicare Part B provider types. In this arrangement, physical and occupational therapists in solo practices or unincorporated partnerships can be recognized as therapists in private practice. These therapists apply for Medicare reimbursement through their regional carrier. They must maintain an independent office to be eligible to be a Medicare provider.

Medicare Part B: Payment Structure

Fee Schedule

The Medicare Part B payment methodology for physical and occupational therapy services is the **fee schedule.** A Medicare fee schedule is a list of procedures with associated payments based on the estimated costs of delivering them. This list of procedures is coded using Current Procedural Terminology, or CPT (American Medical Association 2002). Physical therapists and occupational therapists use codes in the 97000 series, or Physical Medicine and Rehabilitation section of the CPT. Fee schedule payments for each code are determined using a cost-determination method called the Resource-Based Relative Value Scale, or RBRVS. The fee schedule payment for each procedure can be calculated by the following formula (Medicare Program Rule 2000):

[Resource Value Unit for Work x Geographic Practice Cost Index] +
[Resource Value Unit for Practice Expense x Geographic Practice Cost Index]
+ [Resource Value Unit for Malpractice x Geographic Practice Cost Index] x
National Conversion Factor = Fee Schedule Payment

Each year CMS calculates a "value unit" for each procedure that represents the technical ability, knowledge, and skill to perform it. Similarly, value units are determined for the overhead costs necessary to perform the procedure (practice expense and malpractice). Each of these three components of the RBRVS is adjusted for differences in local costs of providing the procedure to beneficiaries. The sum of the adjusted factors is multiplied by a standard national payment amount to determine the fee schedule payment.

Consider the example in Table 8–13. We will use the Physical Therapy Evaluation CPT code to illustrate how a fee schedule payment amount is determined. The occupational therapy evaluation CPT Code (97003) has very similar resource value units. Each relative value unit (RVU) has a factor applied to it that accounts for the work-related and practice-overhead costs associated with the procedure. Each RVU is further adjusted by a local cost index (the GPCI). As can be seen, this adjustment increases the RVU factor in San Francisco as compared to Omaha. The sum total of the adjusted RVUs is multiplied by the national conversion factor to determine the fee schedule amount for this CPT code. The fee schedule payment in San Francisco is about one-third more than a physical therapist in Omaha would expect.

Case Example: Two months after her total hip replacement surgery, Mrs. Miller is still experiencing some hip pain and weakness. Her surgeon sends her to a physical

Table 8–13.   Medicare Part B Reimbursement: Fee Schedule

Physical Therapy Evaluation: CPT 97001

2001 National Conversion Factor: $38.251
Work-related RVU: 1.20
   Geographic practice cost index adjustment
      Omaha (x 0.948) = 1.1376
      San Francisco (x 1.068) = 1.2816
Practice expense RVU: 0.56
   Geographic practice cost index adjustment
      Omaha (x 0.876) = 0.49
      San Francisco (x 1.458) = 0.816
Malpractice expense RVU: 0.10
   Geographic practice cost index adjustment
      Omaha (x 0.430) = 0.043
      San Francisco (x 0.687) = 0.0687
Total relative value units (RVU) = 1.86
   Adjusted total for Omaha = 1.67
   Adjusted total for San Francisco = 2.1663
Fee schedule payment for 97001
   Standard amount (1.86 x 38.2513) = $71.15
   In Omaha (1.67 x 38.2513) = $63.88
   In San Francisco (2.1663 x 38.2513) = $82.86

Source: Medicare Program; Revisions to Payment Policies Under the Physician Fee Schedule for Calendar Year 2001; Final Rule. 65 Fed Reg 65376–66505 (2000).

therapist for an evaluation. The standard fee schedule amount for this examination is $71.15. Mrs Miller pays her physical therapist out of pocket for this examination, with the fee applied to her annual $100 deductible.

Provider Participation

Medicare Part B providers, including physical therapists and occupational therapists in private practice, can elect to accept or not accept the fee schedule amount as payment in full. This is called accepting or declining **Medicare assignment.** A provider that accepts the Medicare assignment agrees to the fee schedule amount as payment in full for the procedure less the deductible and 20 percent coinsurance that is the responsibility of the beneficiary. A provider who does not accept Medicare assignment can still obtain Part B reimbursement but agrees to accept a 5 percent payment reduction from the Medicare fee schedule reimbursement. This provider can charge the beneficiary the full charge for the procedure up to 15 percent limit over the fee schedule amount. The difference between the fee schedule amount and the provider charge along with the deductible and coinsurance is the responsibility of the beneficiary.

Case Example: Mrs. Miller receives one month of outpatient physical therapy from a physical therapist in private practice. The Medicare fee schedule amount for this therapy is $500. Mrs. Miller's physical therapist participates in the Medicare Part B program and accepts Medicare assignment. Medicare reimburses the physical therapist $376.92 (80% of $471.15). Mrs. Miller owes the first $28.85 of the physical therapy as the remainder of her annual deductible and the 20 percent coinsurance amount ($94.23) for a total out-of-pocket cost of $194.23 for her outpatient physical therapy (total therapy cost: $571.15).

Medicare Part C

The Balanced Budget Act of 1997 created a new part of the program: Part C. Part C reorganized and expanded the Medicare-managed care programs and choices for beneficiaries. Currently, most beneficiaries can choose either to continue with traditional Medicare (Parts A and B) or receive their Medicare benefits through a range of managed care options (Part C). All Part C plans provide a benefit package similar to Parts A and B except for hospice services. Additional benefits (e.g., outpatient prescription drugs), may be offered in Part C plans that are not available in Medicare Parts A and B. These benefits are attractive to beneficiaries who cannot purchase supplemental insurance (Luft, 1998).

About 6.2 million Medicare beneficiaries receive their benefits through a Medicare HMO (HCFA Fact Sheet 2000). Part C Medicare plans most commonly are offered through a form of managed care (i.e., a health maintenance organization, preferred provider organization, or provider-sponsored organization). Medicare Part C plans are licensed in their states of operation and assume the financial risk of providing the mandated benefits. In return, Part C plans are paid a capitated monthly payment from HCFA for each enrolled beneficiary. This payment is based on the average per beneficiary cost in their market areas minus a government discount.

The introduction of Medicare Part C plans has been challenging. Local experience with private managed care plans has influenced the acceptance of Part C Medicare (Brown and Gold 1999). Favorable selection has been identified as a problem in Medicare-managed care plans (Morgan et al. 1997). Many beneficiaries have been forced to find new plans or convert to traditional Medicare as managed care plans exited the Part C program due to inadequate reimbursement rates (Medicare News 2000; Laschober et al. 1999; Morgenstern, Gonzales, and Anderson 2000).

Private Health Insurance and Medicare

As was explained above, the Medicare program provides many insurance benefits for beneficiaries but also has significant deductibles and co-payments. In addition, the benefit package does not cover outpatient prescription drugs, foreign medical care services, and some preventive health care services. As a result, some private insurance companies offer a Medicare supplemental, or **Medigap,** policy that beneficiaries can purchase to cover these other expenses. Ten Medicare supplemental plans are defined in Medicare law.

Quality and Medicare

The Medicare program ensures quality health care services through three primary processes: provider certification, utilization review, and oversight by peer review organizations (PROs). All providers must submit an application to CMS in order to participate in the Medicare program. **Certification** ensures that providers are licensed and meet other minimum requirements for participation. For hospitals, accreditation by the Joint Commission on Accreditation of Healthcare Organizations (JCAHO) is evidence of certification. CMS independently surveys a small percentage of JCAHO-accredited hospitals each year. Besides providers, CMS also certifies managed care organizations.

Utilization review is a process of internal audit and review of the processes of care received by beneficiaries, primarily in hospitals. Health care professionals audit patient records, discuss the plan of care with the health care team, and make recommendations regarding the appropriateness of the level of care. Utilization review committees regularly review the quality and appropriateness of care.

Utilization review is also performed by external organizations, including intermediaries, carriers, and **peer review organizations** (PROs). Intermediaries and carriers routinely monitor Medicare claims and investigate possible fraud (see below). PROs independently contract with CMS to perform two primary functions. First, PROs conduct beneficiary protection and education functions (e.g., utilization review, investigation of providers, beneficiary complaint hotlines). Second, PROs conduct special quality-improvement projects focusing on problem-prone areas of concern.

Fraud and Abuse

Medicare fraud and abuse is a multibillion-dollar problem. Much of this fraud and abuse can be attributed to unethical and illegal provider behavior, and some can be attributed to complex and confusing program rules. The Health Insurance Portability and Accountability Act of 1996 strengthened the ability of the government to find and prosecute fraud and abuse by establishing the Medicare Integrity Program. The most common forms of Medicare fraud are listed in Table 8–14. In addition to these types of fraud, provider waivers of beneficiary payment of the Medicare deductible or co-insurance are another form of Medicare fraud.

Fiscal intermediaries, carriers, and "program safeguard contractors" perform routine and special audits of many types of provider activities, including practice patterns. Utilization review by these organizations has three levels. Level I reviews the utilization pattern against an "edit" (i.e., a defined number of visits or days of treatment used to initially screen claims for appropriateness). A Level II review is a focused review by a health professional (e.g., an occupational therapist or physical therapist), who reviews the documentation to determine whether the care meets Medicare guidelines for appropriateness (e.g., a skilled vs. non skilled service, presence of physician certification). A Level II review may result in a denial of payment on a Medicare claim or referral to a Level III review. A Level III review is an onsite review of patient care documentation and Medicare billing records. In response to the increased efforts of the government to reduce Medicare fraud and abuse, compliance programs are being established by providers in order to avoid allegations of fraud. These programs emphasize timely and accurate documentation and the avoidance of improper business relationships between Medicare providers and contractors.

Table 8–14.   Most Common Types of Medicare Fraud

- Billing for services not furnished
- Misrepresenting the diagnosis to justify payment
- Soliciting, offering, or receiving a kickback
- Unbundling or "exploding" charges
- Falsifying certificates of medical necessity, plans of treatment, and medical records to justify payment
- Billing for a service not furnished as billed (i.e., upcoding)

Source: Medicare Definition of Fraud. Accessed at *http://www.hcfa.gov/medicare/fraud/DEFINI2.HTM* on November 11, 2000.

Medicare Reform

Reform of Medicare has been ongoing since the program's inception. The first 15 years of the program were marked by an expansion of eligibility (e.g., persons with disabilities or end-stage renal disease) and program benefits (the program has funded numerous medical innovations, e.g., joint replacements). Since 1983, the Medicare program has implemented multiple cost-restraint initiatives. In its 35-year existence, Medicare has become the largest funder of the health care system.

Bruce Vladeck (1999), a former administrator of HCFA, described the relationship between the growth of the Medicare program and the U.S. medical care system in the last quarter-century as the development of a "Medicare-industrial complex." The strength of Medicare has a direct effect on the viability of the overall medical care system. Medicare is not a pre-funded program but a "pay as you go" funding system. Current payroll taxes, general federal revenues, and beneficiary contributions fund the program.

In the mid-1990s, concerns were raised about the financial viability of the Hospital Insurance Medicare trust fund. These concerns fostered the Balanced Budget Act of 1997 legislation. The 2000 report of the Hospital Insurance trust fund stated that tax revenue for the Part A program is now expected to exceed disbursements until 2017 and the program is solvent until 2025. The Supplemental Medical Insurance trust fund (for Part B) is solvent into the "indefinite future," although the trustees are concerned about program cost inflation rates higher than the overall inflation rate (Medicare trustees 2000). The SMI trust fund receives 25 percent of its revenue from beneficiary contributions and most of the remainder of its funding from general tax revenues.

Wilensky and Newhouse (1999) outline several major challenges for Medicare in the future. First, the current system of controlled pricing is inefficient and difficult to administer. This adds significant indirect costs to the system. Second, the benefits package has not been comprehensively updated since the program's inception and is out of date. This has created a large market for Medigap plans that are often too expensive for the poor and other vulnerable populations. Persons without Medigap coverage face significant out-of-pocket expense and, as a result, probably do not have access to necessary services. Third, the aging of the baby boom generation will put additional strain on the program to deliver benefits while the number of Americans paying into the system in relation to those receiving benefits declines.

To face these challenges, Congress has so far primarily employed provider payment restrictions. These are politically acceptable because they affect few beneficiaries, but they are bureaucratic, do not address beneficiary utilization rates, and reinforce interest group politics. Other proposals for reform include means-testing the program, similar in principle to Medicaid, and raising the age of eligibility. Means-testing program eligibility or benefits is unpopular for some people because Medicare has gained general acceptance as an earned benefit and is not viewed as a welfare program. Raising the eligibility age is politically unpopular and transfers the cost of health care for persons currently covered by the program (at age 65) to the private sector, which is becoming increasingly reluctant to bear the costs of health care (e.g., the widespread acceptance of managed care).

A more radical reform proposal would change Medicare from a "defined benefit" plan to a "defined contribution" plan. A **defined contribution** plan would set government contributions to the Medicare program at a predetermined level. Beneficiaries would receive a voucher to purchase a privately-organized Medicare plan that provides a set of minimum benefits. **Defined benefit** plans would likely increase the out-of-pocket costs to beneficiaries but limit the costs to the taxpayer.

Medicare reform is likely to continue into the next decades as Congress and the president struggle with rising the demand for health care by elderly and disabled Americans as the numbers of workers who pay into the program declines. Physical therapy and occupational therapy will be affected by whatever changes are enacted in the future.

Conclusion

Medicare is the largest, single source of funding for medical care in the United States. It was established in 1965 as a federal entitlement program, Title XVIII of the Social Security Act. It has three parts: hospital insurance, supplementary medical insurance and managed care plans. Medicare Part A covers inpatient hospital stays and services, home health care/hospice and short term skilled nursing facility care. Medicare Part B covers outpatient services, including physical therapy and occupational therapy. Medicare Part C provides a range of managed care options for benificiaries. Medicare has been effective in improving the quality of life for persons over age 65 and for persons with permanent disability or end stage renal disease. It has revolutionized reimbursement systems for providers by defining provider types and implementing cost-based reimbursement models, prospective payment systems, and the fee schedule. As the population ages, Medicare will continue to grow in importance as a major influence on the health care system.

CHAPTER REVIEW QUESTIONS

1. Describe the social and political reasons for the development of Medicare.
2. Define the three parts of Medicare.
3. Who is eligible for Medicare Part A?
4. Define and describe the services of Medicare Part A.
5. What is cost-based reimbursement? Prospective payment?
6. Identify the patient classification systems used for
   a. inpatient hospital care
   b. skilled nursing facility care
   c. home health care
   d. inpatient rehabilitation hospital care
7. What three factors determine a prospective payment rate?

8. Who is eligible for Medicare Part B?
9. Define and describe the services of Medicare Part B.
10. Define the types of therapy providers in Medicare Part B.
11. What is a fee schedule, and how are fee schedule payments determined?
12. Who is eligible for Medicare Part C plans and what are the benefits offered?
13. Describe how the Medicare program assures the quality of its health plans.
14. Define the most common forms of Medicare fraud and abuse.
15. Review the challenges that will confront the Medicare program in the next decade.

CHAPTER DISCUSSION QUESTIONS

1. Medicare's founders have stated that the Medicare program is one step toward national health insurance. From your understanding of the program, what would be the advantages/disadvantages of using the Medicare model as a template for national health insurance?
2. Discuss how the policy decision to pay for Medicare services based on a case rate or capitated basis vs. the fee-for-service method affects the practice of physical therapy and occupational therapy.
3. Consider the examples of Medicare fraud and abuse. Discuss how you can practice so as to avoid committing Medicare fraud.

REFERENCES

American Medical Association. 2002. Current Procedural Terminology: CPT. Chicago: American Medical Association.

Ball, R. M. 1995. What Medicare's architects had in mid. *Health Affairs* 14(4): 62–72.

Blaisdell, F. W. 1992. The pre-Medicare role of city/county hospitals in education and health care. *J Trauma* 32(2): 217–28.

———. 1994. Development of the city/county (public) hospital. *Arch Surg* 129(7): 760–64.

Board of Trustees of the Federal Hospital Insurance Trust Fund. 2000. Annual Report. April 2000. Accessed at *http://www.hcfa.gov/pubforms/tr/hi2000/hi.pdf* on November 10, 2000.

Board of Trustees of the Federal Supplementary Medical Insurance Trust Fund. 2000 Annual Report. April 2000. Accessed at *http://www.hcfa.gov/pubforms/tr/smi2000/smi.pdf* on November 11, 2000.

Brown, R. S. and M. R. Gold. 1999. What drives Medicare managed care growth? Local forces may explain why the Medicare managed care market has not developed as the optimists predicted. *Health Affairs* 18(6): 140–49.

Center for Medicare and Medicaid Services. 2001. Overview of the prospective payment system for inpatient rehabilitation hospitals and rehabilitation units. Accessed at *http://www.hcfa.gov/medicare/irfover2001.htm* on August 23, 2001.

Chaix-Couturier, C., I. Durand-Zaleski, D. Jolly, and P. Durieux. 2000. Effects of financial incentives on medical practice: Results from a systematic review of the literature and methodological issues. *Int J Qual Health Care* 12(2): 133–42.

Clancy, T., S. Kitchen, P. Churchill, D. Covington, J. Hundley, and J. G. Maxwell. 1998. DRG reimbursement: Geriatric hip fractures in the community hospital trauma center. *South Med J* 91(5): 457–61.

Davis, M. H. and S. T. Burner. 1995. Three decades of Medicare: What the numbers tell us. *Health Affairs* 14(4): 231–43.

Forgione, D. A. and C. M. D'Annunzio. 1999. The use of DRGs in health care payment systems around the world. *J Health Care Fin* 26(2): 66–78.

Friedman, E. 1995. The compromise and the afterthought. Medicare and Medicaid after 30 years. *JAMA* 274(3): 278–82.

Gilman, B. H., J. Cromwell, K. Adamache, and S. Donoghue. 2000. *Study of the Effect of Implementing the Post-Acute Care Transfer Policy under the Inpatient Prospective Payment System.* Waltham, MA: Health Economics Research Institute.

Health Care Financing Administration. 1998. Program Memorandum (Intermediaries/Carriers), HCFA Pub. 60AB, Transmittal No. AB-98–18, April 1, 1998.

———. 1998. Medicare Home Health Benefit: The Balanced Budget Act of 1997: Financing Shift of Home Health Services from Medicare Part A to Part B. Transmittal No. A-98-49. December 1998.

———. 1999. *Medicare and You, 2000.* Publication No. HCFA-10050.

———. 1999. *Medicare and You: Medicare Questions and Answers.* Publication No. HCFA-10117.

———. 2000. *Home Health Agency Manual.* Accessed at *http://www.hcfa.gov/pubforms/11%5Fhha/hh00.htm* on November 2, 2000.

———. 2000. Hospice. Accessed at *http://www.hcfa.gov/medicaid/hospice/hospice.htm* on November 2, 2000.

———. 2000. *Skilled Nursing Facility Manual.* Accessed at *http://www.hcfa.gov/pubforms/12%5Fsnf/sn0%2Dfw.htm* on November 2, 2000.

———. 2001. Fact Sheet. Protecting Medicare beneficiaries after Medicare+Choice organizations withdraw. Accessed at *http://www.hcfa.gov/medicare/mcfactf.htm* on November 10, 2000.

Laschober, M. A., P. Neuman, M. S. Kitchman, L. Meyer, and K. M. Langwell. 2000. Medicare HMO withdrawals—what happens to beneficiaries? Most "orphaned" Medicare beneficiaries have been able to find new coverage arrangements, but many now pay more and have fewer benefits. *Health Affairs* 19(1): 263.

Levit, K., C. Cowan, H. Lazenby, A. Sensenig, P. McDonnell, J. Stiller, and P. Martin. Health Accounts Team. 2000. Health spending in 1998: Signals of change. *Health Affairs* 19(1): 124–32.

Luft, H. S. 1998. Medicare and managed care. *Ann Rev Public Health* 19: 459–75.

Medicare News. 2001. Statement by Nancy-Ann DeParle, Administrator, Health Care Financing Administration. Medicare+Choice Plan Nonrenewals. Accessed at *http://www.hcfa.gov/medicare/mcstate.htm* on November 10, 2000.

Medicare Program. 1998. Changes to the Inpatient Hospital Prospective Payment Systems and Fiscal Year 1998 Rates, Final Rule. 42 CFR Parts 410 et.al., 63 Fed Reg 26318–26360.

————. 1998. Prospective Payment System and Consolidated Billing for Skilled Nursing Facilities; Final Rule, 42 CFR Parts 409 et.al., 63 Fed Reg 26252–26316.

————. 2000. Prospective Payment System for Home Health Agencies; Final Rule. 42 CFR Parts 409, 410, 411, 413, 424 and 484, 65 Fed Reg 41128–41214.

————. 2000. Prospective Payment System for Inpatient Rehabilitation Facilities; Proposed Rule, 42 CFR Parts 412 and 413, 65 Fed Reg 66304–66442.

————. 2000. Revisions to Payment Policies Under the Physician Fee Schedule for Calendar Year 2001; Final Rule. 65 Fed Reg 65376–66505.

Menke, T. J., C. M. Ashton, N. J. Petersen, and F. D. Wolinsky. 1998. Impact of an all-inclusive diagnosis-related group payment system on inpatient utilization. *Med Care* 36(8): 1126–37.

Morgan, R. A., B. A. Vernig, C. A. DeVito, and N. A. Persily 1997. The Medicare-HMO revolving door: The healthy come in and the sick go out. *N Engl J Med* 337(3): 169–75.

Morgenstern, N. E., R. Gonzales, and R. Anderson. 2000. Involuntary disenrollment from a Medicare managed care plan at an academic medical center: Effect on patients. *J Am Geri Soc* 48(9): 1151–56.

Office of the Inspector General. 1999. Early Effects of the Prospective Payment System on Access to Skilled Nursing Facilities. DHSS OEI-02-99-00400. August.

————. 1999. Early Effects of the Prospective Payment System on Access to Skilled Nursing Facilities: Nursing Home Administrators Perspective. DHSS OEI-02-99-00401. August.

————. 1999. Physical and Occupational Therapy in Nursing Homes: Medical Necessity and Quality of Care. DHSS OEI-09-97-00121. August.

————. 2000. Medicare Beneficiary Access to Home Health Agencies: 2000. DHHS OEI-02-00-00320. September.

Reynolds, P. P. 1997. The federal government's use of Title VI and Medicare to racially integrate hospitals in the United States, 1963 through 1967. *Am J Pub Health* 87 (11): 1850–58.

Rothman, D. J. 1993. A century of failure: Health care reform in America. *J Health Polit Policy Law* 18(2): 271–86.

Russell, L. B. and C. S. Burke. 1978. The political economy of federal health programs in the United States: A historical review. *Int J Health Serv* 8(1): 55–77.

Stineman, M. G., J. J. Escarce, J. E. Goin, B. B. Hamilton, C. V. Granger, and S. V. Williams. 1994. A case mix classification system for medical rehabilitation. *Medical Care* 32(4): 366–79.

Takemura, Y. and J. R. Beck. 1999. The effects of a fixed-fee reimbursement system introduced by the federal government on laboratory testing in the United States. *Rinsho-byori* 47(1): 1–10.

Vladeck, B. 1999. The political economy of Medicare. *Health Affairs* 18(1): 22–36

Whetsell, G. W. 1999. The history and evolution of hospital payment systems: How did we get here? *Nurs Adm Q* 23(4): 1–15.

Wilensky, G. and J. P. Newhouse. 1999. Medicare: What's right? What's wrong? What's next? *Health Affairs* 18(1): 92–106.

9

Medicaid, SCHIP, and Military/ Veterans Medical Insurance

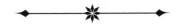

CHAPTER OBJECTIVES

At the conclusion of this chapter, the reader will be able to:

1. Describe the statutory authorization, size, and purpose of the Medicaid program.
2. Identify and relate the criteria for eligibility for Medicaid benefits.
    a. Discuss the impact of welfare and immigration reform on eligibility for Medicaid benefits.
3. Describe the services covered by the Medicaid program.
4. Describe the organization of services in the Medicaid program.
    a. Medicaid managed care
    b. Medicaid waiver programs
5. Describe the statutory authorization, size, and purpose of the State Children's Health Insurance Program.
6. Relate the eligibility criteria and health insurance benefits for active military and veterans health benefit programs.

KEY WORDS: Categorical Eligibility, Dual Eligibility, Means-tested, Medically Needy Eligibility, Personal Care Services, Presumptive Eligibility, Safety-Net Provider, Spend-Down, State Option, Waiver Program

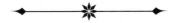

Introduction

The preceding three chapters introduced and described several large insurance mechanisms that finance much of the health care system. In Chapter 6, we discussed the purpose of insurance and introduced several ways that health insurance products are organized. In Chapter 7, we learned about managed care, the dominant form of private health care insurance today. In Chapter 8, we considered Medicare, an example of social insurance, and the largest insurance program, in terms of dollars spent, in the world. In this chapter, we turn our attention to other governmental health care insurance programs: Medicaid, the State Children's Health Insurance Program (SCHIP), and insurance for active military personnel and veterans.

These insurance programs target populations that either have historically not been able to obtain private health care insurance or, as in the case of the military, for whom the government has a direct responsibility for the health care of plan members. Medicaid and SCHIP serve a large and vulnerable component of our society—the poor, persons with disabilities, women, and children. The structure of Medicaid and SCHIP displays the societal tension concerning the roles of government and the private sector in providing solutions to the dilemma of access to health care insurance for everyone in the country. Both programs are federal-state partnerships. Eligibility requirements are sophisticated and limited to certain groups. Benefit packages are generous but are increasingly relying on managed care and private insurance contracting to deliver the services.

First, we will consider Medicaid, the largest health care insurance plan, in terms of persons served, in the United States. The increasing number of uninsured children spawned the State Children's Health Insurance Plan in 1997, an effort to improve health care for poor children in the United States. Finally, we will explore the Veterans' Health Plan and TRICARE, a major source of funding for active and retired military beneficiaries.

Medicaid

What Is Medicaid?

Medicaid is a joint federal-state medical insurance program designed to meet the health care needs of people who meet certain low-income requirements, have high medical costs, or are in certain defined, disadvantaged populations (e.g. low-income pregnant women and children). Medicaid is a **means-tested** program. Historically, eligibility for Medicaid was closely tied to welfare. Unlike Medicare, a beneficiary must qualify by demonstrating a level of need usually based on income, personal assets, or life situation. Medicaid insures more Americans, about 40 million persons, than any other health care insurance program in the country.

Medicaid was established in 1965 as Title XIX of the Social Security Act. It replaced the small medical insurance programs for indigent persons that were offered by several states with one large national program. Medicaid insurance has improved access to medical care for poor families (Newacheck et al. 1998). Medicaid was one of the cornerstones of President Lyndon Johnson's Great Society program.

All 50 states participate in the Medicaid program. The federal government shares with the states the cost of providing a defined package of medical care benefits. The federal share of a state's program ranges from at least 50 percent up to 76 percent of the total program cost (Department of Health and Human Services 2000). Poor states pay less than wealthy states. For many states and territories, these shared payments for the Medicaid program are the largest grant they receive from the federal government, and the cost of the program is one of the largest annual expenditures of state funds.

The total cost of the Medicaid program in 1998 was $170 billion (Levit et al. 2000). Of this amount, $100 billion was paid by the federal government (59%), and $70 billion was paid by state governments (41%). Medicaid program costs have increased more than twofold in the last 10 years. The distribution of Medicaid reimbursements is skewed to certain segments of the population. About three in four Medicaid service dollars are spent on care for the elderly and persons with disabilities. Medicaid is the largest purchaser of long-term care in the United States (Health Care Financing Administration 1999). Children, the largest group of Medicaid beneficiaries, account for about 25 percent of program spending (Kaiser Commission on Medicaid and the Uninsured 1999).

Children comprise 50 percent of the Medicaid beneficiary population (Kaiser Commission on Medicaid and the Uninsured 1999). Most of the remaining 50 percent of Medicaid beneficiaries is made up of elderly people (10%), blind or disabled people (15%), and adults in families (20%). The segments of the population served by Medicaid have been changing in the last 20 years. Congressional action in the 1980s and 1990s increased the number of children covered by Medicaid and reduced the number of adults.

Who Is Eligible for Medicaid?

Eligibility for the Medicaid program is a complicated process that is determined by meeting one or more sets of criteria: **categorical eligibility, medically needy eligibility,** and Medicare-Medicaid **dual eligibility.** Unlike Medicare, Medicaid is a means-tested government program. Potential participants must demonstrate that they meet certain income/assets criteria in order to receive benefits. In general, single men and childless couples are not eligible for Medicaid. Participation in the Medicaid program has been significantly affected by welfare and immigration reforms enacted in the mid-1990s. We will have more to discuss about the effect of these governmental actions on Medicaid after we introduce the basic eligibility criteria.

Table 9–1 summarizes the basic qualifications for Medicaid benefits. The first six items outline the criteria for becoming a categorically eligible beneficiary. All

Table 9–1.   Medicaid Eligibility

Mandatory Categories
1. Low-income families with children
2. Recipients of Supplemental Security Income payments
3. Infants born to Medicaid-eligible women
4. Children under age 6 and pregnant women whose family income is at or below 133 percent of the federal poverty level
5. Recipients of foster care and certain adoptions
6. Working poor who exceed income guidelines (for a transition period)

Medically Needy
1. Spend-down programs

Medicare-Medicaid Eligibility
1. Dual-eligibles—must be Medicare eligible
   a. Qualified Medicare beneficiary
      (1) Low income: <= 100 percent of the federal poverty level
      (2) Limited personal assets: twice the limit for SSI eligibility
      (3) Pays Medicare A and B premiums, deductibles, and co-insurance
      (4) May or may not have access to full state Medicaid benefits
   b. Specified low-income Medicare beneficiary
      (1) Low-income: 100–120 percent of federal poverty level
      (2) Limited personal assets: twice the limit for SSI eligibility
      (3) Pays Medicare B premiums only
      (4) May or may not have access to full state Medicaid benefits

Source: Health Care Financing Administration, 2000. *Medicaid Eligibility.*

states must cover individuals who meet the criteria for one of these categories. This type of eligibility defines the criteria that qualify many poor women, infants, and children for Medicaid benefits. Many people with disabilities receive Supplementary Social Income payments (SSI) from the Social Security program that qualify them to also receive Medicaid. Wards of the state are included in these criteria. Besides these basic eligibility requirements, the federal government will match state costs for more liberal program-eligibility qualifications. For example, many states increase the opportunity for Medicaid eligibility by raising the family income level to 185 percent of the federal poverty level for infants in poor families.

The medically needy eligibility criteria are a **state-option** that can be included or not included in each state's Medicaid program. As an example, the criteria used in Nebraska are provided in Table 9–2. These criteria allow individuals with high medical care expenses to **spend down** their assets to a certain level, after which the Medicaid program will pay for the continuing costs of care. This qualification enables many elderly persons and persons with disabilities who have high medical costs and limited private insurance to access medical and long-term care insurance benefits.

In order to qualify, one must meet two sets of financial criteria. Personal assets must be used to pay for medical care expenses until a financial threshold is

Table 9–2.   Medically Needy Criteria For Medicaid Benefits—Nebraska (2000)

1. Able to maintain $4,000 in assets/$6,000 per couple
   a. Home is exempt until the patient leaves it for a nursing home
   b. $1,500 in life insurance/$3,000 per couple
   c. One car
   d. $3,000 in a burial expense account/$6,000 per couple
   e. If one
2. Meet monthly income guidelines: Must be less than
   a. Single person—$687
   b. Couple—$922
3. If one married spouse enters a nursing home, up to $168,240 of the couple's assets are divided in half. The spouse entering the nursing home uses his/her personal assets to pay for expenses until the $4,000 threshold is reached.

Source: Nebraska Health and Human Services System, 1999. *Aged and Disabled Meicaid.*

reached (in Nebraska, $4,000). The person's monthly income must also be below another threshold value (in Nebraska, $687 per single/ $922 per couple). Once both these criteria are met, the person qualifies as a medically needy Medicaid beneficiary. The spend-down provision requires the person in need of care to use up personal assets first, but in most instances protects some assets and the income of a surviving spouse. For years, couples and families attempted to protect more of an individual's personal assets from being spent on expensive long-term care. Recent legislation has limited these options. States are now able to prevent the transfer of assets to children, recover some previously transferred assets, and recover expenses by applying a lien on the assets of an estate in probate.

To see how the medically needy eligibility provision works, consider this example. A member of a married couple in rural Nebraska experiences a catastrophic medical event that incurs $5,000 in monthly long-term care expenses that lasts for 20 months. This will total $100,000 in medical care expenses. The couple has a home, which is the residence for the other spouse, and one car. The couple's savings and investments total $50,000. In addition, each member of the couple has established a $2,500 prepaid burial account with a local mortuary. Under the Nebraska law, the at-home spouse does not have to sell the home or car to pay for long-term care expenses and can keep $25,000 of the couple's savings and investments. The burial accounts for both persons are not considered assets to be used for paying for long-term care. These asset types are protected from the spend-down provision. As a result, the first $21,000 in long-term care expenses is paid by the remaining assets that are designated to the spouse residing in the nursing home. The spouse residing in the nursing home will continue to have $4,000 in protected personal assets. The remaining $79,000 in long-term care costs is paid by the state Medicaid program.

The final method of obtaining Medicaid coverage is by qualifying for dual eligibility, which allows a low-income Medicare beneficiary to qualify for Medicaid payment of Medicare deductibles and co-insurance. Lamphere and Rosenbach

(2000) have found that many dual-eligible beneficiaries do not take advantage of this benefit because they are unaware that they qualify and the eligibility process is quite complex. In some cases, dual-eligible beneficiaries have access to benefits not covered by the Medicare program, such as prescription drugs and dental care. Examples of dual-eligible status are persons who are "qualified Medicare beneficiaries" or "specified low-income Medicare beneficiaries" (see Table 9–1).

The eligibility criteria for the Medicaid program define who can participate and the size of the program. The Health Care Financing Administration (1999) reported that nearly two in three Medicaid beneficiaries qualified for program benefits based on categorical eligibility in 1996. The remaining Medicaid participants are eligible based on being medically needy or a Medicare-Medicaid dual-eligible. Eligibility for Medicaid has been affected by two major public policy decisions in the 1990s: welfare reform and immigration reform.

Until 1997, persons and families who qualified for welfare benefits under the Aid for Families with Dependent Children program (AFDC) automatically qualified for medical care insurance under Medicaid. In 1996, Congress enacted and the president signed the Personal Responsibility and Work Opportunity Reconciliation Act. This law replaced a federal welfare-entitlement statute. This law established a block grant program to the states with a mandate to time-limit welfare benefits and require people on welfare to return to work. This new program is called Temporary Assistance to Needy Families or TANF (Families USA 1999).

With TANF block grants, the incentive for states is to reduce the number of people on the welfare rolls and return them to work. The decoupling of welfare and Medicaid has had the unintended effect that fewer people are insured in the Medicaid program (Weissman et al. 1999; Chavkin, Romero, and Wise 2000; Garrett and Holahan 2000; Short and Freedman 1998). The decline in insurance coverage is primarily attributed to state strategies to limit enrollment in TANF (Chavkin, Romero, and Wise 2000) and to a lack of access to private health care insurance in low-paying jobs often occupied by persons leaving welfare (Garrett and Holahan 2000). Employed persons who meet the eligibility criteria for Medicaid continue to qualify for the program, but the mechanisms to identify and enroll them are incomplete.

Immigration reform enacted in the same 1996 welfare reform package limited the eligibility of immigrants to participate in the Medicaid program. Table 9–3 lists the critieria for aliens who qualify and do not qualify for participation in the Medicaid program. Recent immigrants have traditionally been much more likely not to be insured than most Americans (Thamer and Rinehart 1998). Medicaid reform of immigrant eligibility is expected to increase the lack-of-insurance trend among recent immigrants (Thamer and Rinehart 1998; Ellwood and Ku 1998; Huang 1997).

Medicaid Services

State agreement to participate in Medicaid and acceptance of matching federal funds mandates the provision of a basic set of benefits in state Medicaid programs. The Medicaid program offers a three-tier package of benefits. A basic benefit pack-

Table 9–3.   Medicaid Eligibility and Immigration Status

1. Qualified Aliens
    a. Veterans or persons on active military duty
    b. Refugees, asylees
    c. Lawful permanent residents with at least 40 quarters of participation in the Social Security program
    d. Canadian-born immigrants of at least 50 percent Native American heritage
    e. Immigrants residing in the United States prior to August 22, 1996 (state option)
2. Non-Qualified Aliens
    a. Temporary resident status
    b. Temporary protected status
    c. Humanitarian status
    d. Pending application for status
    e. Undocumented immigrants

Source: Families USA, 1999. *Immigrants and the Medicaid and CHIP Programs.*

age is established for states that only offer Medicaid benefits to categorically eligible populations. An additional benefit package is established for states that offer a medically needy program. Finally, states are able to include several optional benefits at their discretion. Table 9–4 lists the benefit packages offered in Medicaid.

Like other health insurance programs, Medicaid provides insurance coverage for inpatient and outpatient hospital care and physician services. Unlike most private health insurance plans, states are required to provide coverage for skilled nursing facilities for everyone over age 21 (categorical eligibility). Unlike Medicare, many state Medicaid programs provide a prescription drug benefit. Medically necessary physical therapy and occupational therapy are optional services in the Medicaid program. In reality, all states must cover necessary therapy services provided to children in the early and periodic screening, diagnosis, and treatment (EPSDT) program and to categorically eligible persons over age 21 who reside in skilled nursing facilities. These are federally mandated benefits. Some therapy services are commonly covered in the hospital benefit package but the type and intensity of the covered therapy varies. States may or may not pay for outpatient or home health physical therapy or occupational therapy services.

The high cost of institutionalization has encouraged the development of alternatives to expensive skilled nursing facility care. **Personal care services** are an optional Medicaid benefit that provides for payment of a nonrelative to assist with activities of daily living or, in some cases, instrumental activities of daily living in the patient's residence. This service can allow persons with disabilities to leave their homes and be employed or enjoy other community activities. The home- and community-based **waiver program** is a comprehensive state plan to provide a

Table 9–4.   Medicaid Benefits

A. Categorical Eligible Populations
   1. Inpatient and outpatient hospital services
   2. Physician services
   3. Medical/surgical dental services
   4. Nursing facility services for age 21 or over
   5. Home health care for persons eligible for nursing facility services
   6. Family planning
   7. Rural health clinic and federally qualified health center services
   8. Laboratory and X-ray services
   9. Pediatric and family nurse-practitioner services
   10. Nurse-midwife services
   11. Early and periodic screening, diagnosis, and treatment (EPSDT) services
       under age 21
B. Medically Needy Populations
   1. Prenatal care and delivery services for pregnant women
   2. Ambulatory care services for persons under age 18 and persons entitled to
      institutional services
   3. Home health services
   4. Certain services to persons with mental retardation
C. Optional Benefits
   1. Prescription drugs
   2. Rehabilitation therapies
   3. Prosthetics and orthotics
   4. Personal care services

Source: Health Care Financing Administration, 2000. *Medicaid Services.*

benefit package to persons with disabilities in community settings rather than skilled nursing facilities.

Like Medicare, Medicaid pays providers who agree to participate in the Medicaid program for the services they render to Medicaid beneficiaries. States are free to institute utilization-review procedures or other limits on the amount of services a beneficiary receives. In the 1990s, in response to escalating program costs, numerous states began the development of Medicaid-managed care plans. As of 1999, every state except Alaska and Wyoming had started to implement some form of Medicaid-managed care. A dozen states had 75 percent of Medicaid beneficiaries enrolled in a form of managed care (Kaiser Commission on Medicaid and the Uninsured 1999). CMS reported that 54 percent of all Medicaid beneficiaries were enrolled in managed care in 1998 (Health Care Financing Administration 1999).

Medicaid-managed care takes two forms: primary care case management and capitation (Regenstein and Anthony 1999). Primary care case management contracts with physicians who provide routine care and coordinate the referral and utilization of specialty care services. Capitation forms contract with managed care organizations to provide all the services needed by the beneficiary at a predetermined monthly rate.

The trend to Medicaid-managed care places the state in the position of purchaser of health care services vs. self-payer of health care services (Rosenbaum 1998). It also introduces market forces and beneficiary choice of health plan into the insurance purchasing decision. The results of this change are mixed. Rocha and Kabalka (1999) reported beneficiary confusion and impaired access to care in Tennessee's Medicaid program. Others have found little difference between Medicaid fee-for-service and managed care plans on access, quality, and satisfaction with program services (Coughlin and Long 2000; Phillips et al. 2000). A report by the Urban Institute found that Medicaid beneficiaries with disabilities are utilizing managed care (sometimes voluntarily), although the effect of managed care on the access and quality of Medicaid services for this population is unknown (Regenstein and Anthony 1999). The use of managed care principles in the Medicaid program is increasing the financial pressures on **safety-net providers** (Gray and Rowe 2000). Holahan et al., (1998) note that the program goals of restraining growth in costs, improving care, and supporting vital safety-net providers is difficult to balance when using private managed care organizations to coordinate care.

Medicaid is a vital part of the funding of the United States health care system. It provides access to health care insurance for many groups of Americans who would otherwise have impaired access to health care due to a lack of employment-based private insurance. Its existence supports safety-net providers who serve individuals in these communities. It provides a package of medical care benefits and certain social benefits that are not covered in traditional health care insurance plans (e.g., personal care services, long-term skilled nursing facility care). Access to occupational therapy and physical therapy services is mixed and inconsistent between states and sites of service delivery within states. Medicaid is also the best example of the utilization of managed care principles in a public health care insurance program.

State Children's Health Insurance Program (SCHIP)

An estimated 11 million children in the United States lack health care insurance (Kaiser Commission on Medicaid and the Uninsured 2000). Many of these children live in low-income families with two employed parents. The Childrens Defense Fund (1999) reports that uninsured children are at greater risk for preventable illness and will often perform at lower levels in the classroom because they are ill and lack access to adequate health care. About two in three of these uninsured children are eligible for public insurance (American Academy of Pediatrics 1999). In response to this situation, the federal government in 1997 authorized $20 billion for five years with the aim of increasing the number of children living below 200 percent of the federal poverty level who have health care insurance. This program is called the State Children's Health Insurance Program, or SCHIP.

SCHIP offers eligible children a health insurance benefit package that is similar to the health insurance package offered by their state to its employees or by the largest health maintenance organization in the state to its members. States and territories have responded to this new federal initiative by creating new insurance programs aimed at low-income children, expanding existing Medicaid programs, or using a combination of these approaches.

The National Governors Association (2000) reports that the states have increased the income limits for insurance eligibility, especially for teenage children who previously were excluded from many Medicaid programs (Newacheck et al. 1999). The Kaiser Commission on Medicaid and the Uninsured (2000) estimates that 2 million children have health care insurance through the SCHIP in addition to the 21 million children already insured by Medicaid. Despite these accomplishments, many children remain uninsured. A lack of marketing and the complicated enrollment processes for this program have been identified as barriers to enrollment. In response, states have implemented **presumptive eligibility** rules, marketed the program in schools, and streamlined the enrollment process (Health Care Financing Administration 1999).

Veterans Administration and Military Health Insurance Programs

The Veterans Administration (VA) operates the largest health care system in the world. In this section, we will explore the unique eligibility requirements and the benefit package offered to veterans who utilize this system. Veterans' health benefits date to the beginning of the country and the government's sense of responsibility to care for those who have served in the military. Occupational therapists and physical therapists are important members of the VA health care team. Therapists provide services to the thousands of veterans who have experienced disability as a result of military service.

Table 9–5 lists the eligibility categories that qualify an individual for veterans' health benefits. Veterans who meet the criteria for at least one of these categories are eligible for veterans benefits. Veterans with service-related or service-aggravated disabilities are given the highest enrollment priority. Impoverished veterans also receive priority enrollment in the VA system. Non-service-connected veterans are veterans who have not incurred or aggravated a disability while in military service. Non-service-connected veterans typically have to meet income/asset requirements or pay deductibles and co-payments to receive veteran's health benefits.

Eligible veterans are entitled to a comprehensive package of health care benefits. Table 9–6 lists the main components of this benefit package. Physical therapy and occupational therapy are mandated benefits in the VA health plan. In addition, prosthetics and orthotics are routinely covered. The inclusion of these benefits reflects the connection between disability and veterans' health benefits.

This benefit package is not free to all eligible veterans. The VA health plan has established co-payments for prescription drugs, inpatient and outpatient

Table 9–5.　Veterans Administration Health Program Eligibility

A. Priority Group 1
  1. Veterans with at least a 50 percent service-related disability
B. Priority Group 2
  1. Veterans with a 30 percent to 40 percent service-related disability
C. Priority Group 3
  1. Veterans who are former prisoners of war
  2. Veterans who were discharged for disability-related reasons
  3. Veterans with a 10 percent to 20 percent service-related disability
D. Priority Group 4
  1. Veterans who are receiving homebound benefits
  2. Veterans who are classified as "catastrophically disabled"
E. Priority Group 5
  1. Non-service-connected veterans and service-connected veterans rated 0 percent disabled who meet income/asset threshold guidelines
F. Priority Group 6
  1. Certain other veterans who are not required to make required co-payments
G. Priority Group 7
  1. Non-service-connected veterans who do not meet the criteria for the other groups and agree to pay the required co-payment for services

Source: Department of Veterans Affairs. Eligibility. Accessed at *www.va.gov/health/elig/eligibility.html* on July 17, 2000.

hospital services, and nursing home care. Veterans with service-related disabilities do not pay these costs. Non-service-connected veterans are required to meet income and asset thresholds or demonstrate financial hardship to avoid making the required co-payments. The private insurance companies of insured veterans who receive care in VA health care facilities are routinely billed for the services.

　　Active military personnel receive their health care through a system of military hospitals. Certain services or services for eligible dependents, however, are

Table 9–6.　Veterans Health Uniform Benefit Package

A. Inpatient and outpatient hospital care
B. Prescription drugs
C. Physician services
D. Mental health care
E. Home health and hospice
F. Rehabilitation therapies
G. Prosthetics and orthotics

Source: Department of Veterans Affairs. What Is the Uniform Benefits Package? Accessed at *www.va.gov/health/elig/benefits.html* on July 17, 2000.

provided in the civilian health care system. The government insurance plan for active military personnel and their families is called TRICARE. It is a new plan that replaces the Civilian Health and Medical Program of the Uniformed Services (CHAMPUS).

TRICARE consists of three insurance options for military personnel (Department of Defense 1999). TRICARE Prime uses military hospitals and clinics as the primary provider of care. It is provided at no cost to the member and with low co-payments. Access is limited to the military health care system. TRICARE Extra is a preferred provider organization that utilizes contracted civilian providers in the community. Members must use these providers and pay plan deductibles and co-payments. TRICARE Standard is the fee-for-service option. Members have open choice of providers who will accept TRICARE but are responsible for claims management, paying all deductibles and co-payments, and may be responsible for claims above the allowable charge (similar to a Medicare beneficiary utilizing a non-participating Medicare provider).

The introduction of a managed care product into the military health plan has been demonstrated to be effective. Kravitz et al. (1998) found that managed care reduces emergency department costs, especially among repeat users with non-severe illnesses. Zwanziger et al. (2000) concluded that a test of a CHAMPUS health maintenance organization product resulted in lower utilization of services, adequate patient access to services, good patient satisfaction, and little change in the cost to the government.

Conclusion

In this chapter, we have explored health insurance plans other than Medicare that are operated by the federal and state governments. Combined, these governmental plans fund nearly half of the United States health care system. Eligibility for these programs reflects a public consensus that government should provide health insurance for the poor, children, persons with disabilities, active military personnel, and veterans. Because these classifications include so many people of so many different backgrounds, the eligibility criteria, types of included benefits, and provider payment methods are some of the largest and most influential health policy decisions made by government. Recent innovations in these programs highlight the importance of managed care as a defining mechanism for contemporary payment of health care in America.

Although Medicaid is an important source of health care insurance for low-income people with disabilities, the provision of physical therapy and occupational therapy services is a state option. The lack of a consistent national Medicaid policy for the disabled means that many of these individuals lack access to rehabilitation services, especially in community-based environments. For military personnel and veterans, rehabilitation services are a mandated benefit. This provision reflects a belief that government has a responsibility to care for people who have served the society in certain capacities.

CHAPTER REVIEW QUESTIONS

1. Review the history and origins of the Medicaid program.
2. Describe the partnership arrangement between the federal government and states as it pertains to Medicaid.
3. Define the eligibility criteria in order to receive Medicaid benefits.
    a. categorical eligibility
    b. medically needy
    c. Medicare-Medicaid dual-eligible
4. What is included in the Medicaid benefits package?
    a. Define the position of occupational therapy and physical therapy in the Medicaid program.
5. Describe how managed care is utilized in state Medicaid programs.
6. Recall how welfare reform and immigration reform affected the Medicaid program in the 1990s.
7. Define the purpose of the State Children's Health Insurance Program (SCHIP), and describe its effectiveness in achieving this purpose.
8. Identify the eligibility criteria and benefits package for Veterans Affairs health insurance benefits
9. What is TRICARE and how is it organized?

CHAPTER DISCUSSION QUESTIONS

1. Physical therapy and occupational therapy are included as benefits in the Medicaid and Department of Veterans Affairs health insurance programs. Both of these insurance plans serve persons with disabilities. Compare and contrast the benefit packages. What are the reasons for these differences? Do you agree with them?
2. The eligibility criteria for the Medicaid program is a good example of the policy "balancing act" between egalitarian and libertarian views of the role of government in health care. Examine closely the traditional criteria and the recent immigration criteria. Analyze and discuss these criteria from both the egalitarian and libertarian points of view.
3. Managed care is increasingly being used in public insurance programs. Managed care has been more easily implemented in the Medicaid, SCHIP, and TRICARE programs than in Medicare. What are the reasons for this situation? How does this reflect our political and social realities?

REFERENCES

American Academy of Pediatrics. 1999. *Program Eligibility of Uninsured Children under Age 19, 1999 Projections*. Elk Grove Village IL: American Academy of Pediatrics.

Chavkin, W., D. Romero, and P. H. Wise. 2000. State welfare reform policies and declines in health insurance. *Am J Pub Health* 90(6): 900–908.

Children's Defense Fund. 1997. What are the basic facts about uninsured children? Accessed at *www.childrensdefense.org/health _14things2.html* on July 14, 2000.

Coughlin, T. A. and S. K. Long. 2000. Effects of Medicaid managed care on adults. *Med Care* 38(4): 433–46.

Department of Defense. What is TRICARE? Accessed at *www.tricare.osd.mil/tricare/ beneficiary/whatistricare.html* on July 17, 2000.

Department of Health and Human Services. 2000. Federal Financial Participation in State Assistance Expenditures for October 1, 2000 through September 30, 2001. *Federal Register* 65(36): 8979–80. Accessed at *aspe.os.dhhs.gov/health/fmap01.htm* on July 14, 2000.

Ellwood, M. R. and L. Ku. 1998. Welfare and immigration reforms: Unintended effects for Medicaid. *Health Affairs* 17(3): 137–51.

Families USA. 1999. Welfare-Medicaid Links. Accessed at *www.familiesusa.org/whatwelf .htm* on July 14, 2000.

———. 2000. Go directly to work, do not collect health insurance: Low-Income parents lose Medicaid. Accessed at *www.familiesusa.org/pubs/gowrk* on July 14, 2000.

Garrett, B. and J. Holahan. 2000. Health insurance coverage after welfare. *Health Affairs* 19(1): 175–84.

Gray, B. H. and C. Rowe. 2000. Safety-net health plans: A status report. *Health Affairs* 19(1): 185–93.

Health Care Financing Administration. 1998. National summary of Medicaid managed care programs and enrollment. June 30, 1998. Accessed at *www.hcfa.gov/medicaid/ trends98.htm* on July 14, 2000.

———. The Medicaid Program. 2000. Accessed at *www.hcfa.gov/medicaid/mcdsta95.htm* on July 14, 2000.

———. 2000. Medicaid recipients, and vendor payments by maintenance assistance status. Accessed at *www.hcfa.gov/medicaid/2082-2.htm* on July 14, 2000

———. 2000. Medicaid eligibility. Accessed at *www.hcfa.gov/medicaid/meligib.htm* on July 14, 2000.

———. 2000. Medicaid Services. Accessed at *www.hcfa.gov/medicaid/mservice.html* on July 14, 2000.

———. 2000. List and definition of dual eligibles. Accessed at *www.hcfa.gov/ medicaid/bbadedef.htm* on July 14, 2000.

———. 2000. The State Childrens Health Insurance Program: Preliminary highlights of implementation and expansion. Accessed at *www.hcfa.gov/init/who700.pdf* on July 14, 2000.

Holahan, J., S. Zuckerman, A. Evans, and S. Rangarajan. 1998. Medicaid managed care in thirteen states. *Health Affairs* 17(3): 43–63.

Huang, F. Y. 1997. Health insurance coverage of the children of immigrants in the United States. *Matern. Child Health J* 1(2): 69–80.

Kaiser Commission on Medicaid and the Uninsured. 1999. Health coverage for low-income children. Accessed at *www.kff.org/content/ 1999/2144/pub2144.pdf* on July 14, 2000.

———. 1999. Medicaid Facts: The Medicaid program at a glance. Accessed at *www.kff.org/content/archive/2004/pub2004.pdf* on July 12, 2000.

———. 1999. Medicaid: A primer. Accessed at *www.kff.org/content/1999/2161/pub2161 .pdf* on July 12, 2000.

———. 1999. Medicaid and managed care. Accessed at *www.kff.org/content/archive/ 2068/medicaidmanagedcare.pdf* on July 12, 2000.

———. 2000. Enrolling uninsured children in Medicaid and CHIP. Accessed at *www.kff.org/content/2000/2177/pub 2177.pdf* on July 14, 2000.

Kravitz, R. L., J. Zwanziger, S. Hosek, S. Polich, E. Sloss, and D. McCaffrey. 1998. Effect of a large managed care program on emergency department use: Results from the CHAMPUS reform initiative evaluation. *Ann Emerg Med* 31(6): 741–48.

Lamphere, J. A. and M. L. Rosenbach. 2000. Promises unfulfilled: Implementation of expanded coverage for the elderly poor. *Health Serv Res* 35(1 pt. 2): 207–17.

Levit, K., C. Cowan, H. Lazenby, A. Sensenig, P. McDonald, J. Stiller, and A. Martin. 2000. Health spending in 1998: Signals of change. *Health Affairs* 19(1): 124–32.

National Governors Association. 1999. States have expanded eligibility through Medicaid and the State Children's Health Insurance Program. Accessed at *www.nga .org/Pubs/IssueBriefs/1999/990210MCHUpdate.asp* on July 14, 2000.

Nebraska Health and Human Services System. 1999. Aged and disabled Medicaid. Accessed at *www.hhs.state.ne.us/ags/agsmed.htm* on August 3, 2000.

Newacheck, P. W., C. D. Brindis, C. U. Cart, K. Marchi, and C. E. Irwin. 1999. Adolescent health insurance coverage: Recent changes and access to care. *Pediatrics* 104 (2 pt. 1): 195–202.

Newacheck, P. W., M. Pearl, D. C. Hughes, and N. Halfon. 1998. The role of Medicaid in ensuring children's access to care. *JAMA* 280(20): 1789–93.

Phillips K. A., S. Fernyak, A. L. Potosky, H. H. Schauffler, and M. Egorin. 2000. Use of preventive services by managed care enrollees: An updated perspective. *Health Affairs* 19(1): 102–16.

Regenstein, M., and S. E. Anthony. 1998. Assessing the new federalism: Medicaid managed care for persons with disabilities. Accessed at *www.newfederalism.urban.org/ pdf/occal1.pdf* on July 14, 2000.

Rocha, C. J. and L. E. Kabalka. 1999. A comparison study of access to health care under a Medicaid managed care program. *Health Soc Work* 24(3): 169–79.

Rosenbaum, S. 1998. Negotiating the new health system: Purchasing publicly accountable managed care. *Am J Prev Med* 14(3 suppl): 67–71.

Short, P. F. and V. A. Freedman. 1998. Single women and the dynamics of Medicaid. *Health Serv Res* 33(5 pt. 1): 1309–36.

Thamer, M. and C. Rinehart. 1998. Public and private health insurance of US foreign-born residents: Implications of the 1996 welfare reform law. *Ethn Health* 3(1–2): 19–29.

Weissman, J. S., R. Witzburg, P. Linv, and E. G. Campbell. 1999. Termination from Medicaid: How does it affect access, continuity of care, and willingness to purchase insurance? *J Health Care Poor Under* 10(1): 122–37.

Zwanziger, J., R. L. Kravitz, S. D. Hosek, K. Hart, E. M. Sloss, D. Sullivan, J. D. Kallich, and D. P. Goldman. 2000. Providing managed care options for a large population: Evaluating the CHAMPUS reform initiative. *Mil Med* 165(5): 403–10.

10

The Acute Medical Care System

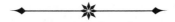

CHAPTER OBJECTIVES

At the conclusion of this chapter, the reader will be able to:

1. Explain the historical development of the hospital.
2. Describe the administrative structure of hospitals.
3. Define a hospital by size, ownership, and scope of services.
4. Compare and contrast primary, secondary, tertiary, and quaternary care.
5. Describe the development of integrated health care systems.
6. Discuss the development and results of physician-hospital integration in the acute medical care delivery system.

KEY WORDS: Hospitals, Integrated Health Care System, Matrix System, Patient-Focused Care, Physician-Hospital Organization, Primary Care, Product-Line Team, Quaternary Care, Secondary Care, Tertiary Care

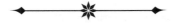

Introduction

In the preceding chapters, we have introduced and focused on health care policy. In Part I of the book, we discussed the principles that guide policymaking and examined policy that specifically addresses disability. In Part II, we discussed reimbursement policy, a powerful force that shapes health care. Many systems, including the health care system, not only proceed from policy decisions made by the public and private sectors, but influence policy decisions as well. In Part III, which begins with this chapter, we will discuss the health care system. Other chapters in this part discuss the post-acute care system (Chapter 11), the various professions that comprise the human workforce in health care (Chapter 12), the mental health system (Chapter 13), and public health (Chapter 14). We begin in this chapter with a discussion of the acute medical care system.

When we think of the U.S. health care system, we commonly break it down into two broad categories—an acute medical delivery system and a post-acute care delivery system (see Figure 10–1). The acute medical delivery system includes primary, secondary, and tertiary care systems. The post-acute care system consists of a mix of sub-acute care, long-term care, outpatient services, home health care, and hospice. This chapter focuses mainly on the acute medical care delivery system and in particular on one of the biggest players in this system, the hospital.

Hospitals are arguably one of the most recognized and least understood entities of the health care system. Hospitals are home to many activities related to health care, including patient care, medical education, and research functions. Additionally, hospitals are usually one of the major employers in a community. In this chapter, we examine hospitals and the acute care medical system more closely and explain their role in the health care system. We discuss the historical development of hospitals, their diverse functions and characteristics, their management structures, and their position within the primary, secondary, tertiary, and quaternary health care system. We will conclude with a discussion of the various forces that both constrain and promote change in the hospital industry. An understanding of the hospital's role in the health care system and the external forces that influence them is critical to therapists because it represents, in large part, the health care environment in which they must interact.

Hospitals

Historical Development

The hospitals that existed in early America were very different from the hospitals that we have today. The first hospitals were primarily charitable religious organizations whose missions were focused more on providing care to those they served than on curing their illnesses (Freymann 1974; Starr 1982). Early hospitals tended to care for and shelter the poor, elderly, orphaned, and homeless, in addition to protecting society from those who were contagious or dangerously insane (Sultz and Young 1999). It may be more accurate to describe early hospitals as nothing more than infirmaries for the sick and the poor. The focus was on caring for individuals and not necessarily curing them. Hospitals were commonly characterized as dirty and overcrowded en-

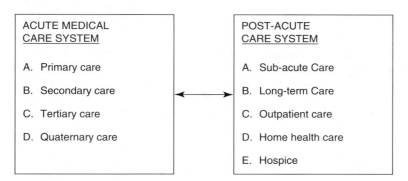

Figure 10–1.   **The United States Health Care System**

vironments with limited medical capabilities. While the early hospitals only served the poor, people with sufficient financial resources received care at home.

From the late 1800s to the early 1900s hospitals began to evolve into the physician's workshop. Advances in biomedical science and technology made it more difficult and complex for physicians to have everything they needed in their "black bags" (Kovner 1995). While earlier hospitals had provided more care than cure, hospitals during this period were better able to provide a cure and a means of intervention. Because of improvements in science & technology, the hospital industry experienced a large growth in the number of hospitals, and by 1909 there were more than 4,300 hospitals, compared to just 178 in 1873 (Stevens 1971).

A second major era of growth took place between 1945 and 1980. Two major events contributed to this growth: (1) federal monies became available to build new hospitals under the Hill-Burton Act, and (2) the rapid growth of hospital insurance, including Medicare and Medicaid, increased the diversity and number of services offered to a hospital's inpatients (Kovner 1995). Without clear and consistent oversight, however, these policies resulted in creating a hospital environment characterized by overbuilding and overcapacity, which resulted in a call for hospitals to become more accountable and efficient. During this era, the number of hospitals grew to more than 6,000.

In part, because of this overbuilding and overcapacity, hospitals in the 1990s experienced consolidation through the formation of networks and through closure. One of the several reasons for these changes included the cost of building and maintaining a hospital, especially in a period of cost control. In some cases, hospitals have closed because of a declining demand for their services. Mergers or consolidations were pursued to establish integrated delivery systems. **Integrated health care systems** are discussed in more detail later in this chapter.

In the next sections, we briefly examine the managerial structure of hospitals and their unique characteristics that help to describe these organizations.

Hospital Structure

Hospitals have a complex administrative structure that is reflective of the growth of hospitals into an established organizational institution. Since physicians have the ability to control the type and amount of services patients consume, physicians have always had, and still do, an important role in the organization and management of hospitals. For years, physicians or leaders of religious organizations managed hospitals. However, the complexity of hospital management has led to the creation of the field of health services management. A traditional hospital structure includes a board of directors, an administrative structure, and a medical staff structure (see Figure 10–2). Physical therapy and occupational therapy services may be positioned under the health services administrator or the medical director.

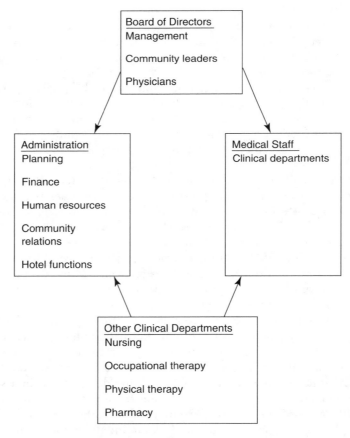

Figure 10–2.   Traditional Structure of Hospitals

A board of directors is selected that retains fiduciary responsibility to manage and govern the hospital. This includes the hiring of a management team. Physicians are commonly represented on the hospital's board of directors. Historically, hospital administrators were primarily responsible for nonclinical matters, such as finance, personnel, community/public relations, and the hospital's "hotel" functions (laundry, housekeeping, etc). However, in today's environment, strategic planning and negotiating ability are critical skills for the successful health care executive.

A hospital structure will also include a medical division, usually headed by a physician known as the chief of the medical staff, who is the liaison to the hospital administration and commonly serves on the board of directors. A medical division is commonly divided into departments by medical specialty (e.g., internal medicine, surgery). The medical division has important oversight over credentialing of health care professionals (i.e., determining their right to admit patients, perform surgery, etc.) and provides consultation about the quality of care in the hospital.

Other clinical professions are represented in various ways. Organizationally, these professions may be placed under the hospital administration component of the structure or under the medical division. The largest unit is usually the nursing division, which is traditionally organized into subunits by types of patient treatment/pathology (e.g., orthopedics, pediatrics). Physical therapy, occupational therapy, and the other rehabilitation disciplines are traditionally organized by discipline.

The development of **patient-focused care** has resulted in a radical reorganization of this system. Patient-focused care organizes providers around perceived patient needs rather than professional disciplines or procedures. This avoids certain problems typical of traditional structures, such as poor communication and redundancy of services. Therapists may be organized into **product-line teams** organized around common patient types (e.g., stroke teams, joint-replacement teams). In this case, occupational therapists and physical therapists may be responsible to a team leader for their activities and performance. In some cases a dual-management structure called a **matrix system** is established whereby a physical therapist may be responsible to a team leader for clinical matters and to a physical therapy manager for nonclinical matters (e.g., personnel issues) (Boissoneau 1983) (see Figure 10–3).

Hospital Characteristics

Hospitals differ along various dimensions, including size and scope, ownership, general vs. specialty hospitals, acute care vs. long-term care hospitals, teaching vs. non-teaching hospitals, and independent hospitals vs. those in multihospital systems or networks. This section explores these issues in greater detail.

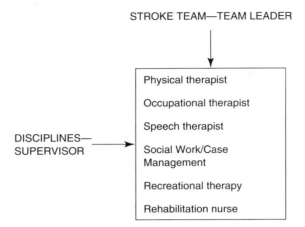

Figure 10–3. "Matrix" Hospital Organizational Structures

Size

The number of inpatient beds that are set up and staffed is one indicator of the size of a hospital. Figure 10–4 shows the distribution of hospitals by bed size. Most hospitals are under 200 beds, but a majority of patients are admitted to the larger

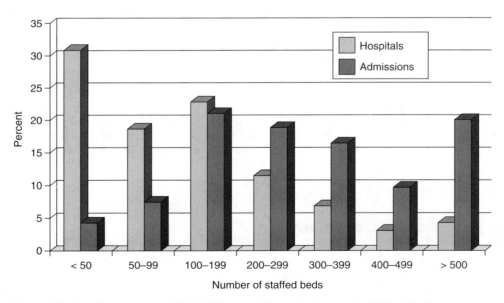

Figure 10–4. Percentage of U.S. Hospitals by Admissions and Bed Size
Source: American Hospital Association, 1998.

hospitals. This is probably due to the greater array of services available in larger hospitals. It is interesting to note the steep increase in admission rates for the largest hospitals. These hospitals most likely represent large tertiary-care centers that care not only for a general population but for a large indigent population and persons in need of advanced specialty services (e.g., trauma care).

Ownership

Hospital organizations generally have one of three types of ownership classification:

1. Hospitals operated by nonprofit organizations are referred to as not-for-profit hospitals.
2. Hospitals owned and operated by profit-making corporations are known as investor-owned or for-profit hospitals.
3. Hospitals owned and managed by either federal, state, or local government bodies are referred to as public hospitals.

Two-thirds of all hospitals are voluntary, not-for-profit organizations that are managed by community boards or religious organizations. For example, religious orders within the Roman Catholic Church operate some of the largest systems of medical care facilities in the United States. These hospitals are more commonly associated with local decision-making and the provision of charity care. In return for their provision of charity care, the federal government has historically granted an exemption from state and federal taxation.

Investor-owned or for-profit hospitals are dominated by national chains (e.g., Tenet Healthcare). Since the 1980s, private investment in hospitals and the development of hospital chains has grown significantly. The net revenue from for-profit hospitals is shared with outside investors who are co-owners of the hospital. Investor participation in the hospital industry increases the amount of private capital available for medical care investment. It also has increased the emphasis on financial management of all hospitals. For-profit companies own approximately 15 percent of the hospitals in the United States.

One of the main distinguishing aspects between for-profit and not-for-profit facilities pertains to how net revenue is used. Whatever its profit status, every hospital must generate some type of profit—the difference is how that profit is used. In a not-for-profit facility, profits are returned to the organization or community, whereas a for-profit organization distributes the profits to its shareholders.

The last type of ownership structure discussed here is the public hospital. The public hospital was the primary source of health care for the poor and indigent before the advent of Medicaid in 1965. Examples of public and government controlled hospitals include city and county hospitals (e.g., Cook County Hospital in Chicago), military hospitals, VA hospitals, and U.S. Public Health Service hospitals (e.g., Indian Health Service hospitals). Public hospitals provide an important safety net for the poor and for populations where private organizations have chosen not to provide services.

In addition to these three distinct categories, a number of hybrid ownership structures exist. Some hospitals have multiple owners. For example, when a not-for-profit hospital is sold to a for-profit company, the not-for-profit organization may retain some ownership short of a majority. Additionally, some local government hospitals may be leased and managed by a for-profit organization while the government retains ownership of the hospital.

General vs. Specialty

A general hospital provides general medical services, such as ambulatory surgery, pediatric inpatient care, rehabilitation outpatient care, emergency services, open heart surgery, angioplasty, obstetric services, and community health promotion. Alternatively, specialty hospitals provide services for either specific diseases or specifically defined populations. Examples of specialty hospitals include children's hospitals, long-term care centers, rehabilitation hospitals, mental health or psychiatric hospitals, and substance abuse centers.

Acute Care vs. Long-Term Care

Many general hospitals are acute care facilities as well. Acute care hospitals serve inpatients who have an average length of stay of no more than 30 days. Most of the patients admitted to these hospitals actually stay for less than 10 days. Patients in these hospitals have acute short-term illnesses, as compared to patients with chronic illness that may require prolonged treatment.

Long-term-care hospitals include such facilities as nursing homes, psychiatric hospitals, and rehabilitation hospitals as well as home health agencies. Long-term care provides care for those experiencing diminishing functional capabilities. The level of functioning may vary across age categories and chronic conditions. Care provided to these individuals may be continuous or intermittent, but will be carried on over a long time or throughout the patient's life (Kane and Kane 1987).

Teaching Hospitals

Teaching hospitals are an important part of America's health care system. In addition to their sophisticated technology and cutting-edge research, they deliver a large percentage of health care services throughout the country (Iglehart 1993). They also deliver a disproportionate share of charity and indigent care. Although only a small percentage of all short-term nonfederal acute care hospitals are classified as members of the Council of Teaching Hospitals and Health Systems (COTH), they represent approximately one-fourth of all the beds and admissions across the country (Luke and Bramble 1996; Moy et al. 1996).

The Council of Teaching Hospitals, part of the Association for Academic Medical Centers (AAMC), specifies (1) that member hospitals must sponsor four approved medical residency programs, and (2) that at least two of the four programs must be either medicine, surgery, pediatrics, family practice, OBGYN, or psychiatry. Teaching hospitals have the additional responsibility of educating our nation's physician base and conduct medical research as well as provide quality patient care. Though other hospitals may participate in training physicians through various residency programs, they have not demonstrated the commitment outlined in the COTH definition.

Multihospital Systems and Networks

According to the American Hospital Association, multihospital systems (MHS) are defined as two or more hospitals that are owned, leased, or contract-managed by the same organization (AHA 1998). These systems can be either for-profit or not-for-profit and may be limited to the local area or part of a national company. The AHA defines alliances as formal organizations that work for the benefits of their members to provide services and products as well as the promotion of activities and ventures. Though many hospitals participate in one or both of these activities, some hospitals remain independent and unaffiliated in any way.

Levels of Care

Hospitals are capable of providing various levels of care. Some hospitals are known as tertiary facilities, while others are primary or secondary care hospitals. In this section, we focus on the three most common levels of care: primary, secondary, and tertiary. The main features of these levels of care are summarized in Table 10–1.

Primary Care

The first level of care in the U.S. health care system is known as **primary care** and represents the main entry point by which most people come into contact with the

Table 10–1. Characteristics of Primary, Secondary, Tertiary, and Quaternary Care

A. Primary care	Treats common, nonchronic, episodic disorders
	Provides care in context of family and community
	Coordinator of care in managed care systems
B. Secondary care	Treats common, chronic-type disorders
	Long-term care required (e.g., diabetes, hypertension management)
C. Tertiary care	Treats complex, acute, and chronic disorders
	Utilizes specialized diagnostic and treatment procedures
C. Quaternary Care	Treats uncommon acute and chronic disorders
	Associated with academic medical centers
	For example, organ transplantation

health care delivery system. It deals with illnesses that are general, episodic, common, and nonchronic in nature. In 1995, the Institute of Medicine offered a revised definition of primary care: "Primary care is the provision of integrated, accessible health care services by clinicians who are accountable for addressing a large majority of personal health care needs, developing a sustained partnership with patients, and practicing in the context of family and community." Note that the central point in this definition is the concepts of access, accountability, and integrated services, all of which are discussed throughout this text.

Primary care provides most of the health care that people usually need. A new purpose of primary care in the age of managed care is to integrate the delivery of health care services. Primary physician care is defined as family medicine, internal medicine, pediatrics, and obstetrics/gynecology.

Secondary Care

Secondary care, like primary care, may be provided in an ambulatory setting or on an inpatient basis. A higher level of care that is more intense than primary care, it often extends over a longer period. Unlike primary care, where illnesses are acute common injuries or illnesses, secondary care focuses on injuries or illnesses that are chronic and require continuing care. Examples of conditions that require secondary care include arthritis, diabetes, and hypertension.

Tertiary and Quartenary Care

The last level of care discussed here is referred to as **Tertiary care.** This is highly specialized, complex, and costly, and delivery takes place in an inpatient setting. Teaching hospitals or academic medical centers were once the main setting for tertiary care services. However, because of the advances being made and the fierce competition among health care providers, many community hospitals can now offer these services. Examples of tertiary care include such procedures as coronary artery bypass grafting and specialized diagnostic devices (Blumenthal et al. 1997). With the continual advances being made, an even higher level of care known as **quartenary care** is available, and is predominantly provided at academic medical centers. Quartenary care services include burn units, trauma centers, transplant services, and so forth.

Hospital Integration

Over the past decade an increase in public awareness of the problems of the uninsured and the costs of health care services coupled with the threat of government reform have set in motion a number of consolidation activities and other market responses from hospital organizations and other health care providers. These responses include outright mergers, vertical integration, and the formation of hospital alliances between various health care organizations (e.g., physician-hospital alliances).

The hospital industry has undergone significant restructuring over the past several decades, beginning with multihospital system growth in the 1970s and 1980s (Ermann and Gabel 1986; Shortell 1988; Alexander and Morrisey 1988) and shifting to local market consolidation in the 1990s (Luke 1991). The formation of local hospital collectives helped hospitals defend themselves against increasingly powerful competitors and improve their market positions relative to such rivals as managed care organizations, consolidating physician populations, active business coalitions, large businesses, and government agencies (Zelman 1996).

Recent efforts to reform the delivery of health care have emphasized the importance of providing cost-effective, comprehensive patient care. One mechanism that has the capability of providing this comprehensive care is the integrated delivery system (American Hospital Association 1992). Integrated delivery systems often consist of a variety of delivery components and payment mechanisms. Many players are involved in the creation of integrated delivery systems, including managed care organizations, which have been a major driving force behind hospital and physician integration (Shortell and Hull 1996; Advisory Board 1993; APM/University Hospital Consortium 1995). Thus, health care providers nationwide are finding themselves in increasingly complex systems that include such organizational structures as integrated delivery systems and strategic alliances (Luke, Olden, and Bramble 1998; Bazzoli et al. 1999; Burns et al. 1997). Many argue that the benefits of joining together in this way include the achievement of greater efficiency.

There are a wide variety of integrated delivery system models. Integrated delivery systems are commonly formed through a process of horizontal or vertical integration (see Figure 10–5). Many of these represent partial integration in organizations in the midst of transition. Horizontal integration occurs when two or more firms producing similar services join to become a single organization (or a strong interorganizational alliance). Hospitals merging or forming strategic hospital alliances (Luke, Olden, and Bramble 1998) and the consolidation of smaller solo practices into larger multi-specialty groups practices (see Kralewski et al. 1999) are examples of horizontal integration.

In the early 1990s, the American Hospital Association advocated the formation of local "integrated delivery systems" (American Hospital Association 1990). These integrated systems were intended to improve the efficiency of care, increasing system accountability for both community needs and health outcomes (American Hospital Association 1992). Although some hospitals have begun to move toward a system that integrates a variety of providers, the most common activity is the horizontal combination of hospitals into local systems of networks within local markets.

There are many reasons why organizations come together to form strategic partnerships. In health care, unique and specific reasons precipitate their formation (Luke, Olden, and Bramble 1998). Foremost is the threat of managed care in the market. As hospitals combine to form local hospital systems and networks, they collectively increase their geographic presence. By thus offering greater spatial cov-

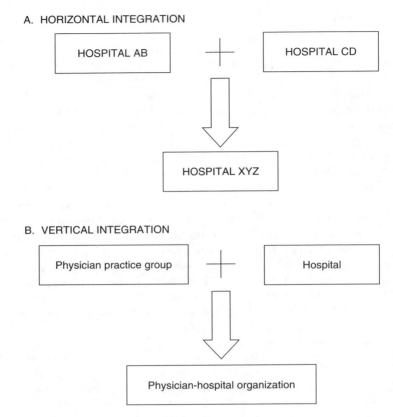

Figure 10–5.   Integrated Delivery Systems

erage, they increase their leverage in negotiations for managed care contracts. Joining together at the local level also allows organizations to develop health care products that enhance their positions in the markets.

In addition to forming horizontal relationships, hospitals are also joining vertically with physician organizations. Physician-hospital relationships are sometimes called **physician-hospital organizations** (PHOs) and represent a vertical integration strategy.

Vertical integration refers to the combination of two or more firms that were previously separate and whose products or services are inputs (or outputs) from the production of another service into a single firm. One possible advantage of these types of integration is transaction cost savings (see D'Aunno and Zuckerman 1987). Combinations of clinical group practices and acute care facilities are examples of vertical integration and represent an essential feature of fully integrated delivery systems. These vertical combinations (i.e., physicians and hospitals) provide a mechanism that aligns incentives among the players and makes it possible to unify marketing efforts directed at managed care organizations (Burns and Thorpe 1995; Morrisey et al. 1999).

Physician-Hospital Relationships

Physician-hospital relationships are defined as the structural mechanism that facilitates the integration of physicians into the management and governance of the hospital as well as the integration of management into the activities of the clinical-medical staff (Alexander, Morrisey, and Shortell 1986). The purpose of these relationships is to link patient entry points to the health care delivery system, forming a continuum of services for the patient (Harris, Hicks, and Kelly 1992). Over the last five years physician-hospital organizations have been cited with increased frequency. In the changing health care environment, physician groups are forging closer ties with hospitals as a means of lowering expenses and taking advantage of managed care contracting opportunities (Gorey 1993).

Having recognized the use of primary care physicians as gatekeepers to manage the entrance of patients into the system (Burns and Thorpe 1993), hospitals are trying to establish linkages with physician groups to ensure a constant flow of patients. Linking up with physician groups increases their leverage over managed care firms by allowing them to pool their contracting activities with other providers to achieve economies and efficiencies of scale (Burns and Thorpe 1993). Hospitals are facing growing competitive threats to their market share and profitability. Large multispecialty group practices are one source of competition. In the face of this threat, hospitals have sought to gain control over the ambulatory care of physicians in the market, thus preempting possible competitive initiatives from physicians.

Physician-system integration and clinical integration include developing mechanisms for joint hospital-physician planning and patient care services. Many new organizations attempt to integrate physicians vertically with acute care facilities, using various mechanisms to achieve this goal. Hospital-physician organizations can be arranged in a variety of ways, and with different types of governance structures in which one or another of the founding entities takes a leadership role. The simplest categorization of these organizations is the four-level model developed by Shortell and his colleagues. The integrated delivery system may be either hospital/health system led, physician/group practice led, insurance company led, or a hybrid model where the hospital organization and the physician groups are co-dominant (Shortell et al. 1994).

A variety of models have been developed for the integration of hospitals and physicians. These include the group practice without walls model (GPWW), the independent practice association (IPA), the management services organization (MSO), the physician-hospital organization (PHO), the salary staff models, the foundation model, and the physician equity model (Conners 1997). While newer terms for these organizations have been introduced, such as joint-operating agreements, franchise agreements, master affiliation agreements, gain-sharing models, and regional service organizations (Alexander et al. 1999), many of the goals and purposes of these organizations remain the same. These goals and purposes include increased leverage in negotiating managed care contracts, capital and information systems sharing, quality improvement and efficiency, creating a broad continuum of care, sharing administrative expenses, and increasing physician involvement in the process of managed care contracting (Coile and Grant 1997; Fine 1997; Burns and Thorpe 1993; Dowling 1995; Shortell et al. 1996).

Conclusion

The twentieth century saw the development of the hospital as the cornerstone of the acute medical care delivery system. Advances in biomedical science and policy decisions to fund hospital services were important catalysts in the development of the hospital. The provision of tertiary and quarternary care was the pinnacle of these twentieth century trends. However, the increasing utilization of hospital services and the high costs associated with hospital growth have factored into the move toward community-based primary care to prevent illness and injury. As a result, the acute medical care delivery system has seen the development of integrated health systems in many markets as providers align with one another both vertically and horizontally to provide services in a more cost-effective manner.

CHAPTER REVIEW QUESTIONS

1. Describe the development of the U.S. hospital in three periods:
   a. pre–1900
   b. 1900–1945
   c. 1945–present
2. How are hospitals administratively organized?
3. Define patient-focused care, product-line teams, and matrix management in a hospital.
4. Identify common characteristic descriptors of a hospital.
5. Define primary care, secondary care, tertiary care, and quarternary care.
6. Describe the incentives for and process of development of integrated health systems in the United States.
7. Summarize the relationship of physicians and hospitals over the last century.

CHAPTER DISCUSSION QUESTIONS

1. Discuss how the administrative structure of hospitals enhances and limits the professional autonomy of occupational therapists and physical therapists. What are the historical reasons for this situation?
2. Clinical occupational therapists and physical therapists working on product-line teams may report directly to a nontherapist supervisor on a regular basis.

Discuss the pros and cons of this form of hospital organization for the role of physical therapists and occupational therapists in a hospital.

3. Integrated health delivery systems that coordinate and, in some cases, consolidate primary, secondary, and tertiary care in a community are a contemporary form of acute medical care delivery. What effect could you expect to observe on small, private-practice providers (e.g., physicians, therapists) in communities with large integrated health delivery systems? Discuss some strategies that would be necessary to compete with such systems.

REFERENCES

Advisory Board. 1993. *The Grand Alliance: Vertical Integration Strategies for Physicians and Health Systems.* Washington DC: Advisory Board.

Alexander, J. A., G. J. Bazzoli, L. R. Burns, and S. M. Shortell. 1999. Measures of physician system integration. Paper presented at the annual meeting of the Association for Health Service Research, Chicago.

Alexander, J. A., M. A. Morrisey, and S. M. Shortell. 1986. Effects of competition, regulation, and corporatization on hospital-physician relationships. *J Health and Soc Behav* 27: 220–35.

American Hospital Association. 1990. *Renewing the U. S. Health Care System.* Washington DC: Section for Health Care Systems, Office of Constituency Sections.

———.1992. *Overview: AHA's National Reform Strategy.* Chicago: American Hospital Association.

———.1998. *AHA Guide, 1999–2000 Edition.* Chicago: American Hospital Association.

APM, Inc. and University Hospital Consortium. 1995. *How Markets Evolve: Hospitals and Health Markets.*

Bazzoli, G. J., S. M. Shortell, N. Dubbs, C. Chan, and P. Kralovec. 1999. A taxonomy of health networks and systems: Bringing order out of chaos. *Health Serv Res* 33(6): 1683–1717.

Boissoneau R. 1983. Matrix management in the health care organization. *Health Care Sup.* 2(1): 22–36.

Burns, L. R., and D. P. Thorpe. 1993. Trends and models in physician-hospital organization. *Health Care Management Rev* 18(4): 7–20.

———.1995. Managed care and integrated health care. *Health care management* 2(1): 101–108

Burns, L. R. G. J. Bazzoli, L. Dynan, and D. R. Wholey. 1997. Managed care, market stages, and integrated delivery systems: Is there a relationship? *Health Affairs* 16: 204–18.

Coile, R. C. and P. N. Grant. 1997. Group practice affiliation structures. In *Integrating the practice of medicine,* ed. R. B. Conners, Chicago: American Hospital Publishing.

Conners, R. B., ed. 1997. *Integrating the Practice of Medicine.* Chicago: American Hospital Publishing.

D'Aunno, T. A. and H. S. Zuckerman, 1987. The emergence of hospital federations: An integration of perspectives from organizational theory. *Med Care Rev* 44(2): 323–43.

Dowling, W. L. 1995. Strategic alliances as a structure for integrated delivery systems. In *Partners for the dance: Forming strategic alliances in health care,* ed. A. D. Kaluzny, H. S. Zuckerman, and T. C. Ricketts, 139–76. Ann Arbor: Health Administration Press.

Fine, A. 1997. Integrated delivery systems. In *Integrating the practice of medicine,* ed. R. B. Conners, 273–87. Chicago: American Hospital Publishing.

Freymann, J. G. 1974. *The American Heatlth Care System: Its Genesis and Trajectory.* New York: Medcom Press.

Gorey, T. M. 1993. Physician organizations and physician-hospital organizations. *Michi Med* 92(9): 34–38.

Harris, C., L. L. Hick, and B. J. Kelly. 1992. Physician hospital networking: Avoiding a shotgun wedding. *Health Care Management Rev* 17(4):17–28.

Iglehart, J. K. 1993. The American health care system: Teaching hospitals. *N Engl J Med* 329(14): 1052–56.

Institute of Medicine. 1995. *Primary Care: America's Health in a New Era.* Washington DC: National Academy Press.

Kane, R. A. and R. L. Kane. 1987. *Long-Term Care: Principles, Programs and Policies.* New York: Springer Publishing Co.

Kovner, A. R. 1995. Hospitals. In *Health care delivery in the United States,* ed. A. R. Kovner, 162–83. New York: Springer Publishing.

Kralewski, J. E., E. C. Rich, R. Feldman, B. Dowd, T. Bernhardt, C. Johnson, and W. Gold. 2000. The effects of medical group practice and physician payment methods on costs of care. *Health Serv Res,* 35(3): 591–613

Luke, R. D. and J. D. Bramble. 1996. COTH hospitals: Building systems in highly consolidating markets. *COTH Reports* 30(2): 1–4.

Luke, R. D., P. C. Olden, and J. D. Bramble. 1998. Strategic hospital alliances: Countervailing responses to restructuring health care markets. In *Handbook of health care management,* eds. W. J. Duncan, L. E. Swayne, and P. M. Ginter, 81–116. Cambridge MA: Blackwell Publishers.

Morrisey, M. A., J. Alexander, L. R. Burns, and V. Johnson. 1999. The effects of managed care on physician and clinical integration in hospitals. *Medical Care* 37(4): 350–61.

Moy, E., E. Valente, R. J. Levin, K. J. Bhak, and P. F. Griner. 1996. The volume and mix of inpatient services provided by academic medical centers. *Acad Med* 71(10): 1113–22.

Shortell, S. M., R. Gilles, and D. Anderson. 1996. *The New American Healthcare: Creating Organized Delivery Systems.* San Francisco: Jossey-Bass.

Shortell, S. M. and K. E. Hull. 1996. The new organization of health care: Managed care integrated health systems. In *Strategic choices for a changing healthcare system,* eds. S. Altman and U. Reinhardt, 101–48. Chicago: Health Administration Press.

Shortell, S. M., R. R. Gilles, and D. A. Anderson. 1994. The new world of managed care: Creating organized delivery systems. *Health Affairs* 13(5): 46–44.

Starr, P. 1982. *The Social Transformation of American Medicine.* New York: Basic Books.

Stevens, R. 1971. *American Medicine and the Public Interest.* New Haven: Yale University Press.

Sultz, H. A. and K. M. Young. 1999. *Health Care USA: Understanding Its Organization and Delivery.* 2nd ed. Gaithersburg MD: Aspen.

11

The Post-Acute Health Care System

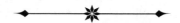

CHAPTER OBJECTIVES

At the conclusion of this chapter, the reader will be able to:

1. Discuss the development of the post-acute health care system in the United States during the last quarter of the twentieth century.
2. Define the main components of the post-acute health care system: informal care and formal care.
3. Discuss the size, importance, and function of the informal care system of post-acute health care.
4. Identify the components, discuss the services, define likely users, and relate the effectiveness of levels of the formal post-acute health care system.
    a. home health care
    b. hospice
    c. adult day services
    d. assisted living
    e. skilled nursing facilities
    f. sub-acute care
5. Define the role of occupational therapy and physical therapy in the post-acute health care system.

KEY WORDS: Custodial Care, Formal Care, Informal Care, Intermediate Care, Level of Care, Swing bed Unit, Voluntary Agency

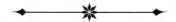

Introduction

Occupational therapists and physical therapists are important providers of rehabilitation services in the post-acute care system. Patients who survive a serious medical illness or an injury often require a lengthy recuperative period. Until the early 1980s, most of this rehabilitation care was provided in inpatient and outpatient hospital environments. The post-acute care environment was limited to nursing homes and a small home health industry. Nursing homes focused on custodial care for persons with chronic disease or illness with little chance for improvement. The increasing incidence of chronic disease and illness and the focus on hospitals as the primary source of care resulted in rapidly rising costs.

The growth and development of a post-acute health care system parallels the policy changes in health care financing and the desire to move away from the hospital to a community-based care system. With the initiation of Medicare Diagnosis-Related Groups prospective payment in 1983, the incentives for extended hospital care decreased. For persons who were medically stable but needed extended treatment for restoration of function, hospitals were viewed as an inefficient and excessively costly place for the delivery of post-acute care. Financial incentives were created to treat individuals as outpatients, in rehabilitation facilities, through home health agencies and in an emerging level of rehabilitation care in nursing homes. The rise of managed care in the late 1980s led to renewed pressure on hospitals and nursing homes from private payers, which resulted in a greater impetus to develop new post-acute alternatives such as sub-acute care and assisted living.

The world of post-acute care has created multiple alternatives for patient treatment after an acute illness or injury. Each **level of care** provides different services and has different costs. The complexity of the system has created a need for a new type of health care professional, the case manager, to assist the patient in navigating the system (see Chapter 7). By 1997, the rapidly increasing costs of post-acute care were evident, and Congress enacted sweeping limits on reimbursement for care provided in all post-acute care venues, to be phased in by 2002 (Balanced Budget Act of 1997). Occupational therapists and physical therapists have felt the effect of this change in limited employment opportunities, changing documentation requirements, and consolidation of the rehabilitation team.

The development of the post-acute care continuum has not been even, complete, or without challenges. The problems include unequal access to care and an inability to finance care. Certain populations continue to lack access to necessary services that would permit full restoration of function. For example, fewer options for long-term care exist in many rural communities. African-Americans are less likely to utilize institutional care and are more likely to use informal care or receive no care at all (Wallace et al. 1997). Simultaneously, Clark (1997) reports that African-Americans are experiencing increasing rates of disability and institutionalization as compared to the majority population. Overall, recent estimates of the unmet long-term care needs of the community-living elderly population range from 2 percent to 35 percent (Williams, Lyons, and Rowland 1997). The financing of long-term-care services has shifted to individuals and local government, and growing federal restrictions on long-term care funding are causing post-acute providers to consolidate and integrate with the acute medical care system (Cohen 1998). The rapid development in the 1990s of large corporations specializing in long-term care climaxed in the bankruptcy of several of these companies in 1999 after the enactment of federal spending limits (Saphir 1999).

The preceding chapter introduced the acute health care system. For patients with chronic disease and disablement, the need for health care extends well beyond the acute health care system. In this chapter, we will explore the multiple levels of care that make up the post-acute care continuum. In the broad sense, the post-acute care continuum has two fundamental components: **informal care** and **formal care** (see Figure 11–1). Informal care consists of the care provided by the family unit. Formal care is a continuum of services that begins with services to supplement informal care (e.g., home health care), extending to services that replace informal care (e.g., skilled nursing facilities, intermediate care for persons with developmental disabilities). Formal care, then, consists of a mix of non-professional services, professional services, and residential care. Physical therapy and occupational therapy are critical professional services on many levels of the formal care continuum. The complexity of each individual patient situation and the availability of services will dictate which level of care is most appropriate. This chapter will explain the structure and services of each level of the post-acute care continuum and what we understand as to each level's effectiveness.

Informal Care

Post-acute care is a system of formal and informal services that provide a continuum of rehabilitation and personal care for people with chronic disease and disabilities. The foundation of long-term care in the United States is the informal care system, namely, the family (Montgomery 1999; Wolf 1999; Robinson 1997). Kennedy et al. (1999) estimate that the number of adults serving as household caregivers numbers over 5 million people. The national economic value of informal caregiving is estimated at $196 billion, which is more than all forms of formal

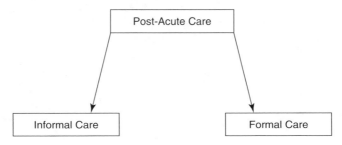

Figure 11–1   The Post-Acute Health Care

long-term care combined (Arno, Levine, and Memmott 1999). This aspect of the informal care system has important social, cultural, and policy implications.

The informal care system (see Figure 11–2) is inexpensive to the larger society and is a desirable alternative to formal care for many persons with chronic disease and disability. It is also heavily dependent on female spouses and adult female children for its implementation. In a study of informal vs. formal care for patients with dementia, Chiu et al. (1999) found that if family labor costs were considered, nursing home care costs would actually be lower than the cost of informal care. One study describing the major values of elderly Americans who are facing the need for long-term care found that a sense of independence and participation in life decisions were important in determining whether to access post-acute care services (Forbes and Hoffart 1998). Among other concerns considered by persons in potential need of informal or formal care were cost, stress on the family, personal preference, and premorbid attitudes about levels of care in the post-acute care continuum (Keysor, Desai, and Mutran 1999). Typically, older Americans prefer to stay at home, but this attitude changes if a significant illness will overburden the informal care system (Fried et al. 1999; Wielink and Huijsman 1999).

Boaz and Hu (1997) report that depending on marital status, networks of family and friends of elderly persons with disabilities can typically provide 10 to 40 hours per week of informal assistance. The burden of informal caregiving typically falls on female spouses and the adult female children of aging relatives (Montgomery 1999; Lee and Tussing 1998). Informal caregivers are mainly older, female, rate their own health as poor or fair, are more likely to be living in poverty, and describe themselves as work-disabled (Kennedy 1999). The family is the predominant source of care for persons with developmental disabilities. Nearly 90 percent of the nation's 3 million people with developmental disabilities are cared for by family members (Fujiura 1998). The experience of providing informal care affects the lives of the caregivers. Parents caring for children with disabilities experience anxiety and increased responsibility for the care of the child (McDermott et al. 1997). For society, the economic and social value of the informal care system is enormous. The development of formal long-term care services (e.g., home health care, skilled

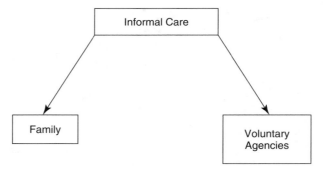

Figure 11–2.   The Informal Care System

nursing facilities) can be traced to the need to bolster the family as primary care-giver for patients with chronic disease and disability. For occupational therapists and physical therapists, this has applications to the design and implementation of intervention plans for patients with chronic disease and disability (e.g., the incorporation of family goals into treatment plans, the development of patient/family education programs).

The family often obtains information and referrals for problems in caregiving through **voluntary agencies.** Voluntary agencies like the American Heart Association or the National Multiple Sclerosis Society provide educational, support, and advocacy services for persons with chronic illness or disease and their families. Typically, these organizations provide health education and health maintenance activities to their constituencies, disease prevention and detection programs to the general public, and advocacy in the area of public and private policy to the government. By their nature, voluntary agencies are not-for-profit organizations that primarily have an educational purpose and provide limited direct patient-care services. It is important for occupational therapists and physical therapists to understand and be involved with these organizations in order to recognize the needs and concerns of people with disabilities and their informal care systems.

Formal Care

Formal care consists of a mix of residential and professional services (see Figure 11–3). Residential services range from facilities that provide supervision and minimal assistance (e.g., assisted living facilities) to facilities that provide multiple medical and rehabilitation treatments (e.g., skilled nursing facilities, sub-acute care units). As we will discover, the deterioration of a person's ability to perceive the

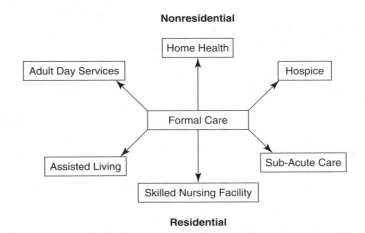

Figure 11–3. The Formal Care System

environment, think, communicate, and perform basic activities of daily living is critical to determining the appropriate level of formal post-acute care.

Home Health Care

Home health care is the "formal, regulated program of care delivered by a variety of health care professionals in the patient's home" (Montauk 1998). In the United States, home health care is a large industry. Growth has been fueled by reimbursement incentives and the emergence of new technologies (e.g., intravenous therapy) that can deliver treatment in the home vs. a hospital. From 1990 to 1996, the number of Medicare beneficiaries using home health care doubled to 10.8 percent and the average number of visits per beneficiary doubled to 73 (Health Care Financing Administration 1999). Employment growth rates in home health care were five times the growth rate of employment in the rest of the health care economy. The growth in the number of home health care agencies peaked in 1997 at nearly 11,000 (Health Care Financing Administration 1997). In 1998, home health care was provided by 9,376 Medicare certified agencies to 4 million Medicare beneficiaries (Health Care Financing Administration 1999). About 250 million home health care visits are provided annually in the United States (Conley and Walker 1998). Fifteen percent of the recipients of home health care have received services for longer than one year (Freedman 1999).

Home health care is provided by non-profit, for-profit, and governmental agencies that are either free-standing organizations or components of an integrated health care system. Home health care agencies provide services to patients who are medically stable but cannot access other community-based resources. For example, home health care is utilized in rural areas where access to physician and hospital services may be more limited (Health Care Financing Administration 1999; Dansky et al. 1998). Home health care has also developed in the gap created by the increasing orientation of medical physicians to high-technology practice environments. It was recently reported that fewer than 1 percent of Medicare beneficiaries receive a home visit from a physician (Meyer and Gibbons 1997).

Home health care is a set of health care services organized and delivered by nurses and rehabilitation professionals under medical supervision. Home health agencies provide a package of skilled services as well as non-skilled services intended for short-term, intermittent needs after an acute illness (see Table 11–1). Skilled services include physical therapy, occupational therapy, nursing, speech-language pathology, dietetics, and pharmacy. Non-skilled services (i.e., homemaking and personal hygiene care) are provided when related to the care and recovery from a medical illness.

Home health care is most beneficial for individuals who need comprehensive care to recover from an illness or injury, desire to live in their home, and have some social support. Intrator and Berg (1998) found that patients who received home health care services after hip fracture were less likely to need rehospitalization or a nursing home admission and were more likely to survive the following year without another Medicare claim. Penrod, Kane, Finch, and Kane (1998) found that the effect

Table 11–1.   Common Services in Nonresidential Sites of the Post-Acute Health Care System

	Skilled	*Nonskilled*
HOME HEALTH	Physical therapy Occupational therapy Nursing Speech/language pathology Dietetics Pharmacy Social work	Homemaking Personal Services
HOSPICE	Medicine Nursing Pastoral care Social work Counseling Rehabilitation therapy Dietetics Pharmacy	Homemaking Personal hygiene Volunteer companions
ADULT DAY SERVICES	Nursing Social work Physical therapy Occupational therapy Recreational therapy	Transportation Meals Personal care

of home health care on functional status was not significant but concluded nonetheless that home health care does help maintain the patient in the home.

Individuals receiving home health care services are homebound, meaning that they are unable to leave their homes except for medical appointments or religious services. Persons most commonly needing home health care services are older (mean age is 75), female, have been recently hospitalized, have limited ability to perform activities of daily living, and can benefit from periodic health care worker visits (Torrez, Estes, and Linkens 1998). The most common medical diagnoses of persons utilizing home health care services are diabetes mellitus, circulatory system disease, and respiratory system disease (Health Care Financing Administration 1999; Diwan, Berger, and Manns 1997). They frequently are also the recipients of informal care for instrumental activities of daily living from family and friends (Diwan, Berger, and Manns 1997).

Patients entering home health care services receive a comprehensive evaluation and care plan developed to meet their needs. This plan of care needs to be certified by the person's physician every 60 days. Discharge from the hospital raises many concerns for patients and their caregivers regarding the procedures to be followed at home, communication with providers, and expectations for the future

(Weaver, Perloff, and Waters 1998). A program of skilled and nonskilled services can ensure a smooth transition to the community after illness.

Overall, the most commonly utilized service in home health care is provided by nonskilled home health aides (Health Care Financing Administration 1999). Home health aides provide assistance with activities of daily living, light housekeeping, and basic medical procedures (e.g., wound-dressing changes). On average, a home health aide will visit six patients per day (Montauk 1998).

Skilled nursing and physical therapy are the professional services most commonly utilized in home health care (Weaver, Perloff, and Waters 1998). Skilled nursing services are closely related to the need for a home health aide and the presence of significant disease (Diwan, Berger, and Manns 1997). Case management, patient education, intravenous therapy, wound care, and pain control are frequently employed nursing procedures (Montauk 1998). Nursing care is limited to no more than eight hours per day, and less than 28 hours per week.

Physical therapy and occupational therapy services are important components of a home health care plan. Payne, Thomas, Fitzpatrick, et al. (1998) studied patterns of home health visit length and found that case management, functional limitations, and clinical instability affected the need for professional intervention. Limitations in performing activities of daily living is the strongest predictor of overall utilization of home health care (Torrez, Estes, and Linkens 1998). Bathing has been identified as the most common ADL limitation in the home health care population (Torrez, Estes, and Linkens 1998). Collins, Beissner, and Krout (1998) reported that patients with musculoskeletal conditions were treated most frequently by physical therapists, followed by neurological and cardiopulmonary problems. Therapists spent an average of 74 minutes per visit, with 35 minutes of that period given to direct treatment of the client. Patients with neurological problems needed longer visits. Travel and documentation were the most common activities performed by the physical therapists. In a study of goal achievement in home health care, O'Sullivan and Volicer (1997) reported that persons discharged to home after total hip replacement who received physical therapy home care were more likely to be discharged with their goals achieved.

Hospice

Hospice services provide care for individuals with terminal illness and their support systems during and after the dying process. The early development of hospice services can be traced to the efforts of volunteers interested in providing services to persons with terminal illness (Petrisek and Mor 1999). The first hospice organization was St. Christopher's Hospice, which opened in London in 1967 (Leland and Schonwelter 1997; Pickett, Cooley, and Gordon 1998). The first hospice in the United States opened in New Haven, Connecticut, in 1974. Today there are approximately 3,000 hospice organizations in the United States (Petrisek and Mor 1999; Leland and Schonwelter 1997; Castle, Mor, and Banaszak Holl, 1997). The Hospice Foundation of America (2000) reports that 540,000 persons were served by hospice care in the United States during 1999.

Hospice is founded on a philosophy of palliative care, not curative medicine. Palliative care focuses on pain management, emotional counseling, and social support (Petrisek and Mor 1999). Byock (1996) has summarized the philosophy of hospice care: "Beyond symptom management, hospice and palliative care intervention can be directed at helping the person to attain a sense of completion within the social and interpersonal dimensions, to develop or deepen a sense of worthiness, and to find their own unique sense of meaning in life(p. 251)." As Leland and Schonwelter (1997) succinctly state, hospice is about "dying well (p. 381)."

Persons in need of hospice care frequently have cancer, heart disease, or pulmonary disease (Emmanuel, Fairclough, and Slutsman 1999; Rasmussen and Sanderson 1998; Haupt 1997). Patient populations are usually older and are equally divided between males and females. The most common physical complaints of patients receiving hospice services include pain, fatigue, anorexia, dyspnea, nausea, confusion, and depression (Ng and von Gunten 1998; Friedrich 1999; Cleary and Carbone 1997). Hospice positively affects the social isolation faced by persons with terminal illness in the hospital (Rasmussen and Sanderson 1998). About two in three hospice patients need help with one activity of daily living and one instrumental activity of daily living. About three in ten hospice patients need assistance to walk (Haupt 1997). Nearly two in three persons need help with transportation, over half with homemaking, and one in four with personal care (Emmanuel, Fairclough, and Slutsman 1999).

The vast majority of hospice services are provided in private residences (Haupt 1997; Emmanuel, Fairclough, and Slutsman 1999). Increasingly, skilled nursing facilities are offering hospice care (Petrisek and Mor 1999; Castle, Mor, and Banaszak-Hull 1997). Some hospice services, including respite care, are provided in special residential hospice facilities (Leland and Schonwelter 1997). Length of stay in hospice varies widely, depending on setting and geographic location in the United States. Stillman and Syrjala (1999) reported that the median length of stay in hospice was 23 days. In skilled nursing facilities, the stay can be much longer. To qualify for hospice benefits, patients with terminal illness are usually expected to die within six months (Petrisek and Mor 1999; Gabel, Hurst, and Hunt 1998).

Hospice services are characterized by a patient-focused, interdisciplinary, coordinated plan of care (see Table 11–1). Besides the family, physicians, nurses, clergy, social workers, home health aides, counselors, and volunteers make up the core of the hospice team.

Occupational therapists, physical therapists, speech/language pathologists, dietitians, and pharmacists are other important contributing professions to hospice care. Hospice care benefits are typically inclusive of necessary prescription drug and durable medical equipment needs. A unique Medicare benefit for hospice services is follow-up bereavement care for family members after the patient's death.

Even with the rapid growth of hospice and its success in meeting the needs of persons with terminal illness, about 55 percent of Americans die in acute care hospitals each year (Gabel, Hurst, and Hunt 1998). This has implications for the social cost of terminal illness, since about one-fourth of Medicare program costs are incurred in caring for people in the last two years of life (McGrail 1997). Many factors explain the relatively low utilization of hospice. Certain populations have less access to hospice services. For example, some patients do not have family to provide hospice care. Haber (1999) found that members of minorities experience greater barriers to access of hospice care. Personal factors can also affect the utilization of hospice services. In a recent study of hospice utilization, Weggel (1999) found that patient and family resistance to acceptance of terminal illness and their unwillingness to give up curative therapy were factors limiting the use of hospice. In some cases, physicians do not provide hospice care as an option for terminally ill patients, primarily due to lack of information about hospice services (Weggel 1999; Miller, Miller, and Single 1997).

Adult Day Services

For the caregivers of adults with chronic disease and disability, the ongoing provision of informal care can be exhausting. A respite from providing care can alleviate this stress and allow for the continuation of informal care. For working caregivers, the ability of an agency to provide services during workday hours allows informal care to continue in the evening or during the weekend. One option in the post-acute care continuum designed to meet these needs is adult day services.

Adult day services provide "community based group programs designed to meet the needs of functionally and/or cognitively impaired adults through an individual plan of care" (National Adult Day Services Association 2000). In the United States, there are approximately 4,000 adult day service providers, and the vast majority of them are not-for-profit agencies. Adult day services provide transportation, meals, social services, personal care, occasional nursing services, rehabilitation services, and activities, usually during normal day business hours, five days per week (see Table 11–1). Adult day services allow for the supervision and care of an adult while the primary caregiver works or is given a respite from daily care.

The National Adult Day Services Association (2000) reports that the typical user of adult day services is a 76-year-old female who lives with a spouse or family and friends. One-half of the recipients of adult day services have a cognitive impairment, over half need help with at least two activities of daily living. The average daily fee for adult day care is $43.13, less than one-half of the daily cost of skilled nursing facility care (National Adult Day Services Association 2000).

The Program of All-Inclusive Care (PACE), is a federal demonstration project designed to increase the availability of adult day care as an option to institutionalization. PACE is organized around the use of adult day care centers, with the aim of reducing the institutionalization of frail elders who would otherwise qualify for skilled nursing facility placement. PACE is unusual in adult day services in that it serves a large minority, low-income population (Irvin, Massey, and Dorsey 1997). It originated in San Francisco's Chinatown in the early 1970s. Recent changes in Medicare law have created expanded opportunities for PACE programs across the country (Lee et al. 1998). In 1998, there were 12 PACE sites nationally, serving 3,600 elderly Americans (MEDPAC 1998).

PACE sites serve 120 to 150 participants who come several times per week to adult day service centers for medicine, nursing, social services, occupational therapy, physical therapy, home care, and other services (Shannon and Van Reenen 1998). The typical PACE participant is a female with three to five limitations in activities of daily living (Mukamel, Temkin-Greener, and Clark 1998; Irvin, Massey, and Dorsey 1997).

Several studies have addressed the effectiveness of adult day services. Travis and MacAuley (1999) found that persons accessing adult day services in rural areas had multiple medical conditions, whereas cognitive problems dominated admissions to similar facilities in metropolitan areas. Zarit et al. (1998) found that the use of adult day services resulted in lowered primary-caregiver stress and improved psychological functioning. Swan (1997) surveyed over 1,000 Oklahomans over age 40 and found that less than 1 percent of the study population had used adult day services but a majority (60%) would use the services if appropriate funding could be found to support the cost of care.

Assisted Living

Assisted living is "a special combination of housing, personalized supportive services and health care designed to meet the needs—scheduled and unscheduled—of those who need help with activities of daily living" (Assisted Living Federation of America 2000). Unlike home health care, adult day care, and many hospice, assisted living facilities provide residential care. Over 1 million Americans live in one of 20,000 assisted living facilities in the United States (Assisted Living Federation of America 2000).

The typical resident is an unmarried woman over 80 years of age. Individuals residing in assisted living facilities need help with activities of daily living, supervision of medications, and may be occasionally incontinent. This level of care is commonly called **intermediate care.** Assisted living facilities usually provide three meals per day, transportation, social activities, assistance with activities of daily living, medication monitoring, and security services (see Table 11–2). Assisted living facilities may be freestanding buildings or, in some cases, are part of a skilled nursing facility. According to the Assisted Living Federation of America, the typical facility has 46 units and charges $66.17 per day. This is about one-half the cost of a day in a skilled nursing facility. Payment is primarily by private funding, although state Medicaid programs are increasingly viewing assisted living facilities as a cost-effective alternative to expensive skilled nursing facility care (Mollica 1998).

Assisted living has been demonstrated to be cost-effective in caring for the population with Alzheimer's disease (Leon and Moyer 1999). Sikorska (1999) interviewed 156 residents of 13 assisted living facilities and found higher rates of resident satisfaction in smaller facilities with limited activities and more personal space. Bishop (1999) reported that assisted living facilities were replacing skilled nursing facilities as the residential choice for persons with minimal disability or post-acute care needs.

Skilled Nursing Facilities

Skilled nursing facilities (SNFs) are the oldest type of long-term care facility. They have been present in the United States in one form or another for over a century. Originally designed to provide long-term **custodial care,** skilled nursing facilities have been transformed in the last two decades into facilities that are a key part of a continuum of care for patients with complex illnesses (American Health Care Association 2000). An indication of this change is the development of specialized units in SNFs for Alzheimer's disease, AIDS, ventilator-dependent patients, and sub-acute care. Reschovsky (1998) classifies persons served by skilled nursing facilities into two types: post-acute and chronic (see Figure 11–4). Post-acute patients receive sub-acute care or skilled services with the anticipation of a community discharge. Chronic patients receive skilled nursing and occasional skilled rehabilitation services to prevent the deterioration of function and health status, with the expectation of long-term residence in the skilled nursing facility.

About 1.5 million Americans reside in over 17,000 skilled nursing facilities in the United States (American Health Care Association 2000). Nationally, occupancy is about 87 percent of capacity (Strahan 1997). Most skilled nursing facilities (52%) are part of a multifacility chain, and two-thirds are for-profit enterprises (American Health Care Association 2000). The average facility numbers 107 beds and consists of resident rooms, dining and activity areas, and therapy space. Skilled nursing facility care is the most expensive site of care in the post-acute care continuum. The average daily cost for a stay in a skilled nursing facility is $112. The federal Medicaid program funds almost seven in ten persons residing in skilled nursing facilities. Largely due to declining length of stays in hospitals, the number of Medicare admissions for short-term post-acute care in skilled nursing facilities doubled between 1990 and 1996 (Health Care Financing Administration 1998).

Skilled nursing facility care is for patients who have complex nursing or rehabilitation needs that cannot be provided in another environment (e.g., home health, assisted living). Persons in skilled nursing facilities typically need help with at least three activities of daily living, and nearly two in three (63%) have cognitive problems

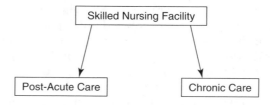

Figure 11–4.   Persons Served in Skilled Nursing Facilities (SNF)

(American Health Care Association 2000). Typically, individuals have complex care needs but are medically stable with regular nursing observation/treatment. Examples of care needs that would qualify an individual for skilled nursing care include daily injections, wound care, tube feedings, needing assistance of more than one person for mobility tasks, help for all personal hygiene cares, and significant confusion.

Four basic services are provided in skilled nursing facilities: nursing and rehabilitation, personal care, residential services, and medical care (American Health Care Association 2000) (see Table 11–2). Each resident receives an individualized plan of care developed by a multidisciplinary team to meet their needs. All facilities have 24-hour nursing services staffed by nurse's aides for personal care, with supervision by licensed practical nurses and registered nurses. Nurse's aides assist with feeding, bathing, dressing, walking, and transfers. Professional nurses provide examination, evaluation, and technical nursing interventions.

Occupational therapists and physical therapists provide evaluation and intervention to improve function and prevent secondary conditions in this population. For patients with short-term, post-acute care needs, Murray et al (1999) found that nursing homes have become important sites to receive rehabilitation therapy services. Over half of the residents in their study of Ohio nursing homes were receiving physical therapy, occupational therapy, or speech/language pathology services (Murray et al. 1999). Rehabilitation in a nursing home typically takes longer, and the post-acute care patients served have more severe deficits. However, one study of nursing home rehabilitation reports that nearly two in three patients ultimately return to the community (Kosasih et al. 1998). Young age, fewer limitations in ADL performance, and rehabilitation therapy are associated with a greater likelihood of community discharge (Mehr, Williams, and Fries 1997).

Restorative care is an important component of rehabilitation services for persons with long-term, chronic disease in nursing homes. Porell et al. (1998) describe how the slow rate of decline in functional task performance among nursing home residents with chronic conditions is exacerbated by serious medical illness (e.g., congestive heart failure, chronic obstructive pulmonary disease, cancer). Restorative care is commonly implemented by a specially trained nursing aide. Training usually encompasses, at a minimum, basic range of motion exercise and ambulation training. Restorative care services are usually overseen by the nursing supervisor. Restorative aides can be a most useful adjunct person for the completion of rehabilitation protocols established by physical therapists and occupational therapists and for providing maintenance therapy, which is not reimbursable as a professional service. An initial evaluation by an occupational therapist or physical therapist to establish a maintenance program in a skilled nursing facility is a Medicare-reimbursable service (see Chapter 8).

For patients with stable but active disease, skilled nursing facilities are an effective site of placement. Patients with chronic obstructive pulmonary disease and dementia are less likely to be admitted to hospitals from nursing homes than from personal homes (Camberg et al. 1997). Still, acute illness rates in a nursing home (e.g., pneumonia, urinary tract infection) average 0.53 episodes per person per month (Alessi and Harker 1998). While medical direction is required in skilled nursing facilities, Katz et al. (1997) found that relatively few physicians spend time caring for residents of nursing homes. The incorporation of primary medical care into skilled nursing facilities has been demonstrated to have a positive impact on preventing hospitalization for acute illness (Joseph and Boult 1998).

The experience of nursing home living is life-changing. The decision to place a family member in a nursing home is usually not pre-planned, is often rushed, and is made at a time of emotional stress for the informal care system (Rodgers 1997). Nearly three in four nursing home admissions are prompted by a hospitalization after a major event, most commonly stroke, hip fracture, congestive heart failure, pneumonia, cancer, or diabetes (Ferruci et al. 1997). Wilson (1997) describes the adjustment to nursing home life for new residents in three phases: overwhelmed, adjustment, and initial acceptance. Fiveash (1998) found that some residents experienced satisfaction with living in a nursing home but others described the experience as limiting and "dehumanizing."

The experience of residential life is very important. Residents place importance on choice and control over bedtime, waking time, food, roommates, care routines, outside trips, use of money, and the telephone (Kane et al. 1997). Residents who are active, have a positive attitude, and believe they have control in their environment make better adjustments to life in a nursing home (Johnson et al. 1998).

Concerns regarding the quality of care in nursing homes have been addressed on several occasions. In the past, nursing homes were criticized for excessive use of restraints. Currently, use of restraints is restricted and must be well documented (Sullivan-Marx et al. 1999). Another chronic problem in skilled nursing facilities is absenteeism and turnover among nursing home workers (Cohen-Mansfield 1997; Parsons, Parker, and Ghose 1998). The Nursing Home Reform Act of 1987 initiated the development of a standardized assessment tool to evaluate the health status and care needs of nursing home residents. Since its implementation in the mid-1990s, the Resident Assessment Instrument (RAI) has resulted in several improvements in nursing home quality. After implementation of the RAI, researchers found improved patient care documentation, better patient care planning, lower use of restraints, fewer hospital admissions from nursing homes, and improvements in ADL function, social interactions, and cognition among nursing home residents (Mor et al. 1997; Phillips et al. 1997; Hawes et al. 1997).

As the decade of the 1990s closed, the for-profit skilled nursing facility industry was rocked by the changes wrought by the Balanced Budget Act of 1997. About two in three nursing homes in the United States are for-profit entities. Prior to 1997, some of these companies engaged in aggressive debt-financed expansion of their chains. Faulting changes in federal reimbursement, some large for-profit nursing home companies filed for federal bankruptcy protection in 1999 (Saphir 1999).

Sub-Acute Care

Sub-acute care is defined as "comprehensive inpatient care designed for someone who has an acute illness, injury or exacerbation of a disease process (American Health Care Association 1995). The National Sub-acute Care Association (2000) defines sub-acute care as a "comprehensive, cost-effective inpatient program for patients who are stable after an acute medical event and need complex medical and rehabilitation treatment." Sub-acute care is intended for the short-term recuperation of a person after a significant illness or injury.

Similar to other levels of care in the post-acute care continuum, sub-acute care experienced explosive growth in the 1990s. Ninety percent of all sub-acute facilities did not exist before 1990 (American Health Care Association 2000). Sub-acute care units have developed both in nursing homes and hospitals. Other locations for sub-acute care units include rehabilitation hospitals and free-standing sub-acute care units. Sub-acute care facilities are licensed as skilled nursing facilities and until 1997 were exempt from Medicare prospective payment limitations. This exemption encouraged hospitals and nursing homes to open sub-acute units to care for patients who were medically stable and in need of rehabilitation but whose acute hospital benefits had been exhausted.

Rousso (1995) and Fogel and Gossman-Klim (1995) have reported that sub-acute care is a cost-effective alternative to hospital care. The American Health Care Association (2000) reports that the cost of sub-acute care is 40 to 60 percent less than hospital care. The conversion of acute care hospital beds to sub-acute beds has been most noticeable in non-profit hospitals (Wheeler et al. 1999). Sub-acute units in hospitals are commonly called **swing bed** units. Utilization of a sub-acute care stay after hospitalization for an acute illness is common. Weaver, Perluff, and Waters (1998) found that over one-third of all inpatient cases in 43 Veterans Administration medical centers contained at least one day in a sub-acute care unit.

Sub-acute care units tend to be organized around patient types (e.g., medically complex, respiratory/ventilator care, post-surgical, stroke or orthopedic rehabilitation, oncology). In contrast to acute hospital care, sub-acute care patients receive a lower intensity of physician and nursing care (see Table 11.2). Physicians typically do not visit on a daily basis; occasionally they visit only weekly. Nursing time is closely monitored and is typically four to seven contact hours per day. In general, physical therapy and occupational therapy services are provided on a daily basis. In contrast to acute medical rehabilitation, sub-acute rehabilitation total therapy time is less than three hours per day. The goal is to move the patient to a less intense level of care (perhaps home or long-term care) as soon as possible. About 50 percent of patients in sub-acute care facilities are discharged to home (American Health Care Association 2000).

Conclusion

In this chapter, we have explored the range of care options for persons in need of rehabilitation and recuperation after serious illness or injury (see Figure 11–5). Given these options, the informal care system remains the largest and most important component of the post-acute care system. The experience of disablement increases the risk of the need for formal post-acute care services. For physical therapists and occupational therapists, the implications of this fact are important.

Table 11–2.   **Common Services in Residential Sites of the Post-Acute Health Care System**

	Skilled	*Nonskilled*
Assisted Living		Meals Transportation Social activities ADL assistance Security
Skilled Nursing Facility	Nursing Physical therapy Occupational therapy Social work Dietetics	Personal hygiene Restorative care
Sub-Acute Care	Medicine Nursing Occupational therapy Physical therapy Speech/language pathology	Personal hygiene

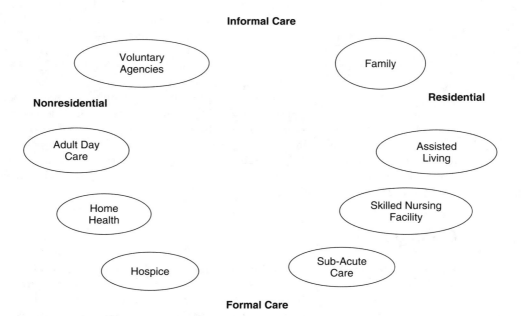

Figure 11–5.   The Post-Acute Health Care System

Therapists make important contributions to reducing the risk of disablement. Rehabilitation services exist to promote and restore the ability to live in the community for patients with chronic disease and disability. For most of them, community living will depend on the strength of the informal care system. The strength of this system is the care provided by parents, female spouses, and adult female children.

The formal care system consists of professional services, non-professional services, and residential care to either support or replace the informal care system. The majority of the residents in formal post-acute care sites are older women, which reflects the longer life span of women and the disproportionate share of informal care provided to males in our society by women. Home health care and adult day services provide professional and nonprofessional services to support the informal care system. Assisted living facilities, skilled nursing facilities, and sub-acute care facilities provide a continuum of residential, professional, and nonprofessional services for the short-term or long-term care of persons with chronic disease and disability.

CHAPTER REVIEW QUESTIONS

1. Consider how the post-acute care continuum evolved over the last 20 years. What are the reasons for these changes?
2. Identify the two components of the post-acute care continuum. Consider how they are related to one another.
3. What are the characteristics of the informal care system? Describe its strengths and weaknesses.
4. Identify the levels of the formal care system. Identify the professional services and residential features, if any, of each level of care.
5. Define home health care. Describe the services common to home health care, the types of patients served, and the effectiveness of home health care.
6. Define hospice. Describe the services common to hospice, the types of patients served, and the effectiveness of hospice care.
7. Define adult day services and the PACE program. Describe the services common to adult day care, the types of patients served, and the effectiveness of adult day care.
8. Define assisted living. Describe the services common to assisted living, the type of patients served, and the effectiveness of assisted living services.
9. Define skilled nursing facilities. Compare and contrast post-acute care services and chronic care services in skilled nursing facilities. Describe the services common to skilled nursing facilities, the types of patients served, and the effectiveness of skilled nursing facility care.
10. Define sub-acute care. Describe the services common to sub-acute care, the types of patients served, and the effectiveness of sub-acute care services.

CHAPTER DISCUSSION QUESTIONS

1. Consider and discuss how societal gender roles have influenced the development of the post-acute care system.
2. Consider the development of the post-acute care continuum in light of the medical and social disability models of disablement. Which model has been most influential in the development of the system to date? Why?
3. A primary purpose of occupational therapy and physical therapy is to promote independence in the living environment. Compare and contrast the settings in the post-acute continuum as they affect the ability of physical therapists and occupational therapists to complete these roles.

REFERENCES

Alessi, C. A. and J. O. Harker. 1998. A prospective study of acute illness in the nursing home. *Aging* 10(6): 479–89.

American Health Care Association. 1999. Todays nursing facilities and the people they serve. Accessed at *www.ahca.org/who/profile3.htm* on April 18, 2000.

———. 1999 National data on nursing facilities. Accessed at *www.ahca.org/who/profile4.htm* on April 18, 2000.

———. 1999 Nursing facilities. Accessed at *www.ahca.org/info/pubthink.htm* on April 18, 2000.

Arno, P. S., C. Levine, and M. M. Memmott. 1999. The economic value of informal caregiving. *Health Affairs* 18(2): 182–88.

Assisted Living Federation of America. 2000. What is assisted living? Accessed at *www.Alfa.org/WhatsAL.htm* on April 17, 2000.

Bishop, C. E. 1999. Where are the missing elders? The decline in nursing home use. 1995. *Health Affairs* 18(4): 146–55.

Boaz, R. F. and J. Hu. 1997. Determining the amount of help used by disabled elderly persons at home: The role of coping resources. *J Gerontol B* 52(6): S317–24.

Brannen, J. J. and E. R. Griemel. 1997. Professional burnout among nursing home personnel: Effects of a training intervention. *Abst Book Assoc Health* 14: 352.

Byock, I. 1996. The nature of suffering and the nature of opportunity at the end of life. *Clin Geriatr Med* 12: 237–52.

Castle, N. G., V. Mor, and J. Banaszak-Hull. 1997. Special care hospice units in nursing homes. *Hosp J* 12(3): 59–69.

Chiu, L., K. Y. Tang, Y. H. Liu, W. C. Shyu, and T. P. Chang. 1999. Cost comparisons between family-based care and nursing home care for dementia. *J Adv Nurs* 29(4): 1005–12.

Clark, D. O. 1997. U. S. trends in disability and institutionalization among older blacks and whites. *Am J Pub Health* 87(3): 438–40.

Cleary, J. and J. Carbone. 1997. Palliative medicine in the elderly. *Cancer* 80(7): 1335–47.

Cohen, M. A., 1998. Emerging trends in the finance and delivery of long term care: Public and private opportunities and challenges. *Gerontologist* 38(1): 80–89.

Cohen-Mansfield, J. 1997. Turnover among nursing home staff. A review. *Nurs Manage* 28(5): 59–62, 64.

Collins, J., K. L. Beissner, and J. A. Krout. 1998. Home health physical therapy: Practice patterns in western New York. *Phys Ther* 78(2): 170–179.

Conley, V. M. and M. K. Walker. 1998. National health policy influence on Medicare home health. *Home Health Care Serv Q* 17(3): 1–15.

Dansky, K. H., D. Brannon, D. G. Shea, J. Vasey, and R. Dirani. 1998. Profiles of hospital, physician and home health service use by older persons in rural areas. *Gerontologist* 38(3): 320–30.

Diwan, S., C. Berger, and E. K. Manns. 1997. Composition of the home care service package: Predictors of type, volume, and mix of services provided to poor and frail older people. *Gerontologist* 37(2): 169–81.

Emmanuel, R. J., D. L. Fairclough, J. Slutsman, H. Alpert, D. Baldwin, and L. L. Emmanuel. 1999. Assistance from family members, friends, paid caregivers and volunteers in the care of terminally ill members. *N Engl J Med* 341(13): 956–63.

Ferruci, L. K., J. M. Guralnik, M. Pahor, M. C. Corti, and R. J. Havlik. 1997. Hospital diagnoses, Medicare charges, and nursing home admissions in the year when older persons become severely disabled. *JAMA* 277(9): 728–34.

Fiveash, B. 1998. The experience of nursing home life. *Int J Nurs Prac* 4(3): 166–74.

Fogel, L. A. and K. Gossman-Klim. 1995. Getting started with sub-acute care. *Healthc Financ Manage* 49(10): 64–65, 68, 70.

Forbes, S. and N. Hoffart. 1998. Elders' decision making regarding the use of long-term care services: A precarious balance. *Qual Health Res* 8(6): 736–50.

Freedman, V. A. 1999. Long term admissions to home health agencies: A life table analysis. *Gerontologist* 39(1): 16–24.

Fried, T. R., C. van Doorn, J. R. O'Leary, M. E. Tinetti, and M. A. Drickamer. 1999. Older persons' preferences for site of terminal care. *Ann Intern Med* 131(2): 109–12.

Fujiura, G. T. 1998. Demography of family households. *Am J Ment Ret* 103(3): 225–35.

Gabel, J. R., K. M. Hurst, and K. A. Hunt. 1998. Health benefits for the terminally ill: Reality and perception. *Health Affairs* 17(6): 120–27.

Haber, D. 1999. Minority access to hospice. *Am J Hosp Palliat Care* 16(1): 386–89.

Haupt, B. J. 1997. Characteristics of hospice care discharges. *Adv Data* 25(287): 1–14.

Hawes, C., V. Mor, C. D. Phillips, B. E. Fries, J. N. Morris, E. Steele-Friedlob, A. M. Greene, and M. Nennstiel. 1997. The OBRA-87 nursing home regulations and implementation of the Resident Assessment Instrument: Effects on process quality. *J Am Ger Soc* 45(8): 977–85.

Health Care Financing Administration. 1998. 1998 Data Compendium. Accessed at *www.hcfa.gov/stats/98datacmp.pdf* on April 18, 2000.

Hospice Foundation of America. 1999. What is hospice? Accessed at *www.hospice foundation.org/virtual_html/whatis.htm* on March 31, 2000.

Intrator, O. and K. Berg. 1998. Benefits of home health care after inpatient rehabilitation for hip fracture: Health service use by Medicare beneficiaries, 1987–1992. *Arch Phys Med Rehabil* 79(10): 1195–99.

Irvin, C. V., S. Massey, and T. Dorsey. 1997. Determinants of enrollment among applicants to PACE. *Health Care Fin Rev* 19(2): 135–53.

Johnson, B. D., G. L. Stone, E. M. Altmaier, and L. D. Berdahl. 1998. The relationship of demographic factors, locus of control and self-efficacy to successful nursing home adjustment. *Gerontologist* 38(2): 209–16.

Joseph, A. and C. Boult. 1998. Managed primary care of nursing home residents. *J Am Ger Soc* 46(9): 1152–56.

Kane, R. A., A. L. Caplan, E. K. Urv-Wong, I. C. Freeman, M. A. Aroskar, and M. Finch. 1997. Everyday matters in the lives of nursing home residents: Wish for and perception of choice and control. *J Am Ger Soc* 45(9): 1086–93.

Katz, P. R., J. Karuza, J. Kolassa, and A. Hutson. 1997. Medical practice with nursing home residents: Results from the National Physician Professional Activities Census. *J Am Ger Soc* 45(8): 911–17.

Kennedy, J., C. Walls, and D. Owens-Nicholson. 1999. A national profile of primary and secondary household caregivers: Estimates from the 1992 and 1993 surveys on income and program participation. *Home Health Care Serv Q* 17(4): 39–58.

Keysor, J. J., T. Desai, and E. J. Mutran. 1999. Elders' preferences for care setting in short- and long-term disability scenarios. *Gerontologist* 39(3): 334–44.

Kosasih J. B., H. H. Borca, W. J. Wenninger, and E. Duthie. 1998. Nursing home rehabilitation after acute rehabilitation: Predictors and outcomes. *Arch Phys Med Rehab* 79(6): 670–73.

Lee, M. and A. D. Tussing. 1998. Influences on nursing home admissions: The role of informal caregivers. *Abstr Book Assoc Health* 15: 55–56.

Lee, W., C. Eng, N. Fox, and M. Etienne. 1998. PACE: A model for integrated care of frail older patients. *Geriatrics* 53(6): 62, 65–66, 69, 73.

Leon, J. and D. Moyer, 1999. Potential cost savings in residential care for Alzheimer's disease patients. *Gerontologist* 39(4): 440–49.

Leland, J. Y. and R. S. Schonwelter. 1997. Advances in hospice care. *Clin Geriatr Med* 13(2): 381–401.

McDermott, S., D. Valentine, D. Anderson, D. Gallup, and S. Thompson. 1997. Parents of adults with mental retardation living in home and out of home: Caregiving burdens and gratifications. *Am J Orthopsychiatr.* 67(2): 323–29.

McGrail, K. 1997. Pattern of health service utilization in the last 24 months of life. *Abstr Book Assoc Health* 14: 293–94.

Medicare Payment Advisory Commission. 1998. Home health utilization. In *Medicare Payment Policy. Report to the Congress: Context for a Changing Medicare Program*, 107–15.

———. 1998. Program of all-inclusive care for the elderly. In *Report to Congress: Medicare Payment Policy*, vol. 2, 111–20

Mehr, D. R., B. C. Williams, and B. E. Fries. 1997. Predicting discharge outcomes of VA nursing home residents. *J Aging Health* 9(2): 244–65.

Meyer, G. S. and R. V. Gibbons. 1997. House calls to the elderly: A vanishing practice among physicians. *N Engl J Med* 337(25): 1815–20.

Miller K. M., M. M. Miller, and N. Single. 1997. Barriers to hospice care: Family physician perceptions. *Hosp J* 12(4): 29–41.

Mollica, R. L. 1998. Managed care and assisted living: Trends and future prospects. *J Health Hum Serv Adm* 20(3): 264–80.

Montauk, S. L. 1998. Home health care. *Am Fam Physician* 58(7): 1608–14.

Montgomery R. J. 1999. The family role in the context of long-term care. *J Aging Health* 11(3): 383–416.

Mor, V., O. Intrator, B. E. Fries, C. Phillips, J. Teno, J. Hiris, C. Hawes, and J. Morris. 1997. Changes in hospitalization associated with introducing the Resident Assessment Instrument. *J Am Geri Soc* 45(8): 1002–10.

Mukamel D. B., H. Temkin-Greener, and H. Clark. 1998. Stability of disability among PACE enrollees: Financial and programmatic implications. *Health Care Fin Rev* 19(3): 83–100.

Murray P. K., M. E. Singer, R. Fortinsky, L. Russo, and R. D. Cebul. 1999. Rapid growth of rehabilitation services in traditional community-based nursing homes. *Arch Phys Med Rehabil* 80(4): 372–78.

National Adult Day Services Association. 2000. Adult day services fact sheet. Accessed at *www.ncoa.org/nadsa/ADS_factsheet.htm* on April 17, 2000.

Ng, K. and C. F. von Gunten. 1998. Symptoms and attitudes of 100 consecutive patients admitted to an acute hospice/palliative care unit. *J Pain Symptom Manage* 16(5): 307–16.

O'Sullivan, M. J. and B. Volicer. 1997. Factors associated with achievement of goals for home health care. *Home Health Care Serv Q* 16(3): 21–34.

Parsons, S., K. P. Parker, and R. P. Ghose. 1998. A blueprint for reducing turnover among nursing assistants: A Louisiana study. *J La State Med Soc* 150(11): 545–53.

Payne, S. M., C. P. Thomas, T. Fitzpatrick, M. Abdel-Rahman, and H. L. Kayne. 1998. Determinants of home health visit length: Results of a multisite prospective study. *Med Care* 36: 1500–14.

Penrod, J. D., R. L. Kane, M. D. Finch, and R. A. Kane. 1998. Effects of post-hospital Medicare home health and informal care on patient functional status. *Health Serv Res* 33(3 pt. 1): 513–29.

Petrisek, A. C. and V. Mor. 1999. Hospice in nursing homes: A facility level analysis of the distribution of hospice beneficiaries. *Gerontologist* 39(3): 279–90.

Phillips, C. D., J. N. Morris, C. Hawes, B. E. Fries, V. Mor, M. Nennstiel, and V. Iannacchione. 1997. Association of the Resident Assessment Instrument with changes in function, cognition and psychosocial status. *J Am Ger Soc* 45(8): 986–93.

Pickett, M., M. E. Cooley, and D. B. Gordon. 1998. Palliative care: Past, present and future perspective. *Sem Oncol Nurs* 14(2): 86–94.

Porell, F., F. G. Caro, A. Silva, and M. Monane. 1998. A longitudinal analysis of nursing home outcomes. *Health Serv Res* 33(4 pt. 1): 835–65.

Rasmussen, B. H. and P. O. Sanderson. 1998. How patients spend their time in a hospice and in an oncological unit. *J Adv Nurs* 28(4): 818–28.

Reschovsky, J. D. 1998. The demand for post-acute and chronic care in nursing homes. *Medical Care* 36(4): 475–90.

Robinson, K. M. 1997. The family's role in long term care. *J Gerontol Nurs* 23(9): 7–11.

Rodgers, B. L. 1997. Family members' experiences with the nursing home placement of an older adult. *Appl Nurs Res* 10(2): 57–63.

Rousso, S. M. 1995. Managing financial pressures with sub-acute care. *Healthc Financ Manage* 49(10): 88–90, 92.

Saphir, A. 1999. Monstrous problems: Medicare's not the only bogeyman haunting the long term care industry. *Mod Healthcare* 29(30): 30–33.

Sikorska, E. 1999. Organizational determinants of resident satisfaction with assisted living. *Gerontologist* 39(4): 450–56.

Stillman, M. J., and K. L. Syrjala. 1999. Differences in physician access patterns to hospice care. *J Pain Symptom Manage* 17(3): 157–63.

Strahan, G. W. 1997. An overview of nursing homes and their current residents: Data from the 1995 National Nursing Home Survey. *Adv Data* 23(280): 1–12.

Sullivan-Marx, E. M., N. E. Strumpf, L. K. Evans, M. Baumgarten, and G. Maislin. 1999. Predictors of continued physical restraint use in nursing home residents following restraint reduction efforts. *J Am Geri Soc* 47(3): 342–48.

Torrez, D. J., C. Estes, and K. Linkens. 1998. The impact of a decade of policy on home health care utilization. *Home Health Care Serv Q* 16(4): 35–56.

Travis, S. S. and W. J. McAuley. 1999. Preexisting medical conditions in adult day services: An examination of nonmetropolitan and metropolitan admissions. *J Gerontol A* 54(5): M262–M266.

Weaver, F. M., L. Perloff, and T. Waters. 1998. Patients' and caregivers' transition from hospital to home: Needs and recommendations. *Home Health Care Serv Q* 17(3): 27–48

Weggel, J. M. 1999. Barriers to the physician decision to offer hospice as an option for terminal care. *WMJ* 98(3): 49–53.

Wielink, G. and R. Huijsman. 1999. Elderly community residents' evaluative criteria and preferences for formal and informal in-home services. *Int J Aging Hum Dev* 48(1): 17–33.

Williams, J., B. Lyons, and D. Rowland. 1997. Unmet long term care needs of elderly people in the community: A review of the literature. *Home Health Care Serv Q* 16(1–2): 93–119.

Wilson, S. A. 1997. The transition to nursing home life: A comparison of planned and unplanned admissions. *J Adv Nurs* 26(5): 864–71.

Wolf, D. A. 1999. The family as provider of long-term care: Efficiency, equity and externalities. *J Aging Health* 11(3): 360–82.

Zarit, S. H., M. A. Stephens, A. Townsend, and R. Greene. 1998. Stress reduction for family caregivers: Effects of adult day care use. *J Gerontol B Psychol Sci Soc Sci* 53(5): S267–77.

12

Health Care Personnel

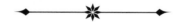

CHAPTER OBJECTIVES

At the conclusion of this chapter, the reader will be able to:

1. Discuss the scope and a classification system for health care personnel in the United States.
2. Describe the role and characteristics of occupational therapists and physical therapists in the health care system.
3. Summarize the role and characteristics of the rehabilitation team in the health care system.
   a. speech/ language pathologists
   b. orthotists and prosthetists
   c. recreational therapists
   d. social workers and psychologists
4. Discuss the scope, role, and characteristics of the medicine and nursing professions in the health care system.
5. Define the features of these exercise-related occupations:
   a. athletic training
   b. personal trainers
   c. kinesiotherapists
6. Discuss the scope and characteristics of providers of complementary and alternative medicine.
   a. chiropractors
   b. massage therapists
   c. homeopaths and naturopaths
7. Outline future directions for health care personnel in the twenty-first century.

KEY WORDS: Allied Health Profession, Allopathic Medicine, Chiropractic, Homeopathy, Naturopathy, Osteopathic Medicine

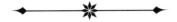

Introduction

In the preceding two chapters, we introduced and described the organizational components of the acute and post-acute health care systems. In this chapter, we turn our attention to the human component of the health care delivery system. The personal nature of health care and the technological sophistication of health care delivery make health care labor unique. Personal contact and technical excellence are hallmarks of effective practice (see Chapter 4). First, health care is a labor-intensive industry. The comprehensive care of persons with illness or injury requires many skilled personnel to provide timely and effective interventions. Second, the complexity of the patient problems and of the system itself requires specialized health care labor. Technology has a unique effect on the need for health care labor. New technology uncovers illnesses that were previously unknown and saves lives that were previously lost. Technology also creates new treatment options for patients. Unlike other areas in the economy, health care technology increases rather than decreases the demand for greater numbers and more specialized types of health care workers (see Chapter 3).

The purpose of this chapter is to explore the human component of the health care delivery system, with special attention to the workers who provide services to patients with chronic disease and disability. After we explore the size, scope, and a conceptual definition that classifies health care labor, we will discuss the educational background and scope of practice for the following occupations:

- Occupational therapy
- Physical therapy
- The rehabilitation team
- Medicine and nursing
- Exercise-related occupations
- Alternative and complementary medicine providers

Physical therapists and occupational therapists encounter many of these providers each day. On completing this chapter, you will have an understanding of each of these health care occupations that will enable you to interact in the system to the advantage of your patients. Before we begin, let us examine and discuss the size and scope of this labor force. Its enormous size requires us to introduce a classification system to better understand the different roles fulfilled by members of the health care team.

The Health Care Labor Force

About 8.5 million Americans were employed in health care in 1998. This accounted for 6 percent of total national employment (Bureau of Labor Statistics 1999). Between 1988 and 1998, the growing United States economy added 20 million jobs. This trend is expected to continue through 2008 (Bureau of Labor Statistics 1999). The national workforce is expected to become more culturally and racially diverse, older, better educated, and equally divided between men and women (Bureau of Labor Statistics 1999). The service-producing sector of the economy is expected to account for nearly all of this growth (Bureau of Labor Statistics 1999). Health care services are a crucial component of this portion of the national economy. Health care is anticipated to add 2.8 million jobs over the next decade (Bureau of Labor Statistics 1999). The current health care labor force is large and expected to expand in coming years.

The demand for health care personnel is affected by social needs and policy decisions. Changes in population characteristics affect the demand for goods and services in the economy. Over the last two decades, the increasing incidence of chronic disease and the aging of the population have changed the nature of disease, disability, and treatment. One hundred years ago, acute illness and private physician practice dominated the delivery of health care. Today, a team of health care workers with differing but complementary skills is needed to meet the complex care needs of the population.

Policy decisions, especially insurance funding of health care services, affects the supply and demand for health care. Public and private decisions to improve access to health care by developing insurance programs increased the demand for health care. To meet this demand, an expansion of educational and research programs in academic medical centers occurred, resulting in an increasing supply of health care workers. Conversely, private and public decisions to restrain the growth in health care costs during the 1990s slowed the growth in demand for health care workers as the twentieth century closed.

Classification of Health Care Employment

In order to understand the scope of this large labor force, it is helpful to classify health care workers by responsibilities and duties. The United States Department of Labor (1999) classifies health care workers into four categories:

- Health diagnosing occupations
- Health assessment and treating occupations

- Health technicians and technologists
- Health service occupations

Two of the categories occupy the professional classification: health diagnosing (e.g., physicians, dentists, podiatrists) and health assessment and treating (e.g., physical therapists, occupational therapists, registered nurses). An estimated 3.75 million persons are employed as health care professionals. Another 4.75 million Americans are employed in technical and supportive health care occupations (e.g., dental hygienists, opticians, therapy assistants, ambulance drivers).

Physical therapists and occupational therapists are considered to be members of the **allied health professions**. The term "allied health profession" was originated in the 1960s by the federal government to define, support, and expand educational programs for many occupations needed by the growing health care industry. The Health Resources Services Administration (1999) defines allied health as "a cluster of health professions, encompassing as many as 200 occupational titles, exclusive of physicians, nurses and a handful of others . . . involved with the delivery of health or related services pertaining to the identification, evaluation, and prevention of diseases and disorders; dietary and nutritional services; rehabilitation and health systems management, among others." This definition includes health assessment and treating occupations (e.g., physical therapy and occupational therapy) as well as some health service occupations (e.g., cytotechnology).

Occupational Therapists

Occupational therapists (see Table 12–1) act to "help people improve their ability to perform tasks in their daily living and working environments" (Bureau of Labor Statistics 2000). The history of occupational therapy can be traced to efforts to improve treatment for persons with mental illness in the early part of the twentieth century. The ideas and activities of pioneers like Susan Tracy, a nurse, and Eleanor Clark Slagle, a social worker, developed the foundational ideas for the usage of occupation as treatment (Friedman 1998). Today, there are 73,000 occupational therapists employed in the United States (Bureau of Labor Statistics 2000).

About 80 percent of occupational therapists are women (AOTA 2000). Occupational therapists find employment in schools, rehabilitation hospitals, psychiatric hospitals, outpatient clinics, nursing homes, community mental health centers and private practice. School-based practice employs the most occupational therapists (22%), followed by hospitals (15%), long-term care facilities (10%), rehabilitation centers (9%), and private practice (9%) (AOTA 2000). About half of practicing occupational therapists have received an entry-level baccalaureate degree education (AOTA 2000). Entry-level education in occupational therapy will be at the post baccalaureate degree level by 2005. An entry-level clinical doctorate in occupational therapy is also emerging (Pierce and Peyton 1998).

Occupational Therapist Assistants and Aides

The Department of Labor (2000) defines an occupational therapist assistant as a person who "works under the direction of occupational therapists to provide rehabilitative services to persons with mental, physical, emotional or developmental impairments." Occupational therapist assistants implement treatment plans and report the status of patients under their care. They are certified for practice after completing an associate's degree in one of 165 accredited programs in the United States. The responsibilities of occupational therapist aides are primarily clerical and patient-transportation functions.

Physical Therapists

Physical therapists (see Table 12–1) emerged as "reconstruction aides" after the First World War. Originally created to treat injured soldiers, the physical therapy profession grew during the poliomyelitis epidemics of the 1940s and 1950s and with the development of the acute medical care system during the last half-century. Today, physical therapists "provide services that help restore function, improve mobility, relieve pain, and prevent or limit permanent physical disabilities of patients suffering from illness or disease. They restore, maintain, and promote overall fitness and health" (Department of Labor 2000). It is estimated that 1 million Americans receive physical therapy services each day (American Physical Therapy Association 1999, p. vii).

In 1998, there were 120,000 physical therapist jobs in the United States. One in four therapists work part-time. Nine in ten physical therapists were employed in

Table 12–1.   Characteristics of Occupational Therapists and Physical Therapists

Characteristic	Occupational Therapist	Physical Therapist
Number	73,000	120,000
Role	Help people to perform every-day tasks	Restore function, relieve pain, improve mobility, disability prevention
Educational level	Bachelor's, master's, clinical doctorate	Master's, clinical doctorate
Practice sites	Schools, rehabilitation hospitals, psychiatric hospitals, outpatient clinics, nursing homes, community mental health centers, private practice, academic institutions	Hospitals, outpatient clinics home health, CORF, SNF, schools, rehabilitation facilities, private practice,academic institutions

health services. About 5 percent of physical therapists are self-employed and 1 percent are employed in government (Bureau of Labor Statistics 1999). Approximately seven in ten physical therapists are women (APTA 2000). The median age of the nation's physical therapists is in the late thirties, and the mean range of years of practice is 11 to 15 (APTA 2000). About four in ten physical therapists in practice have achieved a master's degree or doctorate (APTA 2000). Starting in 2002, all educational programs in physical therapy education began awarding entry-level degrees at the master's degree level. In the early 1990s, the entry-level clinical doctorate in physical therapy emerged as an option for professional preparation in the profession (Threlkeld, Jensen, and Royeen 1999). Clinical specialization is also conferred by the professional association upon demonstration of advanced knowledge and clinical ability.

Two in three physical therapists are employed in a hospital or an outpatient clinical environment (Bureau of Labor Statistics 1999). Other sites of employment include home health agencies, comprehensive outpatient rehabilitation facilities, skilled nursing facilities, schools, rehabilitation centers, industrial practice, community health centers, and academic institutions.

Physical Therapist Assistants and Aides

Physical therapist assistants "perform components of physical therapy procedures and related tasks selected and delegated by a supervising physical therapist" (Department of Labor 2000). In 1998, there were 82,000 physical therapist assistants (PTA) employed in the United States (Department of Labor 2000). Eight in ten physical therapist assistants are women. Seven in ten physical therapist assistants work full-time, and six in ten physical therapist assistants have less than five years employment experience. The average age of physical therapist assistants is in the early thirties. Physical therapist assistants work in the same settings as physical therapists. PTA education is provided in a community college or junior college and generally culminates in an associate's degree after two years of work.

Physical therapist assistants work under the direction and supervision of a physical therapist. They implement treatment programs developed by physical therapists, including exercise, ADL training and modalities, and report the results of their work and the status of the patient's condition to the physical therapist. Specific duties of the physical therapist assistant are regulated by state law. In general, the following tasks are specifically excluded from the practice of a physical therapist assistant: interpretation of referrals; initial examination, evaluation, diagnosis and prognosis; development and modification of a plan of care; delegation of patient care tasks; establishment and documentation of a discharge plan and oversight of documentation.

Physical therapy aides are support personnel who "help make therapy sessions productive . . . keeping the treatment area clean and organized and preparing for each patient's therapy" (Bureau of Labor Statistics 2000). Other tasks of the physical therapy aide include patient transportation and clerical functions. Training as an aide is usually provided at the clinical site by physical therapists. Qualifications for aides vary widely although a minimum of a high school education is usual.

The Rehabilitation Team

We will now introduce other health assessment and treating professionals who work with persons with disabilities:

- Speech-language pathologists
- Orthotists/prosthetists
- Recreational therapists
- Social workers

Each of these occupations has its own professional organization, is licensed in most states, and provides specialized services based on the specific needs of persons with disabilities (see Table 12–2).

Speech-language pathologists and audiologists examine and plan interventions to care for the speech, hearing, and swallowing disorders common to many persons with acquired and congenital disabilities. The primary function of the speech-language pathologist is to assess and treat disorders in the comprehension and production of speech and related language disorders, such as aphasia. Speech-language pathologists also assess and treat dysphagia, or swallowing dysfunction. Audiologists assess and treat hearing loss. Speech-language pathologists and audiologists are employed in schools, hospitals, rehabilitation centers, outpatient clinics, and private practices. The American Speech-Language and Hearing Association (ASHA) accredits the skills of speech-language pathologists and audiologists by awarding a Certificate in Clinical Competence (CCC) after completion of graduate

Table 12–2. Characteristics of Professions in the Rehabilitation Team

Profession	Education	Role
Speech language pathologist	Master's degree	Assess and treat speech comprehension/production problems
Audiologist	Master's degree	Assess and treat hearing problems
Orthotist	Bachelor's degree	Assess and fabricate external braces
Prosthetist	Bachelor's degree	Assess and fabricate replacement limb parts
Recreational therapist	Bachelor's degree	Assess and treat for leisure/recreation issues
Social worker	Master's degree	Counseling/case management

training, passage of a written examination, and completion of a supervised experiential training period (American Speech-Language and Hearing Association 2000).

An orthotist is a professional "specifically trained and educated to provide or manage the provision of a custom-designed, fabricated, modified and fitted external orthosis" (American Board for Certification in Orthotics and Prosthetics 2000). A prosthetist is a professional "specifically trained and educated to provide or manage the provision of a custom-designed, fabricated, modified and fitted external limb prosthesis" (American Board for Certification in Orthotics and Prosthetics 2000). A baccalaureate degree in orthotics and prosthetics or another field with completion of a certificate in orthotics/prosthetics prepares the entry-level practitioner for certification (American Academy of Orthotists and Prosthetists 1994). Individuals may be certified in orthotics (C.O.), prosthetics (C.P), or both fields (C.P.O.). Persons are certified either as practitioners or technicians. Practitioners assess, design, fabricate, and fit prostheses or orthoses. Certified technicians understand the components of an orthosis or prosthesis and can manufacture and repair these adaptive devices.

Recreational therapists provide "treatment services and the provision of recreation services to persons with illnesses or disabling conditions" (American Therapeutic Recreation Association 1987). Recreation therapists work in community settings, hospitals and rehabilitation centers, and long-term care facilities. A baccalaureate degree in therapeutic recreation is usually a prerequisite for employment.

Social workers and psychologists are employed in medical and community-based settings to help people manage complex personal and social situations. Psychologists are master's degree or doctorate trained persons who provide formalized testing and intervention plans for behavioral and cognitive problems. Social workers are employed across the health care system. Examples of areas where social workers provide services are substance abuse, developmental disabilities, aging, and welfare programs (National Association of Social Workers 2000). Social workers provide services to individuals and families through direct counseling, consultation, and care coordination (Bureau of Labor Statistics 2000). A minimum of a baccalaureate degree is required to be a social worker, although a master's degree is generally accepted as the entry-level requirement for employment (National Association of Social Workers 2000).

Medicine

Medicine is the art and science of diagnosing and treating illnesses and deformities caused by disease or injury. Medicine has its roots in antiquity, and physicians are an important part of the contemporary medical care system. Physicians are licensed by the states to practice medicine (see Table 12–3). Licensure requires a medical doctor degree or a doctor of osteopathy degree, completion of a residency, successful passage of a licensure examination, citizenship or resident alien status, certification of moral character, and the payment of a fee. Physicians work in patient care,

Table 12– 3.   Characteristics of Physicians and Nurses

Characteristic	Physicians	Nurses
Number	730,000	2.2 million
Roles	Patient care, administration, research and education, public health	Patient care, administration, research and education, public health
Educational level	Clinical doctorate	Associate degree, bachelor's degree
Practice sites	Clinics, hospitals, government, insurance industry, academic institutions	Hospitals, nursing homes, schools, industrial clinics, private offices, academic institutions, insurance, home health and hospice, government

administration, medical research and education, government, the insurance industry, state and local health departments, and the pharmaceutical industry.

There are about 730,000 physicians in the United States (American Medical Association 2000; American Osteopathic Medicine Association 2000). Physicians are trained in two systems: allopathic medicine (M.D.) and osteopathic medicine (D.O). **Allopathic medicine**, the larger system, is associated with most bioscientific, academic medical centers. **Osteopathic medicine** has its roots in the nineteenth-century manipulative medicine model (similar to chiropractic). In the early twentieth century, osteopaths adopted much of the bioscientific model, and by mid-century the two professions recognized each other's preparation for practice as a medical physician (Gevitz 1993; Frey 1999).

About 35 percent of the nation's physicians practice in primary care, which is defined as internal (adult) medicine, family practice, and pediatrics. About one in three allopathic physicians practice in primary care (Bureau of Labor Statistics 2000). The majority of osteopathic physicians (55%) are in primary care. The remaining 66 percent of the physician labor force practices in a variety of medical and surgical specialties. Obstetrics and gynecology, general surgery, anesthesiology, and orthopedic surgery are among the specialty areas with the highest proportion of members (Bureau of Labor Statistics 2000). Only 1 percent of osteopathic physicians practice primarily in manipulative treatment (American Osteopathic Medical Association 2000). A very small percentage of physicians (0.8%) practice in physical medicine and rehabilitation (American Academy of Physical Medicine Rehabilitation 2000). These specialist physicians, commonly called "physiatrists," can be found in rehabilitation centers, private practice, and other post-acute care environments.

About 60 percent of physicians practice in an office-based practice. Women make up an increasing number of American physicians. In 1970, women comprised 7.5 percent of America's 334,000 physicians. In 1999, women accounted for 23 percent of physicians in the United States (American Medical Association 2000). Four in ten U.S. medical students are women (Barzansky, Jones, and Etzel 1999).

There are 125 medical schools in the United States (Association of Academic Medical Centers 2000). A consensus statement on the status of the physician workforce in the United States notes that the country is "on the verge of a serious oversupply of physicians" (Association of Academic Medical Centers 1997). About 41,000 persons apply to U.S. medical schools each year (Barzansky, Jones, and Etzel 1999), and 97,000 physicians are currently in residency training (Miller, Dunn, and Richter 1999).

Nursing

Nurses are the largest and one of the fastest growing classifications of health care personnel in the United States. Nurses comprise about 25 percent of the health care workforce. The American Nurses Association reports that 2.2 million Americans are licensed as registered nurses, and about 1.85 million registered nurses are employed in the country (American Nurses Association 1999). Registered nurses are expected to be one of the top ten occupations in new job growth over the next ten years (Bureau of Labor Statistics 2000).

Ninety-five percent of nurses are women, and about 10 percent of nurses are from minority backgrounds (Bureau of Health Professions 1996). Sixty percent of nurses find employment in hospitals (Bureau of Labor Statistics 2000). Other sites of employment are in nursing homes, schools, public health agencies, industrial clinics, private offices, educational institutions, the insurance industry, and private duty. Registered nurses perform nursing examination, intervention, and care coordination functions for patients in acute and post-acute care environments. Licensed practical nurses, or LPNs, provide basic and routine nursing care services. Rehabilitation nurses provide specialized care for persons with serious disabilities.

Registered nurses are educated in two-year associate degree programs, three-year diploma programs, and four-year baccalaureate degree programs. The majority of registered nurses have less than a baccalaureate degree education (Bureau of Health Professions 1996). Nearly 700,000 persons are employed as LPNs in the United States (Bureau of Labor Statistics 2000). Education to become an LPN consists of one year of classroom and clinical study.

Registered nurses have four categories of advanced practice: nurse practitioner, certified nurse midwife, clinical nurse specialist, and certified registered nurse anesthetist (American Nurses Association 2000). Nurse practitioners act as primary care providers in a number of settings. They usually specialize in one area of practice (e.g., pediatrics) and act to diagnose and treat minor medical conditions. In many states, they can prescribe medications. Certified nurse midwives deliver about one in 33 babies in the United States. Practice is primarily in "well-woman gynecological and low-risk obstetrical care." Clinical nurse specialists have master's or doctoral degrees and are recognized as experts in a specialized area of practice. Certified registered nurse anesthetists provide anesthesia care, especially in rural settings.

Exercise-Related Occupations

Occupational therapists and physical therapists encounter many other health care workers in their professional practice. Laboratory technicians, radiological technologists, emergency medical technicians, dietitians, and medical assistants are but a few of the many occupations employed in the health care system. In this section, we will briefly introduce several other occupations that use exercise to assess and treat people with injuries or perform wellness activity functions (see Table 12–4).

An athletic trainer is a certified health care provider who delivers care to athletes in schools, sports clinics, and sports programs (National Athletic Trainers Association 2000). Trainers are involved in the prevention, evaluation, field care, and rehabilitation of athletic injuries. Some athletic trainers are involved in administration, and many provide education to students. Athletic trainers use taping and bandaging to prevent athletic injuries and are responsible for providing emergency care on the field. Athletic trainers have at least a baccalaureate degree education and have received extensive supervised clinical experience to achieve certification. Education is provided in more 100 universities in the United States. To be certified, a prospective trainer must pass a written examination administered by the National Athletic Trainers' Association Board of Certification. There are about 16,000 certified athletic trainers in the United States, of which 40 percent are women (National Athletic Trainers Association 1997).

Exercise physiologists and fitness trainers (see Table 12–4) are commonly employed in community fitness environments and in cardiopulmonary rehabilitation. To date, neither of these worker classifications has achieved licensure in any state. A number of organizations have developed criteria for certification in these fields. The American College of Sports Medicine, with 18,000 members, is perhaps the best-known in medical circles and has an interdisciplinary focus that includes medicine and the allied health fields (American College of Sports Medicine 2000).

Table 12–4. Characteristics of Exercise-Related Occupations

Occupation	Educational Level	Role
Certified athletic trainer	Bachelor's degree	Assess and treat athletic-related injuries
Fitness trainer	High school diploma/certification	Provide personal wellness/fitness services
Kinesiotherapist	Bachelor's degree	Assess and treat disabling conditions

The American Council on Exercise sponsors certification for personal-fitness trainers, certified exercise specialists, group-fitness instructors, and lifestyle and weight-management consultants (American Council on Exercise 2000). Certification can be achieved by taking an examination after studying a number of home-study publications. Minimum qualifications include being 18 years of age and CPR-certified, and paying the fee. The National Strength and Conditioning Association provides certification programs resulting in recognition as a certified strength and conditioning specialist or a certified personal trainer (National Strength and Conditioning Association 2000). Individuals desiring the CSCS must have a baccalaureate education. Certified personal trainers must have a high school diploma.

Kinesiotherapy is "the treatment of the effects of diseases, injury and congenital disorder by the use of therapeutic exercise and education" (American Kinesiotherapy Association 2000). This field was established in the post–World War II period to work with injured veterans in military hospitals. The American Corrective Therapy Association (which later became the American Kinesiotherapy Association) was founded in 1953, and a process of credentialing was established. Kinesiotherapists must complete a baccalaureate degree, pass a certification examination, and complete an internship before professional recognition. The field is small, with about 125 kinesiotherapists graduating each year. Many kinesiotherapists are employed in the Veterans' Administration health system, although they are also found in other medical and educational environments.

Complementary and Alternative Medicine Providers

The National Center for Complementary and Alternative Medicine (NCCAM) of the National Institutes of Health (2000) has defined seven categories of complementary and alternative medicine:

- mind-body systems
- alternative medicine
- lifestyle and disease prevention
- biologically based therapies
- manipulative systems
- biofield
- bioelectromagnetics

Some of these methods and procedures (e.g., yoga) are utilized in conventional medical and therapeutic practice. Other methods are common to certain socioeconomic or cultural groups (e.g., traditional Native American medicine). Many of these methods are commonly used by the general population (e.g., dietary supplements and lifestyle management). In this section, we will explore four providers who can be considered practitioners of complementary or alternative medicine: chiropractors, massage therapists, homeopathic physicians, and naturopathic physicians.

Chiropractic medicine (see Table 12–5) is defined as a manipulative and body-based system of alternative medicine (NCCAM 2000). Chiropractic medicine originated in Davenport, Iowa, in the late nineteenth century as a system of manipulative medicine. Chiropractors employ a noninvasive, drug-free, holistic approach to the management of the musculoskeletal system (American Chiropractic Association 1999). There are between 55,000 and 70,000 practicing chiropractors in the United States. Chiropractic education is provided in 16 educational institutions in the United States.

The philosophy of chiropractic medicine centers on self-healing of the body and the use of natural approaches to healing (Mootz and Phillips 1997). Similar to naturopathy and contrary to the allopathic philosophy, chiropractic does not emphasize the identification of external agents causing disease, but instead focuses on strengthening the body's capabilities to maintain and restore normal function. The importance of the nervous system in good health is at the core of chiropractic practice. Manipulation of individual spinal segments to alleviate malalignment of the spine and abnormal pressure on spinal nerves is intended to maintain and restore good health. Chiropractors who practice using only manipulation procedures are called "straights." Chiropractors who incorporate modality treatment, nutrition, and lifestyle counseling into their practices are commonly referred to as "mixers" (Mootz and Phillips 1997).

Chiropractic education consists of four years of professional training that includes clinical experiential periods. The typical first-year curriculum focuses on the basic sciences, the second and third years are spent on clinical sciences, and the fourth year is a clinical experiential year (Coulter, Adams, and Sandefur 1997). Chiropractors are licensed to practice and regulated in all 50 states and the District of Columbia (Sandefur and Coulter 1997). Private insurance companies as well as the major social insurance programs, Medicare and Medicaid, reimburse for chiropractic services (Jensen, et al. 1997).

Massage and bodywork is another subclassification of a manipulative body-based system of alternative medicine (NCCAM 2000). Massage therapy has been defined as the application of "manual techniques" and "adjunctive therapies" to

Table 12–5.   Characteristics of Selected Alternative Medicine Providers

Provider	Education	Role
Chiropractor	Clinical doctorate	Assess and treat using the manipulative model of treatment
Massage therapist	High School diploma/ certificate	Use manual techniques to improve health
Naturopathic physician	Clinical doctorate	Assess and treat using naturopathic model of treatment
Homeopathic physician	Clinical doctorate	Assess and treat using homeopathic model of treatment

improve the health and well-being of the patient (American Massage Therapy Association 1999). Massage therapy is regulated in 26 of the 50 states; 19 states license massage therapists. The American Massage Therapy Association and the National Certification Board for Therapeutic Massage and Bodywork certify therapists in massage therapy. A typical educational requirement is 500 hours of classroom preparation or experiential training.

Homeopathic and naturopathic physicians are other examples of alternative medicine providers. **Homeopathy** can be traced to the late eighteenth- and early nineteenth-century advocacy of Samuel Hahnemann (Gevitz 1993). Homeopathic physicians employ strategies to restore the homeostasis of the whole person who is ill or injured. The philosophy of homeopathy holds that substances that create symptoms in normal persons can be used to treat similar symptoms in persons with disease. Small doses of these substances are used to treat illness and disease (Frey 1999a). Naturopathic providers emphasize prevention, patient education, and the body's natural healing capabilities (vitalism) in treatment (Frey 1999b). Nutrition, herbalism, detoxification, and acupuncture are common treatment modalities employed by naturopaths.

In the nineteenth century, manipulative medicine, homeopathy, and **naturopathy** were competing systems with allopathic medicine. The successes of the bioscientific model in diagnosing and treating illness and injury (e.g., the development of microbiology) led to the rapid growth of allopathic medicine and the slow growth or decline of these other systems (chiropractic is a notable exception). Today, the limitations of the allopathic model in treating some forms of chronic disease have brought about a renewed interest in complementary and alternative medicine models.

Future of Health Care Personnel

The Department of Labor estimates that 14 percent of all wage and salary jobs created between 1998 and 2008 will be in health care (Bureau of Labor Statistics 2000). As a result, a 26 percent increase in total health care employment through 2008 is expected (Bureau of Labor Statistics 2000). The aging of the population and emerging technologies are expected to be the catalyst for job growth in health services. Many of these jobs will be in technical positions. Change is on the horizon for health care professionals. The rise of managed care and the budget challenges in social insurance programs are creating uncertainty for the future of health care professionals.

Occupational therapy and physical therapy are good examples of this trend. Until the late 1990s, occupational therapy and physical therapy had experienced increasing employment opportunities for nearly 40 years. This was fueled by the growth in reimbursement and the post-acute health care system. Cuts in rehabilitation reimbursement in the Medicare program changed the picture by early 1999 (Saphir 1999). By mid-1999, data from an American Physical Therapy Association survey indicated that 3.2 percent of the nation's physical therapists were unemployed, up from 1.2 percent in 1998 (Goldstein 1999). In April 2000, the unemployment rate had fallen below 3 percent. The outlook in the present decade is more positive. Recent government estimates indicate that "although the effects of federal limits on reimbursement for therapy services will cause keen competition for jobs during the first half of the projection period, employment is expected to increase over the 1998–2008 period" (Bureau of Labor Statistics 1999, 205).

These changes and the increased uncertainty of some health care professionals have fostered a new trend: unionization. From 1996 to 1999, the Service Employees International Union doubled its medical care membership to nearly 600,000 members (Jaklevic 1999). In 1999, the American Medical Association and the American Nurses Association both formed bargaining groups for members (Jaklevic 1999). Unionization is an option only for workers who are employees of businesses. Therapists in private practice are excluded from unionization because of antitrust concerns. Currently, unionization activity in occupational therapy and physical therapy is minimal (Tumolo 1999).

In the future, health care personnel will need to adapt to the changing health care delivery environment. In the 1990s, the California-based Pew Healthcare Trust organized a commission to study the future needs of the health care workforce. Among other things, it recommended that the workforce become more sensitive to the needs of the contemporary health care system, improve ties between health care providers and the public, and require assurance of the continuing competence of all health care providers (Pew Health Professions Commission 1999). The educational system should consider the number of educational programs it implements in light of the number of practitioners needed in a community. The regulatory system should provide for public representation on health profession licensing boards, and a system of continuing competence assessment needs to be implemented. For individual providers, the Pew Commission outlined "21 Competencies for the Twenty-First Century" health care professional practice. These are listed in Table 12–6.

Conclusion

The health care workforce is large and diverse. Teams of workers are organized to treat medical problems that range from acute injury to chronic disease and disability. The increase in the number and type of workers in the health care workforce is tied to the aging population, the rising incidence of chronic disease and disability, the expansion in insurance funding for health care services, and increased public support for the educational preparation of health care workers. In this chapter, we introduced several health care occupations that are frequently encountered by occupational therapists and physical therapists. The future of health care personnel will be affected by both an increased demand for services for an aging population and the need to be cost-efficient with economic resources.

Table 12–6.   Pew Commission: 21 Competencies for the Twenty-First Century

1. Embrace a personal ethic of social responsibility and service.
2. Exhibit ethical behavior in all professional activities
3. Provide evidence-based, clinically competent care
4. Incorporate the multiple determinants of health in clinical care.
5. Apply knowledge of the new sciences.
6. Demonstrate critical thinking, reflection, and problem-solving skills.
7. Understand the role of primary care.
8. Rigorously practice preventive health care.
9. Integrate population-based care and services into practice.
10. Improve access to health care for those with unmet health needs.
11. Practice relationship-centered care with individuals and families.
12. Provide culturally sensitive care to a diverse society.
13. Partner with communities in health care decisions.
14. Use communication and information technology effectively and appropriately.
15. Work in interdisciplinary teams.
16. Ensure care that balances individual, professional, system, and societal needs.
17. Practice leadership.
18. Take responsibility for quality of care and health outcomes at all levels.
19. Contribute to continuous improvement of the health care system.
20. Advocate for public policy that promotes and protects the health of the public.
21. Continue to learn and help others learn.

Source: Pew Health Professions Commission, 1998. *Recreating health professional practice for a new century: Executive summary.* Used by permission

CHAPTER REVIEW QUESTIONS

1. Review the classification of health care personnel used by the federal government. Define the position of physical therapy and occupational therapy in this framework.
2. Define the role and responsibilities of occupational therapy and physical therapy in the health care system. Correlate educational preparation to these responsibilities.
3. Summarize the characteristics and responsibilities of other professions in the rehabilitation team (i.e., speech/language pathology, orthotics and prosthetics, recreational therapy, psychology, social work).
4. Describe the educational preparation, role, and responsibilities of the professions of medicine and nursing.
5. Summarize the educational preparation and characteristics of the occupations of athletic trainer, personal trainer/fitness specialist, massage therapist, and kinesiotherapist.

6. Define complementary and alternative medicine.
7. Discuss the history, philosophy, and practice principles of chiropractic, homeopathic medicine, and naturopathic medicine.
8. Describe the future of healthcare personnel in the twenty-first century.

CHAPTER DISCUSSION QUESTIONS

1. Turf battles are common to the health professions and occupations. What do you believe is (are) the source(s) of conflict between health care providers? Are these conflicts constructive or counterproductive to the professions and occupations? To the public?
2. Compare and contrast the philosophics of allopathic medicine and complementary/alternative medicine. Describe the practice of physical therapy and occupational therapy in the context of these differing philosophies.
3. Review the "21 Competencies for the Twenty-First Century" in Table 12–6. Identify the three competencies that you believe are most important. Discuss how you will implement these priority competencies in your practice group.

REFERENCES

American Board for Certification in Orthotics and Prosthetics. 1999. Practitioner certification—traditional pathway. Accessed at *www.opoffice.org/abc/pcbookofrules.htm* on May 26, 2000.

American Chiropractic Association. 1999. What is chiropractic? Accessed at *www.amerchiro.org/about_chiro/index.html* on May 26, 2000.

American College of Sports Medicine. 1999. Fact Sheet. Accessed at *www.acsm.org/media.htm* on May 26, 2000.

American Council on Exercise. 1999. Background sheet. Accessed at *www.acefitness.org/media/backround.cfm* on May 26, 2000.

American Kinesiotherapy Association. 2000. Our history: Employment and practice. Scope of practice. Accessed at *www.akta.org* on May 26, 2000.

American Massage Therapy Association. 1999. AMTA definition of massage therapy. Massage therapy facts for physicians. Accessed at *www.amtamassage.org/about.htm* on May 26, 2000.

American Medical Association. 2000. Nonfederal physicians in the United States and possessions by selected characteristics. Accessed at *www.ama-assn.org/physdata/physnow/nowgraf1.htm* on May 25, 2000.

———. 1999. U.S. physician population approaches 700,000. Accessed at *www.ama-assn.org/ad-com/releases/1996/pcd96.htm* on May 25, 2000.

American Nurses Association. 1999 Advanced practice nursing: A new age in health care. Accessed at *www.nursingworld.org/readroom/fsadvprc.htm* on May 25, 2000.

———. 1997. Today's registered nurse: Numbers and demographics. Accessed at *www.nursingworld.org/readroom/fsdemogr.htm* on May 25, 2000.

American Occupational Therapy Association. 2000 member profile.

American Osteopathic Medical Association. 2000. Osteopathic medicine. Accessed at *www.aoa-net.org/Consumers/omed.htm* on April 21, 2000.

American Physical Therapy Association. 1999. *Guide to Physical Therapist Practice.* Alexandria VA: APTA.

————. 2000. The physical therapist assistant: A profile. Accessed at *www.apta.org/About/about_pt/Profile_Asst* on April 24, 2000.

————. 2000. Demographics of the physical therapist assistant. Accessed at *www.apta.org/Research/survey_stat/pta_demo* on April 24, 2000.

————. 2000. The physical therapist: A professional profile. Accessed at *www.apta.org/About/about_pt/profile* on April 24, 2000.

————. 2000. A historical perspective. Accessed at *www.apta.org/About/about_pt/history* on April 24, 2000.

————. 2000. Demographics of the physical therapist. Accessed at *www.apta.org/Research/survey_stat/pt_demo* on April 24, 2000.

American Speech-Language and Hearing Association. 1999. Fact sheet: Speech-language pathology. Fact Sheet: Audiology. Accessed at *www.asha.org/students* on May 26, 2000.

American Therapeutic Recreation Association. 1999. Therapeutic recreation. Educational/career information. Accessed at *www.atra-tr.org/educat.html* on May 26, 2000.

Association of American Medical Colleges. 1997. Consensus statement on the physician workforce. Accessed at *www.aamc.org/meded/edres/workforc/consen.htm* on May 25, 2000.

Barzansky, B., H. Jones, and S. I. Etzel. 1999. Educational programs in U.S. medical schools: 1998–99. *JAMA* 282(9): 840–46.

Coulter, I. D., A. H., Adams, and R. Sandefur. 1997. Chiropractic training. In *Chiropractic in the United States: Training, practice and research,* chap. 3, 17–28. AHCPR Pub. No. 98–N002.

Frey, R. J. 1999a. Homeopathic medicine. In *Gale encyclopedia of medicine,* vol. 3, 1467–70. Detroit: Gale.

————. 1999b. Naturopathic medicine. In *Gale encyclopedia of medicine,* vol. 4, 2029–32. Detroit: Gale

Friedland, J. 1998. Occupational therapy and rehabilitation: An awkward alliance. *Am J Occup Ther* 52: 373–80.

Gevitz, N. 1993. Unorthodox medical theories. In *Companion encyclopedia of the history of medicine,* ed. W. F. Bynum and R. Porter, vol. 1, 603–33. London: Routledge.

Goldstein, M. 1999. Changes in the employment market. *PT Magazine.* 7(4): 20–22.

————. 1999. The effect of the Balanced Budget Act on employment of physical therapists. *PT Magazine* 7(11): 22–24.

Jaklevic, M. C. 1999. AMA to wear union label. *Mod Healthcare,* vol. 29, 2–3. June 28.

————. 1999. Associations join pro-union ranks. *Mod Healthcare,* vol. 29, 6–7. July 5.

Jensen, G. A., R. D. Mootz, P. G. Shekelle, and D. C. Cherkin. 1997. Insurance coverage of chiropractic services. In *Chiropractic in the United States: Training, practice and research,* ed. D. C. Cherkin and R. D. Mootz, 39–48. AHCPR Pub. No. 98–N002.

Miller, R. S., M. R. Dunn, and T. Richter. 1999. Graduate medical education 1998–99: A closer look. *JAMA* 282(9): 855–60.

Mootz, R. D., W. C. Meeker, and C. Hawk. 1997. Chiropractic in the health care system. In *Chiropractic in the United States: Training, practice and research,* ed. D. C. Cherkin and R. D. Mootz, 49–66. AHCPR Pub. No. 98–N002.

Mootz, R. D. and R. B. Phillips. 1997. Chiropractic belief systems. In *Chiropractic in the United States: Training, practice and research,* ed. D. C. Cherkin, and R. D. Mootz, 9–16. AHCPR Pub. No. 98–N002.

National Association of Social Workers. 1999. Social work careers. Accessed at *www.naswdc.org/PRAC/career.htm* on May 26, 2000.

National Athletic Trainers Association. 1999. NATA history. What is an athletic trainer? Accessed at *www.nata.org/brochures* on May 26, 2000.

National Center for Complementary and Alternative Medicine. 2000. Classification of complementary and alternative medicine practices. Accessed at *www.nccam.nih.gov/nccam/fcp/classify/index.html* on April 21, 2000.

National Strength and Conditioning Association. 1999. The certified strength and conditioning specialist credential. The NSCA-certified personal trainer credential. Accessed at *www.Nsca-cc.org* on May 26, 2000.

Pew Health Professions Commission. 1998. Recreating health professional practice for a new century: Executive summary. Accessed at *www.futurehealth.ucsf.edu/pdf_files/rept4.pdf* on April 24, 2000.

Polsdorfer, J. R. 1999. Osteopathy. In *Gale Encyclopedia of Medicine,* ed. D. Olendorf, C. Jeryan, and K. Boyden, vol. 4: 2113–15. Detroit: Gale.

Saphir, A. 1999. How far they have fallen. *Modern Healthcare* 29: 12–13. April 12.

Simon, C. I., D. Dranove, and W. D. White. 1998. The effect of managed care on the income of primary care and specialty physicians. *Health Serv Res* 3(Pt. 1): 549–69.

Tumolo, J. 1999. Will PTs unionize? *Advance for physical therapists and PT assistants* 10: 25–26.

U.S. Department of Health and Human Services. 1996. Bureau of Health Professions, Division of Nursing. Notes from the national sample survey of registered nurses, March 1996. Accessed at *http://158.72.83.3/bhpr/dn.survnote.htm* on May 25, 2000.

U.S. Department of Labor, Bureau of Labor Statistics. 2000. Tomorrow's jobs. In *Occupational Outlook Handbook, 2000–2001.* Accessed at *www.stats.bls.gov/oco/oco2003.htm* on April 24, 2000.

———. 2000. Employment projections. Accessed at *www.bls.gov/news.release/ecopro.t01.htm* on April 24, 2000.

———. 2000. Health services. In *Occupational Outlook Handbook, 2000–2001.* Accessed at *www.stats.bls.gov/oco/oco2003.htm* on May 26, 2000.

———. 2000. Occupational data: National industry-cccupation employment matrix. Accessed at *www.bls.gov/empoils.htm* on April 24, 2000.

———. 2000. Occupational therapists. In *Occupational Outlook Handbook,* 2000–2001, 202–203. Accessed at *www.bls.gov/oco/ocos80.htm* on April 24, 2000.

———. 2000. Occupational therapy assistants and aides. In *Occupational Outlook Handbook,* 2000–2001, 345–46. Accessed at *www.bls.gov/oco/ocos80.htm* on April 24, 2000.

———. 2000. Physical therapists. In *Occupational Outlook Handbook,* 2000–2001, 205–207. Accessed at *www.bls.gov/oco/ocos80.htm* on April 24, 2000.

———. 2000. Physical therapist assistants and aides. In *Occupational Outlook Handbook,* 2000–2001, 345–46. Accessed at *www.bls.gov/oco/ocos80.htm* on April 24, 2000.

———. 2000. Physicians. In *Occupational Outlook Handbook,* 2000–2001, 193–96. Accessed at *www.bls.gov/oco/ocos80.htm* on April 24, 2000.

———. 2000. Licensed practical nurses. In *Occupational Outlook Handbook,* 2000–2001, 227–28. Accessed at *www.bls .gov/oco/ocos80.htm* on May 25, 2000.

———. 2000. Registered nurses. In *Occupational Outlook Handbook,* 2000–2001, 210–13. Accessed at *www.bls.gov/oco/ocos80.htm* on May 25, 2000.

———. 2000. Recreational therapists. In *Occupational Outlook Handbook, 2000–2001,* 209–10. Accessed at *www.bls.gov/oco/ocos80.htm* on May 26, 2000.

———. 2000. Social workers. In *Occupational Outlook Handbook,* 2000–2001, 161–63. Accessed at *www.bls.gov/oco/ocos80.htm* on May 26, 2000.

———. 2000. Speech-language pathologists and audiologists. In *Occupational Outlook Handbook,* 2000–2001, 214–16. Accessed at *www.bls.gov/oco/ocos80.htm* on May 26, 2000.

13

Mental Health Practice and Public Policy

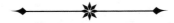

CHAPTER OBJECTIVES

At the conclusion of this chapter, the reader will be able to:

1. Describe the history of mental health policy in America from the perspective of occupational therapy practice.
2. Relate important perspectives of public policy and mental health policy.
3. Describe potential mental health practice settings

KEY WORDS: Deinstitutionalization, Holistic, Nontraditional Practice

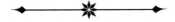

Introduction

No textbook about public policy would be complete without considering mental health practice. Since the inception of the occupational therapy field, occupational therapists have always worked in mental health practice. As the practice of occupational therapy has always been linked with mental health practice, this chapter will address mental health practice and public policy from the perspective of occupational therapy.

Historical and Policy Aspects
of Mental Health Practice

To place this discussion about public policy, mental health, and occupational therapy practice in context, it is beneficial to first overview some key perceptions about public policy. Ellek (1991) reflects that mental health policies often represent the values of society about mental illness, rather than an underlying theory of justice. Thus, this discussion will demonstrate how different values about mental illness have influenced key mental health policies, such as institutionalization and **deinstitutionalization**.

Another perspective we will consider is that the development of public policy is rarely sudden; rather, public policy is evolutionary over a long period of time (Grob 1991). The change in America's mental health system from a system of institutionalization to a community-based system reflected a slow, evolutionary process. Finally, trends in the overall health care environment, especially about reimbursement, influenced mental health practice. For example, the growth of managed care in the 1980s and the 1990s greatly influenced all aspects of the health care environment, including mental health practice.

To integrate these key concepts which shape the practice of mental health occupational therapy practice, we will continue with a discussion of the evolving philosophies of practice. During the early twentieth century, the moral, or humane, philosophy of treatment of persons with mental illness emerged. This paradigm encouraged the growth of occupational therapy. Occupational therapy was founded on the principles of a **holistic** approach to health care as depicted by the philosophy of pragmatism. This philosophy was dominant at the beginning of the twentieth century. Pragmatism considers the person's mind and body, temporal and spatial aspects, as well as social context (Breines 1995).

The arts and crafts movement, a part of the moral/ humane movement, was used as a treatment approach to help cure people. This movement, a counter-reaction to the industrialization of society, proposed a return to a more simple approach to life. Early occupational therapy mental health treatment also included "habit training," which involved scheduling people in very structured activities throughout the day (Zimke 1994). Additionally, from the beginning of the occupational therapy field, therapists treated people with physical and mental diagnoses in work programs (Lohman and Peyton 1997). Over the years, the profession moved away from this holistic perspective and became increasingly influenced by the biomedical model (see Chapter 1). The dominance of the medical model peaked in different historical periods, in particular between 1950 and 1980. In recent years, a holistic perspective has re-emerged with the development of the neuro-occupation and occupational science philosophies (Padilla and Payton 1997; Clark, Wood, and Larson 1998).

In the early to mid-twentieth century, societal policies encouraged state institutionalization of people with chronic mental conditions. As a result of these external, societal influences, many occupational therapists found employment opportunities in hospitals and state mental institutions. Mental hospitals exemplified society's moral response to care for the mentally ill. People with mental illness were viewed as having character deficits beyond their control (Grob 1991). Although humanitarian concerns were behind the original premise to provide state funds for mental institutions, economic considerations played a more paramount role (Grob 1992). Prior to the turn of the century, caring for the mentally ill was funded by local and state funds. With state legislation to fund institutions, local governments were more than willing to switch funding sources to the states. For example, state acts reclassified persons with Alzheimer's disease as having a psychiatric diagnosis and the institutional populations included patients who suffered from organic disorders (Grob 1992). Other researchers provide additional perspectives on the trend toward increased institutionalization of the mentally ill members of society. Ellek (1991) believes that institutionalization was based on the premise that mentally ill people were to be feared by society and thus needed to be protected by institutions. Camann (1996) reflects that institutionalization created an "out of sight, out of mind" mentality for families embarrassed by a mentally ill relative (p. 480).

Other historical events continued to influence the practice of occupational therapy. During World War I and World War II, the physical rehabilitation aspect of occupational therapy developed to meet the needs of injured soldiers. Occupational therapists did, however, continue to provide mental health treatment to soldiers. Mental health practice remained the largest area of occupational therapy practice during this time (Reed 1993). A holistic approach toward treatment continued with the development of rehabilitation practice after World War II (Cynkin 1995). However, by the 1950s, mental health practice had strongly separated from physical rehabilitation practice. After World War II, the recognition of mental illness as a problem grew. This awareness occurred after almost 2 million soldiers were rejected for service based on mental illness (Greene 1984). The National Mental Health Act (NMHA) of 1946 (Public Law 79–487) provided government funding for research, training, and the establishment of community clinics (Grob 1991). The NMHA also created the National Institute of Mental Health (NIMH), an organization that advocates for mental health concerns (Ellek 1991).

The 1950s was also a time of growth for medicine, and correspondingly, it has been described as an era of reductionism for occcuptional therapy as medical approaches came to dominate practice. The 1950s were perceived as a period of polar opposites in mental health practice, as represented by the dominant treatment perspectives of the time: psychoanalysis and behaviorism (Cynkin 1995). Occupational therapy treatment took place in public and private institutions. It was very common in the 1950s for occupational therapists to be employed by large state mental health institutions.

The influence of medicine, seeded in the 1950s, continued strongly with the impact of specialization on the field of occupational therapy between 1960 and 1980. Occupational therapists referred to themselves as specialists, such as mental health occupational therapy practitioners (Punwar 1994). The 1960s brought about much reform in the health system, as evidenced by the public policies of Medicare and Medicaid (Titles 18 and 19 of the Social Security Act, respectively).

Both acts helped to hasten the deinstitutionalization of elders from hospitals to nursing homes (Grob 1992). The Medicare Act, which covers inpatient and limited outpatient service, includes mental health practice. In fact, some of the initial Medicare language in the occupational therapy section of the Medicare Act used examples of mental health practice to illustrate treatment approaches. For example, the Medicare law mentions that occupational therapists may use the therapeutic activity of sewing with a person diagnosed with schizophrenia to help "reduce confusion and restore reality orientation" (Article 3101.9, Medicare Guidelines for Occupational Therapy Services). Occupational therapy mental health practice continues to be covered by Medicare. However, the Medicare law is regulated so that treatment is reimbursed based on the clinical setting. Thus, mental health occupational therapy treatment should be provided in mental health settings only. This perspective may have promoted a division between physical rehabilitation and mental health occupational therapy practice, rather than a holistic treatment approach.

The 1960s brought new and significant public policies that led to the deinstitutionalization of persons with mental illness and the growth of community-based mental health treatment. Deinstitutionalization was prompted by the Mental Health Centers Act of 1963 (Public Law 88–487). In the next decade Public Law 88–164, which provided funding for community mental health centers, further influenced deinstitutionalization (Punwar 1994). Deinstitutionalization was also strongly affected by the development of psychotropic medications, the overall economic impact of treating persons with mental illness (Ellek 1994), and the national mood of concern about the civil rights of persons with mental illness. This civil rights movement was influenced by a strong media campaign highlighting the poor conditions in mental institutions (Grob 1991; Punwar 1994). Other influences included a shift of thinking to consider socio-environmental factors and an increased awareness of community and outpatient treatment approaches from World War II. Psychiatrists who had served in the military later promoted deinstitutionalization and community-based practice (Grob 1991). Furthermore, the belief in prevention through early intervention in the community, and the enhanced social welfare role of the federal government diminished the authority of state governments and encouraged deinstitutionalization (Grob 1992).

The original goal of deinstitutionalization was to integrate those with chronic mental illness back into the community. However, as a result of inadequate funding for treatment, lack of aftercare services by state hospitals, and the focus of community mental health centers on acute conditions and prevention (Ellek 1994), people with chronic mental illness dropped out of the system and lost necessary services. Ignoring people with chronic mental illness was a paradoxical switch in values from the beginning of the century, when public policy had promoted taking care of the chronically mentally ill in institutions. At the time of deinstitutionalization, it was believed that chronic mental illness was caused by environmental and biological factors (Grob 1991). Thus, providing community-based centers based on a social model and moving the person with chronic mental illness back to the community was viewed by American society as a solution to this difficult problem. The reality was that community mental health centers did not address the needs of a chronic mentally ill population perceived to be untreatable, and instead focused on more treatable and varied conditions (Grob 1991). An unfortunate result of this policy change is that many people with chronic mental illness ended up among the homeless members of our society (Punwar 1994).

In the mental health arena, occupational therapists were slow to respond to the trend toward community practice, and many therapists continued to work in institutions and hospital-based programs (Adams 1993; Moeller 1993; Punwar 1994). Suggested reasons for why occupational therapists did not transition into the community mental health arena include insufficient understanding of community mental health practice and a lack of confidence in change (Moeller 1993). Meanwhile, the occupational therapy literature encouraged practitioners to develop community mental health resources (Adams 1993; Dasler 1984; Stokebrand et al. 1996). As Dasler (1984, 2b) stated, "Like their patients, OTs must break away from the security offered by institutional practice. For patients, the price of institutional security is loss of freedom. For our profession, the price is dilatation of the ability to move patients towards meaningful activity by continuing to use the artificial environment of residential facilities for training (p. 26)."

Corresponding to the major changes in the health care system during the 1970s and 1980s, occupational therapy grew in physical rehabilitation practice while the mental health practice area diminished. For the first time in the history of the field, physical rehabilitation and pediatrics dominated practice. Between 1973 and 1996, mental health practice by certified occupational therapists in psychiatric facilities decreased from 22 percent of total practice to 1.8 percent (Member Data Survey Update 1996). There is no simple explanation for the decline of mental health occupational therapy practice. Some of the factors mentioned in the literature are restricted reimbursement from managed care providers, unclear practitioner roles, and lower salaries in mental health practice (Gibson 1993). Other explanations are lack of research about the efficacy of practice (Bonder 1997), the elimination of positions, and smaller numbers of occupational therapy students choosing mental health practice because of a lack of exposure in their preparatory fieldwork (Kautzmann 1995; Price 1993). In addition, the societal stigma of working with persons with mental illness strongly influenced the decline in mental health practice (Paul 1996; Slady 1994).

Many occupational therapists who remained in mental health practice worked in traditional settings, such as acute care inpatient units, state institutions, or private hospitals (Adams 1993). While many state institutions closed down as a result of deinstitutionalization, new areas of occupational therapy mental health practice developed, such as working with alcohol- and drug-abuse programs, eating disorders, halfway houses, and residential treatment centers (Gibson 1993; Punwar 1994). These new areas reflected the movement toward outpatient and community services (Grob 1992).

A positive development for the field during the 1980s was the growth of theory in all areas of occupational therapy practice (Cynkin 1995). This brought about a return to viewing patients holistically and a theory-based approach to practice. Correspondingly, the new public policies on the national level (Community Support Programs and the Omnibus Budget Reconciliation Act of 1981) increased funding to community centers. These efforts attempted to meet the needs of the previously ignored population with chronic mental illness (Punwar 1994). At the same time, managed care grew in all areas of health care, including mental health practice.

During the 1990s, the number of occupational therapists working in mental health continued to decrease, perhaps because of unclear role definitions (Walens et al. 1998). In addition, mental health practice became more business-focused because of the strong influence of managed care. Therapists, however, began to develop new and unique areas of practice, such as working in the criminal justice system (Dressler and Snively 1998), vocational programming (Jeong 1998), and consumer-focused community rehabilitation programs (Feder 1998). Advocacy and leadership roles were encouraged for mental health practitioners (Dressler and MacRae 1998; Walens et al. 1998). The movement toward community-based and **nontraditional practice** continued to grow.

Another societal movement that encouraged persons with disabilities to remain in or enter the workplace resulted in the Americans with Disabilities Act (ADA) (see Chapter 5). This law guards against job discrimination and is considered to be a civil rights act for the disabled (Schneider 1998). It covers physical as well as mental disabilities and allows for "reasonable accommodations" on the job.

The American Occupational Therapy Association (AOTA) supports legislation related to mental health parity, or equal coverage of medical/surgical and mental health services. In 1996 the Mental Health Parity Act was passed. This law, valuing the importance of mental health care, requires lifetime dollar limits for mental health insurance coverage that are equal to those for medical and surgical services (AOTA 1998). Several states have enacted or are considering parity legislation (Metzler 2000), but there continue to be concerns about private system compliance with this law (Johansson 2000).

Practice Sites for Mental Health

Thus far, this chapter has addressed the growth of mental health policy and how the many changes have influenced occupational therapy practice. It is also helpful for practitioners to become more familiar with current mental health practice options. There are multiple options for occupational therapists interested in mental health practice, ranging from traditional hospital programs to nontraditional community-based programs. Each of these sites has its own philosophy of treatment.

State Institutions for Mentally Ill

The most traditional mental health treatment settings are large public institutions. Programming at these sites is often specialized by age groups or addictions (Punwar 1994), and in accordance with current trends in the health care environment, patients do not stay as long as in the past. As mentioned, these sites are currently not as prevalent because of deinstitutionalization. Occupational therapists employed by these facilities often do group-oriented treatment and community re-entry programs.

Hospitals

Treatment for mental health conditions in hospitals takes place in specialized units of general hospitals or in private psychiatric hospitals. The specialized mental health unit in a general hospital treats the most acutely disturbed people, often admitted for crisis intervention, after being triaged from the emergency room (Barry 1998; Dunton 1986). Admission can be voluntary or court-ordered. It is important for therapists to be familiar with mental health legislation related to hospital admissions. Overall treatment is based on the medical model, with a strong emphasis on pharmacological interventions. Thus, clients are regulated on medication to help them function better. Programming and the unit environment are planned to meet the needs and safety concerns of very disturbed clients in crisis, who are often violent or very disorganized (Richert and Gibson 1993). With the growth of managed care, the average stay in the hospital is very short, and patients who need additional support are often triaged to community support systems (Richert and Gibson 1993). Occupational therapists practicing on these units need to be flexible, prompt, accountable, and good communicators (Denton 1986). Since stays are so short they need to work on assessment for additional intervention, function, and self-esteem issues (Mosey 1986). Private hospitals primarily service individuals with adequate insurance or who are able to pay out of pocket for treatment. Sometimes these hospitals are specialized, such as providing treatment for addiction conditions.

Partial-hospitalization programs provide a less expensive alternative than inpatient hospitalization. These programs render support and medication monitoring to keep clients in their normal environment rather than be hospitalized. Recently discharged people from inpatient hospitals, people requiring crisis intervention, and community-living persons with chronic mental illness are helped by partial-hospital programs (Barry 1998). Usually there is a comprehensive program involving a multidisciplinary team, and there can often be role-blurring (Richert and Gibson 1993). Occupational therapy treatment focuses on home and community living skills, stress reduction, vocational skills, and social skills.

Community Health Centers

Community health centers developed because of the Community Mental Health Act of 1963 and are the largest treatment provider for people with mental illness (Punwar 1994). These facilities receive federal and state funding and therefore may receive guidance from community citizen boards (Richert and Gibson 1993). The goal of these facilities is to maintain people with mental health concerns in the community in their contextual surroundings rather than in hospitals (Mosey 1986). Table 13–1 lists required and optional mental health services for community health centers based on the Community Mental Health Act. If a community

TABLE 13–1.   Basic and Optional Services in a Community Mental Health Center
Based on the Community Mental Health Act

Basic Services	Optional Services
Comprehensive Community Health Center	
Inpatient	Diagnostic
Outpatient	Rehabilitation
Partial hospitalization	Precare and aftercare
Emergency services	Professional and staff training programs
Consultation and education to community, organizations, groups, and residents	Research and evaluation

Adapted from: Barry, 2002.

center offers all 10 services, and is located in a community with a population between 75,000 and 200,000, it is titled a "comprehensive community mental health center" (Barry 2002).

Programs in community health centers are becoming more consumer-driven than professionally driven. This emphasis helps to empower the clients (Feder 1998). Services offered by these centers address all age groups and may include outpatient therapy, medication supervision, chemical-dependency services, health prevention, and crisis intervention. Programming may occur during the day or evening. Occupational therapists employed by these facilities work with clients on community-living skills and social skills, and may perform case-management roles (Richert and Gibson 1993). Usually, far fewer people actually receive interventions from these centers than the number who need them (Abrams, Beers, and Berkow 1995).

Clubhouse Models

Clubhouse models, or community rehabilitation programs, are another interesting mental health alternative. These programs focus on skill acquisition for reentry into society and are based on a social rather than medical model. Thus, programming may include vocational skills, independent living skills, social skills, and stress-reduction skills (Richert and Gibson 1993). For example, clients adapting to community living may learn shopping skills, money-management skills, and transportation skills.

Adult Day-Care Programs

Adult day-care programs service people who require supervision during the day but can spend their evenings with supervised help in the community (Abrams, Beers, and Berkow 1995). We introduced this concept in Chapter 11. Day programs offer very structured environments providing group and individual interventions (Hooper 1998). Some adult day-care programs focus specifically on community-dwelling persons with mental illness, especially elders (Coveinsky and Buckley 1993). In spite of funding and regulation issues, adult day-care centers continue to increase (Abrams, Beers, and Berkow 1995).

Home-Care Programs

Home care is a growing area of mental health intervention. Treatment takes place in the home and is based on a social model rather than a medical model (Barry 1998). A multidisciplinary team, including occupational therapy and physical therapy, provides intervention. Occupational therapists working in this setting focus on maintaining the client's independent living and community-living skills.

Nursing Homes

Some elders with mental illness, often deinstitutionalized elders, are found in nursing home settings. Regrettably, for many elderly persons with mental illness who have been reinstitutionalized in nursing homes, there are no structured programs to address many of their mental health concerns. This could be a growth area for occupational therapy mental health practice.

Another growing population found in nursing home are elders with Alzheimer's disease. These individuals require specialized services, often offered in nursing home programs. Some programs focus on the continuum of specialized care designed to accommodate the residents' changing needs as they progress through the stages of dementia. For clients with Alzheimer's disease, Medicare will reimburse for therapy if there is a change in status or a skilled need–for example, if a client falls and breaks a hip. Practitioners can assume consultative roles in these units. Therapists have skills to adapt activities and address activities of daily living at the client's functional level, to develop and/or provide group programming, and to consult about environmental adaptations and behavioral concerns.

Geriatric Psychiatric Units

Geriatric psychiatric units address mental health concerns and the overall medical needs of elders. These units provide comprehensive, coordinated care of elders with major mental health concerns, such as major depression, psychotic disorders, and dementia with behavioral problems. Often these units include traditional rehabilitation services reimbursed by Medicare.

Nontraditional Settings

In addition to the traditional settings, occupational therapists are branching out into nontraditional community settings. Examples of nontraditional mental health settings are correctional centers, residential settings for people with mental illness, community programs for people on Medicaid (Kautzmann 1998; Wilberding 1993), health-promotion programs in community businesses (Maynard 1993), and occupation-based programs in independent living facilities (Clark et al. 1998).

Conclusion

As evidenced by this discussion, over the past 100 years the mental health treatment arena has gone through numerous changes. Much of the discussion has been about occupational therapy practice, and it is impossible to separate out the history of occupational therapy from the overall history of health care and the influence of public policy. Occupational therapists who work in mental health practice and want to continue to grow professionally need to keep abreast of policy changes and the multiple perspectives about public policy. By keeping aware, therapists will have a proactive rather than a reactive approach to policy and related historical events.

CHAPTER REVIEW QUESTIONS

1. Define the effects of pragmatism and holism on occupational therapy mental health practice.
2. Define institutionalization and deinstitutionalization as they affect mental health practice.
3. How has occupational therapy practice in mental health changed in the last century? What are the reasons for these changes?
4. Describe the persons served and the services provided in these traditional mental health practice settings:
   a. state institutions
   b. hospitals
   c. community health centers
   d. clubhouse model
   e. adult day care facilities
   f. home care
   g. nursing homes
   h. geriatric psychiatric centers
5. Identify two nontraditional mental health practice settings for occupational therapists.

CHAPTER DISCUSSION QUESTIONS

As a small group of four to six people, discuss one of these questions in depth. Choose a moderator who will share the result of the discussion with the class.
1. What societal values influenced institutionalization?
2. What societal values influenced deinstitutionalization?

3. What do you believe is current society's values toward persons with mental illness?
4. Provide several examples of how mental health policies often represented the values of society about mental illness rather than an underlying theory of justice.
5. Explain the concept that public policy is not sudden but rather a slow evolution.
6. Describe reasons why occupational therapy mental health practice was slow to move into community practice and how this influenced a decrease in mental health practice.

REFERENCES

Continuum of Care. 1995. In *The Merck manual of geriatrics,* ed. W. B. Abrams, M. H. Beers, and R. Berkow, 2nd ed. Whitehouse Station NJ: Merck Research Laboratories.

Article 3101.0 Medicare Guidelines for Occupational Therapy Services. Department of Health and Human Services: Health Care Financing Administration.

Adams, R. 1993. The role of occupational therapists and community mental health. In *Psychosocial occupational therapy: Proactive approach,* ed. R. P. F. Cotrell. Bethesda MD: American Occupational Therapy Association.

Barry, P. D. 2002. *Mental health and mental illness,* 7th ed. Philadelphia: Lippincott.

Bonder, B. R. 1987. Occupational therapy in mental health: Crisis or opportunity? *Amer J Occup Ther* 49: 495–99.

Breines, E. B. 1995. *Evolution, Adaptation, and Culture.* Occupational Therapy: A Self-Study series. Bethesda, MD: American Occupational Therapy Association.

Camann, M. A. 1996. Family-focused mental health care policy issues. *Ment Health News* 17(5): 479–86.

Clark, F. A., S. P. Azen, R. Zemke, J. Jackson, M. Carlson, D. Mandel, J. Hay, K. Josephson, B. Cherry, C. Hessel, J. Palmer, and L. Lipson. 1997. Occupational therapy for independent-living older adults. *JAMA* 278: 1321–26.

Clark, F., W. Wood, and E. A. Larson. 1998. Occupational science: Occupational therapy's legacy for the 21st century. In *Willard & Spackmans's Occupational Therapy,* ed. M. E. Neistadt and E. B. Crepeau, 9th ed. Philadelphia: Lippincott.

Coviensky, M. and V. C. Buckly. 1993. Day activity programming: Surveying the severely impaired chronic client. *Psychosocial occupational therapy: Proactive approach,* ed. R. P. F. Cotrell. Bethesda MD: American Occupational Therapy Association, 177–81.

Dasler, P. J. 1984. Deinstitutionalizing the occupational therapist. *Occup Ther Health Care* 1: 31–40.

Dressler, J. and A. MacRae. 1998. Advocacy, partnerships and client centered practice in California. *Occup Ther Mental Health* 14: 35–43.

Dressler, J. and F. Snively. 1998. Occupational therapy in the criminal justice system. In *Psychosocial occupational therapy: A clinical approach,* ed. E. Cara and A. Macrae. Albany NY: Delmar Publishers.

Dunton, P. 1993. Occupational therapy practice in acute care: Changes, challenges, and coping strategies. In *Psychosocial occupational therapy: Proactive approach*, ed. R. P. F. Cotrell. Bethesda MD: American Occupational Therapy Association.

Ellek, D. 1991. The evolution of fairness in mental health policy. *Amer J Occup Ther* 45: 947–51.

Feder, J. 1998. Bridging the gap: Integration of consumer needs into a psychiatric rehabilitation program. *Occup Ther Mental Health* 14: 89–95.

Friedlob, S. A., G. A. Janis, and C. Deets-Aron. 1993. A hospital connected halfway house program for individuals with long-term neuropsychiatric disabilities. In *Psychosocial occupational therapy: Proactive approach*, ed. R. P. F. Cotrell. Bethesda MD: American Occupational Therapy Association.

Greene, B. 1984. Evolving mental health policy. *J Health Adm Ed* 2: 193–200.

Grob, G. N. 1992. Mental health policy in America: Myths and will and realities. *Health Affairs*, 11(3): 7–22.

Hooper, J. B. 1998. Out of the ashes. *Occup Ther Mental Health* 14: 57–65.

Jeong, G. 1998. Vocational programming. In *Psychosocial occupational therapy: A clinical approach*, ed. E. Cara and A. Macrae. Albany NY: Delmar Publishers.

Johansson, C. 2000. Mental health care still limited, GAO says. www.aota.org accessed September 15, 2000.

Kautzmann, L. N. 1995. Alternatives to psychosocial fieldwork: Part of the solution or part of a problem? *Amer J Occup Ther* 49: 266–68.

Kautzmann, L. N. 1998. Contributing to system change in Kentucky: Occupational therapy in an evolving program of Medicaid managed behavioral healthcare. *Occup Ther Mental Health* 14: 21–28.

Lohman, H. and C. Peyton. 1997. The influence of the conceptual models of work in occupational therapy history. *Journal of Work* 9: 209–19.

Maynard, M. 1993. Health promotion through employee assistance programs: A role for occupational therapy's. In *Psychosocial occupational therapy: Proactive approach*, ed. R. P. F. Cotrell. Bethesda MD: American Occupational Therapy Association.

Metzler, C. and C. Willmarth. 2000. *The American Occupational Therapy Association (2000): Public Policy 101*. Bethesda MD: American Occupational Therapy Association.

Member data survey updates. 1996. Bethesda MD: American Occupational Therapy Association.

Moeler, P. 1993. The occupational therapist as case manager and community mental health. In *Psychosocial occupational therapy: Proactive approach*, ed. R. P. F. Cotrell. Bethesda MD: American Occupational Therapy Association.

Mosey, A. C. 1986. *Psychosocial components of occupational therapy*. New York: Raven Press.

Paul, S. 1996. Mental health: An endangered occupational therapy specialty. *Amer J Occup Ther* 50: 65–68.

Price, S. 1993. New pathways for psychosocial occupational therapist. *Amer J Occup Ther* 47: 557–59.

Reed, K. L. 1993. The beginnings of occupational therapy. In *Willard and Spackman's occupational therapy*, ed. H. L. Hopkins and H. D. Smith, 8th ed. Philadelphia: J. B. Lippincott Co.

Richert, G. Z. and D. Gibson, 1993. Practice settings. In *Willard and Spackman's Occupational Therapy*, H. L. Hopkins and H. D. Smith 8th ed. Philadelphia: J. B. Lippincott Co. 546–51.

Schneider, D. 1998. When do I disclose? ADA protection and your job. *Occup Ther Mental Health* 14: 77–87.

Sladyk, K. 1994. Are some occupational therapist and physical disability practice settings hastening extinction of mental health practice? *Amer J Occup Ther* 48: 174–75.

Stokebrand, K. S., K. A. Balckman, J. M. Madigan, and S. H. Cash. 1996. Can we influence practice preference? Examining the factors in seeking solutions. *Amer J Occup Ther* 50: 152–53.

Wilberding, D. 1993. The quarterway house: More than an alternative of care. In *Psychosocial occupational therapy: Proactive approach,* ed. R. P. F. Cotrell. Bethesda MD: American Occupational Therapy Association, 127–38.

14

Public Health

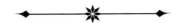

CHAPTER OBJECTIVES

At the conclusion of this chapter the reader will be able to:

1. Define public health and discuss the role of public health services within the overall health care system.
2. Describe the levels of organization of public health services:
   a. international
   b. federal
   c. state
   d. local
3. Describe the delivery of public health services:
   a. assessment
   b. policy development
      1. Healthy People 2010
   c. assurance of access to health care services
4. Discuss the opportunities for physical therapist and occupational therapist involvement in public health activities.

KEY WORDS: Epidemiology, Public Health Model

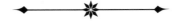

Introduction

For most of this book, we have been discussing the largest component of the health care system: personal health care services. Personal health care provides services to individuals who have acute and post-acute illness and injury. In this chapter, we will discuss another component of the health care system: public health. The public health system has existed in the United States since colonial times. The Maritime Health Service was established by the Congress in the late nineteenth century to prevent the spread of infectious disease from incoming ships and sailors (Sultz and Young 1999). Today, the public health system consists of a complex array of governmental agencies and services that not only measure and control communicable disease but are actively involved in the prevention of chronic disease and in the promotion of healthy lifestyles. Because their professional development has taken place within the medical model, physical therapists and occupational therapists have traditionally had limited involvement with public health activities. Most therapists are currently employed in the personal health care system. However, increased attention to chronic disease and the health of populations will create opportunities for rehabilitation therapists in public health settings.

We have several objectives to accomplish in this chapter. First, we will define and describe the function of the public health system. Second, we will examine the organizational scope of the public health system on the international, federal, state, and local levels. Third, we will explore the three fundamental roles of public health organizations: assessment, policy development, and assurance of health care services to their communities. Finally, we will explore opportunities for occupational therapists and physical therapists in public health.

What Is Public Health?

Public health is a system of surveillance and services to a population that are intended to identify and reduce mortality, morbidity, and disability due to illness, injury, and disease. Table 14–1 defines public health and lists 10 essential public health services that have been identified by the Public Health Functions Steering Committee (1994), a coalition of public health and governmental agencies. As can be seen from this definition of public health, the emphasis is on community action, prevention, and health promotion. These 10 public health services have been further subdivided into the three major roles of public health agencies as defined by the Institute of Medicine (1988): assessment, policy development, and assurance. We will explore these functions of public health agencies in more detail later in the chapter.

Public health services differ from personal health care care primarily because of their emphasis on populations, not individuals. Many of the major achievements in individual health and longevity can be traced to improvements in public health practices (see Table 14–2). Bunker and colleagues (1994) calculated that 25 years of the 30-year gain in age longevity during the twentieth century could be attributed to improved public health practices. Early and significant gains in public health focused on the identification and control of infectious disease (e.g., cholera, poliomyelitis). Today, the increased incidence of chronic disease is creating new public health challenges to prevent and control disablement. This situation is creating population-based practice opportunities for occupational therapists

Table 14–1.   What Is Public Health?

Public Health

1. Prevents epidemics and prevents the spread of disease.
2. Protects against environmental hazards.
3. Prevents injuries.
4. Promotes and encourages healthy behaviors.
5. Responds to disasters and assists communities in recovery.
6. Assures the quality of life and accessibility of health services.

Essential Public Health Services

Assessment

   1. Monitor health status to identify community health problems.
   2. Diagnose and investigate health problems and health hazards in the community.
   3. Evaluate effectiveness, accessibility, and quality of personal and population-based health services.
   4. Research for new insights and innovative solutions to health problems.

Policy Development

   5. Develop policies and plans that support individual and community health efforts.
   6. Mobilize community partnerships to identify and solve health problems.
   7. Assure a competent public health and personal health care workforce.

Assurance

   8. Inform, educate, and empower people about health issues.
   9. Enforce laws and regulations that protect health and ensure safety. Link people to needed personal health services, and assure the provision of health care when otherwise unavailable.

Adapted from: Public Health in America (Fall 1994), accessed at *www.health.gov/phfunctions/public.htm* on June 12, 2000.

and physical therapists in such areas as reducing repetitive workplace injuries (Keller, Corbett, and Nichols, 1997), developing fall-prevention programs (Gillespie et al. 2000; Harada et al. 1995), and designing health-promotion interventions for persons with disabilities (Rimmer 1999; Buning 1999).

Given the past accomplishments and future challenges of public health, the amount of money spent on public health services is only a small percentage of what is spent on all health care services (see Figure 14–1). In 1998, total national spending on health care services was $1.1 trillion. Government public health services accounted for $36 billion, or about 3 percent of national health care expendi-

Table 14–2. Twentieth-Century Achievements in Public Health

1. Vaccination
2. Motor vehicle safety
3. Safer workplaces
4. Control of infectious diseases
5. Decline in deaths from coronary heart disease and stroke
6. Safer and healthier foods
7. Healthier mothers and babies
8. Family planning
9. Fluoridation of drinking water
10. Recognition of tobacco as a health hazard

Source: Centers for Disease Control, *Ten great public health achievements: United States, 1900–1999* (1999).

tures. Spending on research, another role of public health, added $19.9 billion, or about 2 percent of national health care spending. Together, the nation spent about $56 billion, or 5 percent of total national health care expenditures, on public health. In contrast, Americans spent over $1 trillion, 95 percent of national health care expenditures, on personal health care services. The ramifications of this situation are that Americans value personal health care services more than public health care interventions. Note, too, that the personal health care service emphasis on cure of active pathology is much more expensive than prevention efforts advocated by public health agencies. One of the challenges for the public health system in the coming decades will be to increase public support and partici-

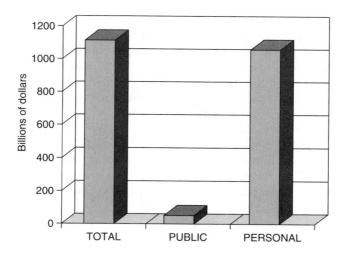

Figure 14–1. Spending on Public Health vs. Personal Health, 1998
Source: K. Levit et al., Health spending in 1998 (2000).

pation in effective public health promotion and disease-prevention activities. The governmental response to the terrorist strikes of September 2001 has highlighted the importance of a strong public health infrastructure in the United States.

Organization of Public Health Services

Public health is organized and delivered by different levels of government. Internationally, the World Health Organization is the public health agency of the United Nations. On the national level, the Public Health Service is a major component of the United States Department of Health and Human Services. Each state has a public health department. Many counties and cities have their own public health organizations. Rural or poor communities may lack a local public health organization. Sometimes certain responsibilities of public health are integrated within other governmental agencies. For example, management of toxic wastes may be the responsibility of an environmental department.

The World Health Organization (WHO) was created as a branch of the United Nations in 1948 (WHO 2000). The purpose of the WHO is "the attainment by all peoples of the highest possible level of health" (WHO 2000). The responsibilities of the WHO are listed in Table 14–3. These responsibilities include the surveillance of disease, development of policy, and implementation of basic health procedures for persons around the world, especially in Third World countries. In addition, the WHO has an important consultative function with governments. Among its major accomplishments are the worldwide eradication of smallpox and the near-eradication of poliomyelitis and leprosy through extensive immunization programs.

Table 14–3. Objectives and Functions of the World Health Organization

1. To assist governments, upon request, in strengthening health services.
2. To establish and maintain such administrative and technical services as may be required, including epidemiological and statistical services.
3. To provide information, counsel, and assistance in the field of health; to stimulate the eradication of epidemic, endemic, and other diseases.
4. To promote improved nutrition, housing, sanitation, working conditions, and other aspects of environmental hygiene.
5. To promote cooperation among scientific and professional groups that contribute to the enhancement of health.
6. To propose international conventions and agreements on health matters; to promote and conduct research in the field of health.
7. To develop international standards for food, biological, and pharmaceutical products.
8. To assist in developing an informed public opinion among all peoples on matters of health.

Source: World Health Organization, About WHO: Objectives and functions, accessed at *www.who.int/aboutwho/en/objectiv/htm* on June 12, 2000.

The U.S. Department of Health and Human Services is the primary federal agency with responsibilities for public health (Department of Health and Human Services 2000). The department has two major operating divisions: the Public Health Service and Human Services. The most extensive function of the Human Services division has already been explored in our discussion of the activities of the Center for Medicare and Medicaid Services (see Chapters 8 and 9). The Public Health Service has eight agencies (see Figure 14–2). These agencies are involved in support and delivery of a significant portion of the nation's agenda for health care research, education, and services to vulnerable, underserved communities.

The National Institutes of Health (NIH), with a budget of nearly $18 billion, is the largest medical research organization in the world. NIH has "centers" of research for major public health problems (e.g., neurological diseases, stroke, aging). The National Center of Child Health and Human Development includes the National Center for Medical Rehabilitation Research. This center is an important source of federal research planning and funding for occupational therapy, physical therapy, and rehabilitation research. The Food and Drug Administration (FDA) has primary public health responsibilities for the safety of food, pharmaceuticals, and medical devices, including therapy equipment. The FDA assesses and develops policy for assuring safety in many everyday products used by most Americans. The Centers for Disease Control and Prevention is the primary federal epidemiological research organization, responsible for surveillance and control of communicable disease and more recently, injuries. The CDC maintains extensive laboratories for the identification of infectious agents.

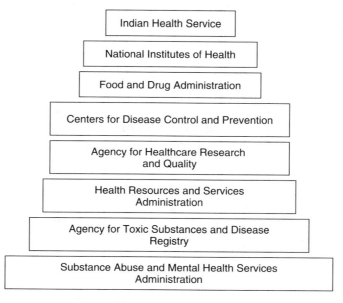

Figure 14–2.   Agencies of the U.S. Public Health Service

The Indian Health Service and the Health Resources Services Administration have important responsibilities to help improve the health of disadvantaged communities. The Indian Health Service provides primary health care services, including occupational therapy and physical therapy, for nearly 1.5 million American Indians and Alaskan natives in both rural reservations and urban environments (Indian Health Service 1999). The Health Resources and Services Administration provides grant funding to establish educational programs that will improve access to health services for people in underserved communities. Federal agencies provide direct services to the public and grant funding to state and local public health departments, universities, tribes, and other organizations to address public health problems in communities.

States have the primary constitutional responsibility for the health of their populations. Policy development is an important function of state public health agencies. Each state has a public health agency. In some instances it is an independent department, in others its public health functions are integrated within other state agencies (e.g., environmental quality). Many counties and cities have public health agencies that perform assurance and assessment functions at the local level. Some large local public health organizations participate in policy development.

This multilevel system of public health provides for the development and employment of extensive resources against public health problems. It also creates a complicated bureaucracy that has been criticized for being ineffective, excessively political, and reactive to public needs. The resources provided to public health agencies, however, are generally viewed as inadequate to manage the problems faced by these organizations. In the next section, we will discuss how public health organizations manage these challenges by functioning in their assessment, policy development, and assurance roles.

Assessment

Epidemiology is the foundational science of public health. The purpose of epidemiology is to identify the threats to a population and to devise a control strategy to reduce them. This is done by routine surveillance, which includes gathering vital statistics (birth and death records), analyzing water quality analysis and investigating disease outbreaks (e.g., the AIDS epidemic in the 1980s, the hanta virus outbreak in the 1990s, anthrax in 2001).

The purpose of epidemiological assessment is to identify the cause of the problem. This is done by investigation, using the **public health model** (see Figure 14–3). This classic epidemiological model is widely utilized to identify the cause of communicable diseases and develop effective control strategies. More recently, it has been applied to the problems of chronic disease and disability (Verbrugge and Jette 1994). In this model, the agent is the factor that is causing the problem. For example, the human immunodeficiency virus (HIV) is the agent causing AIDS. The host is the person who is the target of the agent and is afflicted by the disease or injury process. The environment is the third factor. The environment can posi-

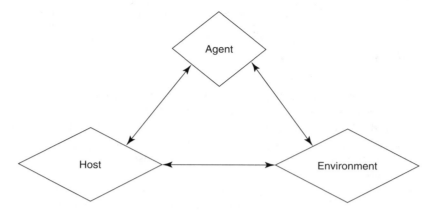

Figure 14–3.   Public Health Model

tively or negatively modify the disease process by affecting either the host or the agent. Strategies aimed at removing the agent, quarantining the host, or modifying the environment are fundamental strategies in managing public health problems.

Policy Development

Policy development is the second purpose of public health agencies. The identification of public health problems and strategies to control them requires planning, coordination, and education. Policy development begins with analysis and interpretation of the data. After this phase is completed, a strategic plan can be developed to address the identified problem areas. A good example of a state policy-development effort in public health is Nebraska's Turning Point program.

Turning Point was developed using grant funds from the Robert Wood Johnson Foundation in order to shape state public health policy in the first decade of the twenty-first century. A broad-based stakeholders group and "policy cabinet" was formed to develop and review this policy initiative. The result is a policy statement that defines the vision for public health in Nebraska and identifies eight strategic objectives for the state (see Table 14–4). The policy statement emphasizes development of a public health infrastructure in this rural state, the need to coordinate public health efforts, and an initiative to reach out to underserved and disadvantaged communities and to demonstrate the effectiveness of public health efforts.

On the national level, the Healthy People Initiative is an excellent example of public health policy. The Healthy People Initiative began after the release of a surgeon general's report in 1979 and has had several iterations over the last 20 years. The newest version, Healthy People 2010, is a "prevention agenda for the nation" (Department of Health and Human Services 1999). Healthy People 2010 was developed by a coalition of 600 governmental and private organizations that estab-

Table 14–4.   Vision and Strategic Directions for Nebraska Public Health

VISION: To have healthy and productive individuals, families, and communities across Nebraska.

STRATEGIC OBJECTIVES:
1. Build the public health infrastructure at local community levels.
2. Develop new and improved partnerships between state and local communities.
3. Build effective strategies to meet the needs of racial/ethnic minorities and create a culturally sensitive and linguistically appropriate public health system.
4. Develop innovative health-promotion and disease-prevention programs in non-traditional settings.
5. Develop more effective monitoring and intervention strategies to protect the public from environmental health hazards and safeguard the natural environment.
6. Build an integrated health and medical system that maintains an adequate safety net and improves access to high-quality services for all people in Nebraska.
7. Improve accountability by developing and monitoring performance-based standards and measures at all levels and in all programs.
8. Develop and implement a promotional campaign to increase the visibility and understanding of various public health activities.

Source: Nebraska Health and Human Services System, Broad strategies for change, accessed at *www.hhs.state.ne.us/puh/Tpstrat.htm* on June 12, 2000.

lished goals in 28 "focus areas" (see Table 14–5). The overall goals of Healthy People 2010 are to (1) increase quality and years of healthy life, and (2) eliminate health disparities between groups in the population. The Healthy People Initiatives include measurement and reporting of progress of the status of these national public health goals. As we will discuss later, the Healthy People Initiative has ramifications for the practice of physical therapy and occupational therapy.

Assurance

Assurance, the third role of public health organizations, is the primary function of local and state public health agencies. Assurance activities measure and determine whether the policy standards and goals are being achieved. In some policy areas, public health agencies have enforcement power. A good example is the regular inspection of restaurants by local public health agencies. A restaurant that does not maintain a clean food-preparation environment can be closed by a public health agency. In another example, the regulatory actions of state licensing boards restrict the professional practice of physical therapy and occupational therapy to qualified practitioners. Licensing boards have enforcement power to revoke the licenses of practitioners who harm patients or otherwise endanger the public health.

Public health organizations also act to provide basic health care services to their communities. On the local level, many public health organizations provide immunization and emergency mental health and dental health screening programs. Some local governments provide health care services to indigent persons through hospitals or long-term care facilities. As mentioned earlier, the Indian Health Service is a federal effort to provide primary health care services to American Indians. Many public health agencies have active health promotion and disease-prevention education programs.

Public Health and Therapy Services

At least 11 target areas of the Healthy People 2010 Initiative have applicability to occupational therapy and physical therapy practice: arthritis, osteoporosis and chronic back conditions, disability and secondary conditions, educational and community-based programs, maternal, infant and child health, mental health and mental health disorders, nutrition and overweight, occupational safety and health, physical activity and fitness, respiratory diseases, heart disease and stroke, and substance abuse (see Table 14–5). Movement-, fitness-, and physical activity-related public health issues are serious national problems. Francis (1999) recently reported that only one of the 13 national physical activity and fitness goals of the Healthy People 2010 Initiative had been met. Therapists, however, have not inte-

Table 14–5.   Healthy People 2010 Focus Areas

Access to quality health services	Injury and violence prevention
Arthritis, osteoporosis, and chronic back conditions	Maternal, infant, and child health
	Medical product safety
Cancer	Mental health and mental disorders
Chronic kidney disease	
Diabetes	Nutrition and overweight
Disability and secondary conditions	Occupational safety and health
Educational and community-based programs	Oral health
Environmental health	Physical activity and fitness
Family planning	Public health infrastructure
Food safety	Respiratory diseases
Health communication	Sexually transmitted diseases
Heart disease and stroke	Substance abuse
HIV	Tobacco use
Immunization and infectious diseases	Vision and hearing

Source: Healthy People 2010, Healthy people in healthy communities, accessed at *http://www.health.gov/healthypeople/About/hpfactsheet.pdf* on June 12, 2000.

grated these vital public health efforts into their everyday practice. For example, Fruth, Ryan, and Gahimer (1998) report that physical therapists provide health-promotion and disease-prevention information infrequently and rarely outside the "physical realm" of health.

The need to consider significant change in practice in light of the pressing public health goals in the area of chronic disease and disability has been advocated. Erikssen and colleagues (1998) found that even small improvements in physical fitness resulted in lower death rates for healthy middle-aged men. Finlayson and Edwards (1997), noting the shift to primary care away from specialty services, encourage occupational therapists to utilize the concept of occupation as a useful template for health-promotion and disease-prevention activities. As an example, Finlayson and Edwards (1995) reported on the Canadian Seniors' Health Promotion Project. This public health effort was implemented in two provinces by occupational therapists and resulted in active therapist involvement in advocacy for transportation services, the development of health-promotion videotapes, and a regular health-promotion column in a newsletter for seniors. Finally, Jette and colleagues (1999) demonstrated that a community-based resistance-exercise program for elderly persons could achieve high rates of compliance, improved lower-extremity strength, and lower rates of disability. This Strong for Life program was advocated as an effective public health strategy.

Conclusion

Public health is the organized program of assessment, policy development, and assurance activities performed to promote health and identify and control disease and injury in a population. Public health activities are performed by international, national, state, and local governmental organizations. Many of the improvements in personal health over the last century can be directly traced to public health efforts. While occupational and physical therapists have not traditionally performed in public health activities, the sedentary nature of American society and the increasing incidence of chronic disease and disability is challenging them to become involved in public health efforts.

CHAPTER REVIEW QUESTIONS

1. Define public health and its purpose in the health care system.
2. Compare and contrast public and personal health care services.
3. Describe the role and function of the World Health Organization.
4. Identify and describe the role of the agencies in the U.S. Public Health Service.
5. Describe the role and function of state and local public health organizations.
6. Define epidemiology and its use in the public health model.
7. What is the Healthy People Initiative?

8. Identify and describe three assurance functions of public health organizations.
9. Describe the involvement of physical and occupational therapists in the public health care system.

CHAPTER DISCUSSION QUESTIONS

1. Review Table 14–1 and Figure 14–1. Do you agree or disagree with current policy decisions regarding the allocation of money for personal health care vs. public health care services. Why do you believe this discrepancy exists? What should be done about it, if anything?
2. Many occupational therapists and physical therapists do not regularly provide health-promotion or disease-prevention information to their patients. What are the reasons for this problem? How can you ensure that each of your patients receives necessary health-promotion and disease-prevention information?

REFERENCES

Buning, M. E. 1999. Physical activity and fitness for persons with disabilities: A call to action. *OT Practice* 4(8): 26–31.

Bunker, J. P., H. S. Frazier, and F. Mosteller. 1994. Improving health: Measuring the effects of medical care. *Milbank Q* 72: 225–58.

Centers for Disease Control. 1999. Ten great public health achievements: United States, 1900–1999. *MMWR* 48(12): 241–43.

Erikssen, G., K. Liestol, J. Bjornholt, E. Thaulow, L. Sandvik, and J. Erikssen. 1998. Changes in physical fitness and changes in mortality. *Lancet* 352(9130): 759–62.

Finlayson, M. and J. Edwards. 1995. Integrating the concepts of health promotion and community into occupational therapy practice. *Can J Occup Ther* 62(2): 70–75.

——— and ———. 1997. Evolving health environments and occupational therapy: Definitions, descriptions and opportunities *Br J Occup Ther* 60(10): 456–60.

Fisher, T. F. 1998. Preventing upper extremity cumulative trauma disorders: An approach to employee wellness. *AAOHN J* 46(6): 296–301.

Francis, K. T. 1999. Special focus series: Health promotion and fitness. Status of the Year 2000 health goals for physical activity and fitness. *Phys Ther* 79(4): 404–14.

Fruth, S. J., J. J. Ryan, and J. A. Gahimer. 1998. The prevalence of health promotion and disease prevention education within physical therapy treatment sessions. *J Phys Ther Educ* 12(1): 10–16.

Gillespie, L. D., W. J. Gillespie, R. Cumming, S. E. Lamb, and B. H. Rowe. 2000. Interventions for preventing falls in the elderly. *Cochrane Library* (Oxford), 1–35.

Harada, N., V. Chiu, J. Damron-Rodriguez, E. Fowler, A. Siu, and D. Reuben. 1995. Screening for balance and mobility impairment in elderly individuals living in residential care facilities. *Phys Ther* 75(6): 462–69.

Indian Health Service. 1999. About the Indian Health Service. Accessed at *www.ihs.gov/aboutIHS/ihsintro.asp* on June 12, 2000

Institute of Medicine. 1988. *The Future of Public Health*. Washington DC: National Academy Press.

Jette, A. M., M. Lachman, M. M. Giorgetti, S. F. Assman, B. A. Harris, C. Levenson, M. Wernick, and D. Krebs. 1999. Exercise: It's never too late: The Strong for Life program. *Am J Pub Health* 89(1): 66–72.

Keller, K., J. Corbett, and D. Nichols. 1998. Repetitive strain injury in computer keyboard users: Pathomechanics and treatment principles in individual and group intervention. *J Hand Ther* 11(1): 9–26.

Levit, K., C. Cowan, H. Lazenby, A. Sensenig, P. McDonnell, J. Stiller, and A. Martin. 2000. Health spending in 1998. *Health Affairs* 19(1):124–30.

Nebraska Department of Health and Human Services. 1999. Turning Point: Nebraska's plan to strengthen and transform public health in our state. Accessed at *www.hhs .state.ne.us/puh/TPtoc.htm* on June 12, 2000.

Public Health Foundation. 2000. Where do the dollars go? Measuring local public health expenditures, 6. Accessed at *www.phf.org/Reports/Expend1/loclexpn.pdf* on July 12, 2000.

Public Health Functions Steering Committee. 1994. Public health in America. Accessed at *www.health.gov/phfunctions/public.htm* on June 12, 2000.

Rimmer, J. H. 1999. Health promotion for people with disabilities: The emerging paradigm shift from disability prevention to prevention of secondary conditions. *Phys Ther* 79(5): 495–502.

Sultz, H. A. and K. M. Young. 2001. *Public health and the role of government in health care.* In *Health care USA: Understanding its organization and delivery*, chap. 14, p. 352. 3rd ed. Gaithersburg MD: Aspen.

U.S. Department of Health and Human Services. 2000. Healthy People 2010. Accessed at *www.health.gov/healthypeople* on June 12, 2000.

Verbrugge, L. M. and A. M. Jette. 1994. The disablement process. *Soc Sci Med* 38(1): 1–14.

World Health Organization. (2000). About WHO: Objectives and functions. Accessed at *www.who.int/aboutwho/en/objectiv.htm* on June 12, 2000.

———. 2000. About WHO: Rapid overview. Accessed at *www.who.int/aboutwho/en/ rapid.htm* on June 12, 2000.

15

Effecting Policy Change:
The Therapist as Advocate

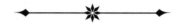

CHAPTER OBJECTIVES

At the conclusion of this chapter, the reader will be able to:

1. Recognize the role of the occupational therapist and physical therapist as an advocate.
2. Discuss the ethical responsibilities of the therapist as a patient advocate.
3. Relate the basic skills of effective advocacy
   a. self-reflection/attitude
   b. knowledge
   c. assertive communication
4. State the responsibilities of the therapist in client advocacy.
5. State the responsibilities of the therapist in advocating in professional organizations.
6. Discuss methods of effective advocacy in the health care environment.
   a. policy analysis
   b. lobbying
   c. legislative process

KEY WORDS: Advocacy, Coalitions, Empowerment, Lobbying, Reflection, Testimony

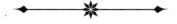

Introduction

Thus far the material in this book has focused on policy and systems. This chapter takes these discussions one step further by emphasizing **advocacy** skills. Therapy practitioners often encounter situations where they can make a difference through the use of advocacy skills. Advocacy involves standing up for clients and advising clients about their rights. It also involves advancing legislation, public policy, and social awareness (Sachs and Linn 1998). Health politics is expected to be one of the top 10 health trends in the twenty-first century(Coile 2000). Therefore it is of benefit for therapists to develop advocacy skills.

There has been very little research on the impact of client advocacy in the rehabilitation fields. Sachs and Linn (1997) studied client advocacy to determine when occupational therapists advocated, and what affected their advocacy behavior. From their qualitative research they identified three advocacy themes. The first advocacy theme was that therapists viewed themselves as "guardians of morals" for individual, professional, and social misbehavior aimed at their clients. The second advocacy theme involved representing the client's functional abilities to health and community agencies. This allowed the therapists to increase public awareness for helping people with disabilities. The third theme was working with the interdisciplinary team, which could be either supportive or restrictive. Thus, as this research study illustrates, advocacy is multileveled.

Advocacy is an important professional skill. It can help clients, be used with peer professionals to advance one's profession, and can bring about changes in public policy. In this chapter we will consider advocacy within all of these areas. First, we will discuss the linkage between advocacy and ethics, and then we will provide an overview of the advocacy skills necessary for therapists.

Advocacy and Ethics

The advocacy process is closely tied to professional ethics. Both the Physical Therapy Code of Ethics (APTA 2002a) and the Occupational Therapy Code of Ethics (AOTA 2000a) address advocacy. The Physical Therapy Code of Ethics (APTA 2000a) and the Guide for Professional Conduct (APTA 2002b) which expand on the code, highlight advocacy in several principles. Principle 1 of the Physical Therapy Code of Ethics states that physical therapists should respect the rights and dignity of all individuals (APTA 2002a, p. 1). This means that "physical therapists shall recognize that each individual is different from all other individuals and shall respect and be responsible to those differences" (APTA 2002b, p. 1). Thus physical therapists should not force advocacy on anyone who does not want it and shall respect personal differences when approaching advocacy. Furthermore, "physical therapists are to be guided at all times by concern for the physical, psychological, and socioeconomic welfare of those individuals entrusted to their care" (APTA 2002b, p. 1). This statement empowers physical therapists to advocate for clients. Principle 4 states that "physical therapists accept responsibility for the exercise of sound judgement" (APTA 2002a, p. 1). This includes referring the client to an appropriate practitioner "if the diagnostic process reveals findings that are outside the scope of the physical therapist's knowledge, experience, or expertise" (APTA 2002b, p. 2) and communicating findings to that practitioner (APTA 2002b). In addition, the Code of Ethics clearly states that physical therapists should address reimbursement concerns by informing patients of any known limitations. This implies advocacy. Principle 7 states that "physical therapists seek remuneration for their services that is deserved and reasonable (APTA 2002a, p. 1). Therefore, on behalf of patients, physical therapists do not "place their own financial interest above the welfare of individuals under their care" or charge unreasonable fees (APTA 2002b). Therapists should not underutilize therapy services because of constraints by third-party insurers. Finally, Principle 10 implies that physical therapists should render pro bono (reduced or no-fee) services to patients who lack the ability to pay for services, as each physical therapist's practice permits (APTA 2002b). Helping people who do not have the means to pay is a strong example of professional advocacy.

The Occupational Therapy Code of Ethics (AOTA 2000a) also emphasizes advocacy and even mentions the word "advocate" in principle 1 and its accompanying subprinciples. Principle 1 states that "occupational therapy personnel shall demonstrate a concern for the well-being of the recipients of their services (beneficence) (AOTA 2000a, p. 1). This is interpreted to mean that "occupational therapy personnel shall make every effort to *advocate* for recipients to obtain needed services through available means" (AOTA 2000a, p. 614). Advocacy also involves respecting the rights of the client, which is clearly stated in principle 3: "Occupational therapy personnel shall respect the recipient and/or their surrogate(s) as well as the recipients' rights (autonomy, privacy, confidentiality" (AOTA 2000a, p. 614.). Principle 4 mentions that "occupational therapy personnel shall achieve and continually maintain high standards of competence (duties)" (AOTA 2000a, p. 615). Therefore providing current and good patient care is a form of advocacy. Principle 5 states that "occupational therapy personnel shall comply with laws and the Association policies guiding the profession of occupational therapy (justice)" (AOTA 2000a, p. 615). Principle 5 clearly refers to policy on the association, local, institutional, state, and federal, levels. By keeping aware of policy on all levels, therapists can be advocates. Finally, principle 7 states that "occupational therapy personnel shall treat colleagues and other professionals with fairness, discretion, and integrity (fidelity)" (AOTA 2000a, p. 615). This principle refers to professional relationships. Being an advocate involves respecting other professionals as well as exposing breaches of the Code of Ethics to the proper boards.

Therapist Skills for Advocacy

In order to advocate, therapists need to have special skills, a correct attitude, and self-understanding. Without a proper attitude, advocacy efforts by therapists will not be successful. A proper attitude involves embracing the idea of being capable of making changes and being proactive with changes. Proactivity rather than reactivity is a very important skill in today's ever-changing health care environment. In addition, therapists need to understand their personal perspective and motivation for approaching client advocacy. Are they concerned about the person's well-being? Are they concerned about quality of care?

Are they advocating because of concerns for the profession? Understanding one's self-motivation requires **reflection**. Perhaps from self-reflection the therapist discovers that the motivation for advocacy comes from a personal reason, such as meeting an unfulfilled need, rather than from a client-centered or professional reason. In that case, the therapist will need to further reflect about his or her motivation for advocacy. Consider the questions in Table 15–1 to better understand personal motivation and advocacy.

In addition to self-understanding, therapists need to be knowledgeable about different systems. For example, to successfully advocate with the legislature, therapists need to understand the legislative process. (Advocacy with the legislature will be discussed later in this chapter.) Furthermore, assertive communication skills are imperative for successful advocacy. Therefore, it is beneficial to review these skills.

Assertive Communication

Assertive communication is empowering. It allows people to speak up for their own rights without stepping on others. To understand what assertive communication is, one must understand what it is not. Assertive communication is not aggressive communication. Aggressive communication is acting out or being angry to get one's way. Aggressive communication does not respect the rights of others. On the other hand, assertive communication is also not being quiet or passive. Being quiet about what is important allows others to achieve what they want to achieve at the expense of one's own position. Assertive communication is not passive-aggressive communication, or undermining others, such as talking about a person without the person being present.

Assertive communication involves clearly expressing one's feelings, beliefs, and attitudes. Different methods for assertive communication are presented in the

Table 15–1.   Reflective Questions for Advocacy: Therapists May Have More Than One Answer

I advocate because of:
  Concern for client's well-being
  Concern for quality of care
  Concern for the profession
  Concern for the health care environment
  Personal reasons
  Other reasons (please list)

Box 15–1   Example of DESC Methodology

<u>D</u>escription: I observed Mr. C. in room 210 eat lunch. He was noted to pocket food in his right cheek and not fully chew his food. In addition, I noted that he would cough with each bite.

<u>E</u>xpression: I feel that Mr. C. might have an aspiration risk.

<u>S</u>pecification of change: Mr. C. would benefit from a swallowing study.

<u>C</u>onsequences: That may prevent him from having an aspiration risk.

---

literature (Alberti and Emmons 1978). Davis (1998) provides one option: the DESC communication model. DESC is an acronym for *describing* the circumstance, *expressing* feelings, *specifying* the change, and identifying the *consequences*. The example of communication between a therapist and a physician in the accompanying box illustrates how a therapist uses the DESC method to advocate for a client who is an aspiration risk.

Assertive communication skills accompany advocacy skills and can be used on the various levels of advocacy. Assertive skills may be used in the health care system to advocate for patients. Patients in the medical system are often in a dependent role and have minimal control. Therapists can advocate, using assertive communication skills, for clients who are vulnerable. Assertive skills can also be used on the professional level. Therapists can advocate for appropriate referrals to help patients when therapy is not being utilized. Assertive communication skills can be used with the legislature to articulate professional concerns. The discussion will now address advocacy skills on these different levels.

Client Advocacy Skills

A traditional view of advocacy involves helping vulnerable people who cannot effectively help themselves (Namerow 1982; Carpenter 1992). Advocacy in this sense involves helping people who lack the ability to advocate on their own behalf, such as children, people with disabilities, or people unaware of available resources (Carpenter 1992). Therapists develop a rapport with clients that allows them to learn about situations that may require advocacy. Reporting someone for elder abuse is an example of advocating for a vulnerable client (Foose 1999).

As discussed, advocacy should be a reflective process. Reflection involves utilizing an in-depth problem-solving or clinical reasoning process. Therapists may ask themselves the following questions:

- Is it necessary that I intervene?
- Does the person want me to intervene?

- Can he or she self-advocate without my help?
- What resources are available to help the person?
- What would empower the person to self-advocate?

These reflective questions bring up an important discussion. When should a therapist intervene, and how can therapists empower clients to be their own self-advocates? Sachs (1989, as cited by Sachs and Linn 1997) found in her study that very few therapists helped patients or families by giving them the necessary information to self-advocate. Sometimes therapists or others may jump in when a person is perfectly capable of self-advocating on his or her own behalf. Allowing people to do their own advocating is empowering. Just providing the resource information may be all that the therapist will have to do. However, advocacy is important for clients who are incapable of self-advocating. Table 15–2 addresses some of the areas in which therapists can help with client advocacy. The list is not all-inclusive, and the reader may identify other areas.

The American Occupational Therapy Association (AOTA) and the American Physical Therapy Association (APTA) have government affairs departments that can help practitioners with client advocacy. Through the Trialliance for Health Rehabilitation Professions, consisting of the presidents of AOTA, APTA, and the American Speech Language and Hearing Association (ASLHA), advocacy efforts have been made to influence health care policy, such as with the Americans with Disabilities Act (ADA) (Evert 1995). Ultimately, these health policies positively in-

Table 15–2. Areas Where Therapists Can Help Clients Through Advocacy

1. Suggesting that a client seek legal advice and where to get it.
2. Providing an explanation of insurance plans.
3. Suggesting that a client seek counseling and where to get it.
4. Providing information to help the client make an informed decision (Sachs and Linn 1998).
5. Suggesting that a client get a referral to a specialist for better medical care.
6. Referring a client to social service for different types of help (e.g., with housing).
7. Providing suggestions of resources to enable a client to remain in his or her home.
8. Providing suggestions to family members for a client who has cognitive and/or communication deficits.
9. Educating clients about their rights to access appropriate health care.
10. Educating clients how to write Congress about key issues.
11. Educating clients how to appeal a denial of coverage.
12. Educating and communicating with managed care organizations (MCOs) on behalf of clients.
13. Acting as an expert witness in court.

fluence client care. In addition, both associations have committed to supporting outcome or efficacy studies that also improve client care.

Professional Level of Advocacy

On the professional level, therapists advocate with peer professionals and with others, such as insurers. There will be times in employment settings that therapists may identify misconduct in the way peer professionals deal with clients. Perhaps a therapist identifies that a physician has made the wrong diagnosis. Or maybe a peer professional has acted rudely toward a client. Or a peer has made the wrong treatment decision. Or the therapist may become aware of a peer acting in an unethical manner. Such matters should be reported to the appropriate agency (e.g., state licensure board) for review. Or perhaps a therapist identifies that therapy is not being given to a client who could benefit from physical or occupational therapy services. In that case the therapist will need to advocate for a referral. Handling situations with peer professionals involves diplomacy and assertive communication skills. Complete Exercise 15–1 to reflect about how you would handle advocacy situations involving peer professionals.

Another key area for professional advocacy is with employers to improve insurance coverage for therapy benefits. Often employers who self-insure do not understand the benefits and cost savings of therapy and may decide not to include it in their employee insurance plan. In such cases, meeting with key employers can make a difference for insurance coverage.

In addition, professional advocacy may involve educating other professionals about the benefits of therapy services, such as with the staff of an MCO. Communi-

---

Exercise 15–1

Answer the following questions as an individual self-reflection or in a group.

1. Describe how you would handle a situation in which a physician has ordered a treatment that is contraindicated. You are aware that this physician does not like to ever be seen as wrong.
2. Describe how you would handle a situation in which you find out that a patient has been misdiagnosed.
3. Describe how you would handle a situation in which you feel that a patient being reviewed on a treatment team would benefit from your therapy services.
4. Describe how you would handle a situation where you observe a peer therapist not providing the best treatment.
5. Describe how you would handle a situation in which you observe a peer engaging in unethical behavior.

cation and education can make a difference with case managers or other MCO representatives.

Advocacy with Professional Organizations

Both APTA and AOTA have legislative bodies that allow professional members to voice their opinions and influence the positions of the organization. The APTA House of Delegates is the organization's deliberative policymaking body. It meets annually to discuss and debate professional issues and to state policy positions of physical therapists to the outside community. AOTA has a legislative body called the representative assembly (RA). It is the governing and policy-making part of the association. "The RA consists of three standing commissions: Education, Practice, and Standards and Ethics and six Standing Committees: Agenda, Bylaws, Policies & Procedures, Credentials Review and Accountability, Nominating, Recognitions, and Strategic Plan (AOTA 2000f, p. 1). Just as in Congress, state representatives debate and vote on important issues at the national AOTA conference. It is important for therapists to communicate their stands on resolutions up for discussion to their state representative prior to the national conference.

Both APTA and the AOTA have government affairs staff to help lobby for issues. The APTA Department of Government Affairs maintains Web-based legislative action centers for both federal and state legislative affairs (APTA 2000c). In addition, an annual Federal and State Government Affairs Forum is held each year to allow members to meet, discuss, and mobilize for legislative action. A federal government affairs committee advises the department on critical legislative and regulatory issues facing the profession. The Physical Therapy Political Action Committee (PT-PAC) is the political fundraising arm of the profession and makes contributions to the political campaigns of candidates running for public office.

APTA supports members "participating in shaping the current and emerging health care environment" (APTA 2000d, p. 10). The association strongly encourages members to become active in other associations. In addition APTA actively works with members of different associations to promote the organization's needs (Connolly 1999). APTA also helps physical therapists on the state level advocate for concerns. For example, the national association provides "Take Action" packets with clear, precise information on advocacy (Griffith 1999; Wynn-Gilliam 2000). These packets provide educational background about issues, relevant APTA documents, and ideas for strategies (Griffith 1999).

AOTA government affairs activities include federal legislative activities, federal and state regulatory activities, and state policy support. AOTA works closely with individual members and state associations on state and national issues pertaining to occupational therapy practice. Legislative updates and calls for action about key legislative concerns are mentioned regularly on the AOTA Website and in AOTA publications. At the annual conference the government affairs staff educates members about important legislative issues.

AOTA also has an AOTAction Network. This network, consisting of contacts in each state, provides a local contact for distributing critical information and spurring action. AOTA sponsors educational activities and information to help occupational therapists learn advocacy skills and informs practitioners of important issues.

In addition AOTA has a political action committee called AOTPAC, or the American Occupational Therapy Political Action Committee. AOTPAC provides financial assistance to House and Senate candidates who support occupational therapy. This coalition helps ensure the visibility of occupational therapy in Washington and in politics.

Advocacy with the Health Care Environment

In the United States, the state and federal legislatures are available systems to allow citizens to advocate for concerns. As Scott Lee (1999, p. 5) states, "The framers of the Constitution believed so strongly in the people's right to participate in government, that they preserved that right, among others, for themselves, their fellow colonials, and the future generations of Americans." Today therapists advocate by lobbying for concerns that have an impact on therapy practice. Advocacy occurs in the legislative process and the regulatory process. Legislative advocacy involves being informed about legislative issues, **lobbying** through personal visits or letters, and being involved in political campaigns. Regulatory advocacy means being involved with providing input when the rules that implement legislation are written. A good example of the legislative advocacy process was the therapist advocacy concerning policies that capped the Medicare Part B reimbursement for therapists. The $1,500 therapy limit was widely recognized as inadequate for providing necessary therapy services. After a massive lobbying effort by the professional organizations along with individual efforts by therapists and clients, a moratorium was placed on it. This example illustrates several principles. First, therapists must stay aware of what happens in the larger health care environment that affects practice. Second therapists can make a difference through advocacy.

Now let us consider a regulatory advocacy example. This author (H.L.) made a difference on the state level by successfully advocating for legislative changes in the state worker's compensation law to increase therapy coverage. After reviewing the state law, she went to the billing officer of the hospital to express her concerns about limitations in therapy payment of key codes for worker's compensation clients. The billing officer immediately connected her with the lawyer for the State Worker's Compensation Court so that she could voice her concerns. From this communication she learned about an upcoming hearing. Along with a representative from the state occupational therapy organization, she prepared and presented testimony that resulted in increased payment for therapy services. Thus, successful changes because of advocacy can and do occur on the state and national levels, and behind every successful advocacy effort is the power of motivation and desire to make changes.

Therapists can advocate with representatives of the state and federal governments to promote issues that help therapy practice. Advocacy is most effective when done in **coalitions** or by groups of people with similar concerns. Although first attempts at advocacy may seem very overwhelming, sometimes just making the effort results in successful changes. Even if changes are not successful, just getting involved is a learning experience. When advocating with the legislature, it is important to understand the bigger picture about the current legislature, or its power structure. Therapists should know the positions of the stakeholders and the majority and minority parties on important health care issues (Callahan, 2000). Timing is essential. Obviously a legislator will be most interested in viewpoints before a vote is taken. The following sequence highlights one method to promote advocacy with state and federal legislatures (Vermithrax 2000). As noted in this discussion, there are many points in the sequence where therapists will need to critically analyze the political process.

Sequence for Advocacy

Step I: Knowledge

Therapists should become aware of key issues that concern state or national therapy practice. Knowledge comes from communication with state and national professional associations, professional news bulletins, professional Internet sites, state agencies, and the media.

Step II: Research

From doing research, therapists determine the key issues involved in the identified legislation so as to develop a clear understanding of the intent of the bill. It helps to understand whether the bill is addressing a feature of a problem or the actual problem (Callahan 2000). In addition, it helps to have an understanding of any previous legislative history (Callahan 2000) and what may be missing from the current legislation. It is also interesting to consider how the issue is being presented by the media (Callahan 2000). Are the real facts being presented, or are biases being presented? Reading the actual legislative language of the bills and comparing similar bills helps to clarify the different opinions. It also helps to be able to understand and articulate the reasons for opposing viewpoints. Therapists need to determine who (i.e. professional organization, coalition, political party) is behind the proposed legislation as well as who is against the proposed legislation, and their viewpoints. This involves identifying the key people involved with the proposed legislation and networking with them. Securing their cooperation as allies helps make successful changes. Attending coalition meetings with them can be very beneficial to clarify the political picture about the legislation. Some members of a coalition may share research about the legislation that benefits all members.

Networking is also done with other rehabilitation professionals. For example, an occupational therapist in charge of legislative issues for a state organization may network with the legislative representative in the state physical therapy association about an issue. Therapists will also need to do additional journal or Internet research to better understand the bill. Internet sites often provide analyses of legislation. However, critical readers will need to consider the source of the information. Is the source supportive of one's viewpoints, and even if it is supportive, does it provide accurate information? This step is completed when therapists are ready to take positive action because they clearly understand all the issues related to a bill.

Step III: Implementing Political Action

In order to implement political action, therapists must identify their state and national legislative representatives and their stances on the legislation. If they do not know this information, awareness can come from many sources, including attending coalitions or getting information from the library, newspaper articles, or Internet sites. The APTA and AOTA sites and other Internet sites have links that make it possible to find out who one's legislative representatives are. Or one can call the U.S. Capitol switchboard at (202) 224–3121 and ask for the office of one's senator and/or representative. Newspaper articles will quote the key players and their stances on the legislation as well as public opinions. The Internet site of one's senator and representative can also help in determining their position on an issue.

Implementing political action involves communicating with the appropriate legislative personnel. A key to successful advocacy is working with the staff people of the legislator. These people are the gatekeepers for the legislative representative and should be treated with respect. Furthermore, therapists should network with representatives from their own constituency. Letters are a popular method for communicating with legislators. Table 15–3 lists hints for writing about a specific act/bill.

A Legislative Visit

Another very successful advocacy technique is scheduling a visit with the federal or state legislator. Ideally, it is helpful to visit someone who supports a bill or who is undecided about an issue. Sometimes meeting with a person who opposes a bill can provide a clearer picture of another perspective, which is important for critical analysis of a bill. This meeting may result in changing the legislator's opinion, or at the very minimum make him/her aware of your concerns. Visiting legislative offices is very important, as legislators are very sensitive to public opinion because of their political needs. Often therapists end up meeting with staff members. However, as stated earlier, never underestimate the power of a staff member. Table 15–4 provides hints for talking with legislative personnel. Legislators on the federal level will always have staff personnel. On the state level, legislators may or may not have a staff representative.

Table 15–3.   Writing a Letter to a Legislator about a Specific Act or Bill

1. Use a professional letterhead. Use personal letterhead if your home is in the legislator's district and the address is in a different district than work.
2. Addressing correspondence:

To a Representative

The Honorable (full name)
__(Rm.#)__(name of)House Office Building
United States House of Representatives
Washington, DC 20515
Dear Representative:

To a Senator

The Honorable (full name)
__(Rm.#)__(name of)Senate Office Building
United States Senate
Washington, DC 20510
Dear Senator:

To a Committee Chair or Speaker

Dear Mr. Chairman or Madam Chairwoman: Or Dear Mr. Speaker:

3. Clearly state in the first paragraph the number and name of bill and your position.
4. Make the letter clear and concise, usually no longer than one page. Limit issues presented.
5. Use specific examples to support your views. If applicable, provide examples from your practice area.
6. Try to use your own verbiage and not to copy a form letter. Accessing a form letter can be a good beginning resource.
7. When representing an organization, it is important that everyone has the same stated stand.
8. Be constructive and provide solutions, not just complaints.
9. The same guidelines apply for writing e-mails to congressional representatives as with writing letters. Remember to keep the e-mails original.
10. Faxes are also an expedient method for communication. Fax numbers can be obtained from the same source as legislative and congressional telephone numbers.

Source: The American Occupational Therapy Association, 2000d *www.learn2.com* or *http://www .propeople.org/advocate.htm* or *http://www.apha.org/legislative/Writingtips.htm*

Appearing at Hearings and Preparing Testimony

Table 15–5 summarizes the legislative process. Prior to appearing at hearings and providing **testimony** therapists should review the legislative process, noting the many points where a bill can be killed. Therapists should also be aware that there can be

Table 15–4. Communicating with Legislators or Staff Members

1. Make an appointment by letter or phone clearly stating the reason for the visit. If telephoning, after identifying yourself briefly state your position on the specific bill.
2. If you receive an appointment with a staff member, ask to meet with the one who handles the issues that you are addressing.
3. Ask for the legislator's position on an issue if you do not know it.
4. Be aware of the timing of congressional recesses, as members often return to the home state during that period and it may be easier to make an appointment.
5. Work as part of the state and/or national therapy association (APTA or AOTA). As discussed, coalitions are more powerful. If going on your own, advise the state and/or national organization, because it can provide valuable resources. Also, members of the organization can advise you on how to present, if your stand differs.
6. Sometimes it helps to attend a meeting along with a coalition of other professionals to coordinate efforts.
7. Be prompt and dress professionally.
8. Be patient and flexible. It is not unusual for a meeting to be interrupted with other business.
9. Have facts clearly outlined on a handout to provide to the legislator or staff member. It is best to research the literature and have clear facts rather than an emotionally-based handout.
10. Stick with the key points on the handout, so that information is clearly presented. Communicating different stories can undermine the power of the coalition.
11. Bring educational materials to the meeting. Often a legislator or staff member is not familiar with the nuances of a situation. Therapy practitioners are experts on the impact of legislation on patient care.
12. Keep the meeting as an equal discussion, not as a lecture. Allow time for questions.
13. Remember the bigger picture by articulating the linkage between your stand and the interests of the legislator's constituency.
14. Describe how you or your professional group can be of help to the legislator.
15. If appropriate, ask for a commitment to your stance.
16. Be polite and respectful. Consider the visit as a beginning of an ongoing relationship, so keep communication channels open.
17. Do not monopolize their time. Plan on 15 minutes, as legislators and their staff members are busy people.
18. Provide a thank-you letter clearly restating the key points covered in the meeting. Include in this mailing any requested materials.

Source: AOTA 2000e, AOTA, *OT Advocate Packet* (2000); D. Vermithrax, Lobbying/advocacy techniques (2000).

Table 15–5.   Legislative Process: How a Federal Bill Becomes a Law

House	*Senate*
1. Bill is introduced in the House Bill is titled HR__.	**1. Bill is introduced in the Senate** Bill is titled S__. (Senate follows the same steps as House, with exception of the "rules" step.)
2. Bill is referred to committee Bill is carefully analyzed. If the committee takes no action, the bill passing is killed.	**2. Bill is referred to committee**
3. Bill is referred to a subcommittee At this point therapists and others can provide testimony at a scheduled hearing. The specialized subcommittee may "mark-up" the bill, or make changes to it, prior to recommending it back to the full committee. If the subcommittee votes not to report legislation to the full committee,the bill is killed.	**3. Bill is referred to a subcommittee**
4. Bill is reported by full House committee After obtaining the subcommittee's report, the full committee may do further study and hearings, which is again a time to testify. The full committee votes, or "orders a bill to be reported," on its recommendations.	**4. Bill is reported by full Senate committee**
5. Written Report Publication After full committee votes favorably to have a bill reported, the chairperson allocates staff to prepare a written report which includes the intent and scope of legislation, influence on existing laws, position of the executive branch, and dissenting views.	**5. Written Report Publication**
6. Rules Committee Action Many bills go to this committee for a "rule" to accelerate floor action and set conditions for discussion and amendments on the floor. Some "privileged" bills go directly to the floor for debate.	**5. Rules Committee Action** In the Senate the "rules" step is skipped. In addition, some bills may skip committee discussions and go to the Senate floor for debate.

7. Debate/Floor Vote
Bill is debated, often amended, or can be killed. If passed it goes on to the Senate to follow the same route.

7. Debate/Floor Vote
Bill now goes on to the next step of conference action.

Conference Action

After the Senate and House have passed related bills, and if the bill is significantly changed, conference occurs with representatives from both divisions to reconcile differences.

If the conference does not reach a compromise, the bill is killed. If differences are reconciled, a written conference report is prepared, which both divisions must approve. Bill is then sent to the president.

Presidential Action

The president has four options:

Option 1: Sign the bill and it becomes law.

Option 2: Take no action for 10 days, while Congress is in session, and the bill automatically becomes law.

Option 3: Veto bill. If the bill is vetoed, Congress can override the veto by a two-thirds vote in both houses.

Option 4: Take no action, after the Congress has adjourned for its second session, and the bill is killed.

Source: APTA, PT advocacy (2000c); AOTA, *OT Advocate Packet* (2000g).

key testimonial times during the process unless the bill is directly marked up to the floor. In addition, legislation can change quickly. Bills can be reintroduced with changes. Therefore it is important to find out if any last-minute changes have occurred. Table 15–6 provides hints for preparing and presenting testimony.

Advocacy on the State Level

Most of what we have discussed applies to advocacy on both the federal and state levels. What is unique about advocacy on the state level is that oftentimes it is easier to get in contact with state personnel about issues. Also unique on the state level is that some public policies, such as Medicaid, are combined federal-state laws. Therefore, state departments will have the responsibility for determining the particular state law. Therapists can have a strong impact when advocating with these agencies on a state level.

Step IV: Reflection

This step involves carefully evaluating what was and was not successful in the advocacy effort. Based on this step, alternative strategies may be tried if the initial effort was unsuccessful (Callahan 2000). Although reflection is written into the ad-

Table 15–6.   Preparation of Testimony

- Testimony involves research and clear facts. Like studying for an examination, therapists need to know their subject.
- Type the testimony and have others review it.
- Role-play presenting the testimony and time it.
- Prepare to answer questions or provide supplementary knowledge. Have someone role-play an advesarial stance to practice answering difficult questions.
- Know the names of all the legislators on the committee and something about their stands. Do your research!
- Address committee chairpersons as Mr. Chairman, Madam Chairwoman, Mr. Speaker, etc., depending on the person.
- Make verbiage clear and to the point. Do not use vague terminology such as "it seems," or "it appears."
- Present what the committee might want to hear, such as fiscal issues.
- Complete a pre-hearing briefing to determine that everything is organized.
- Make sufficient copies of the testimony to bring to the hearing and provide copies to members of the committee before the hearing.

Presentation of Testimony
- Dress professionally.
- Address comments to the members of the committee.
- With your introduction, identify yourself, your professional background, and the organization you represent. Relate the importance of the issue and thank the members of the committee for allowing you time to present. Always be very polite.
- Ask that your testimony be included in the record of the hearing.
- Articulate loudly and clearly. Do not read word-for-word testimony; rather, provide a presentation.
- Do not repeat information that has already been stated in prior testimony.

Answering Questions and Conclusion of the Testimony
- Close the testimony with a brief summary of your position, and offer to answer any questions.
- Be clear and consistent in your answers to questions, and not evasive.
- If you do not know the answer, offer to provide it in writing at a latter specific date.
- Do not appear intimidated.
- Follow-up with members of the committee. Be sure to promptly write thank-you letters. Include in the letters key points covered in the testimony and any requested materials.

Source: D. Vermithrax, Lobbying/advocacy techniques (2000).

Table 15–7. Reflective Questions after an Advocacy Effort

1. Were we proactive rather than reactive with our advocacy efforts?
2. Did we follow the steps for successful advocacy?
3. Which of our efforts worked?
4. What didn't work and why?
5. What would we do differently next time?
6. Who are the key people that we will stay in contact with? Did we properly thank them for their help?

vocacy sequence as a final step, therapists should be critically analyzing the advocacy process throughout. Table 15–7 presents some reflective questions to consider.

Conclusion

Advocacy is an essential skill that therapists should develop on many levels, whether with clients, professional organizations, other organizations, the state legislature, or the U.S. Congress. Even if one does not get involved on a state or national level, advocacy can be done in one's own workplace by helping clients and promoting therapy. Essential to the advocacy process is an understanding of one's own motivation and having assertive communication and critical thinking skills.

Advocacy Resources

Related to the legislative process and contacting senators and representatives

To obtain free copies of up to six federal bills contact:
    Senate Document Room, Rm. B-04 Hart Bldg., Washington, DC 20510– 7106 or
    House Document Room, Rm. B18 Ford Bldg., Washington, DC 20515– 6620.
To call or fax or visit a Website for the U.S. Capitol:
    202–224–3121 (number to get contact phone numbers of senators)
    FAX: 202–456–246
    Website: *http://www2.Whitehouse.gov/site*
To contact the Senate: *http://www.senate.gov/contacting/index.cfm*
To find out who is on specific committees: *http://www.senate.gov/committees/*
To find out the status of a legislative bill: *http://thomas.loc.gov/*
To locate your representative: *http://www.house.gov/house/MemberWWW.html*
To write your representative: *http://www.house.gov/writerep* (Sometimes professional sites like AOTA and APTA have direct links to contact the representative.)

To find out basics about Congress: *http://www.congresslink.org/basics.html*
To find out about current legislation: *http:/www.cspan.org*
To get information about health care policies from the Kaiser Family Foundation: *http://www.kff.org/*
To get information about health care policies from Families USA: *http://www .familiesusa.org*

Exercise 15–2   Advocacy Scenarios: Identify What You Would Do to Advocate in Each Situation.

Scenario 1: Mark works in an outpatient therapy clinic for a private company. He treats a large population of elders, particularly with orthopedic concerns. Mark's main concern is client care, and he does an adequate job rehabilitating the clients. He is, however, ignorant of the changes in the outer health care environment. If asked, he states, "I assume that the company I work for will keep me aware." Therefore, Mark is caught totally unaware when health care changes result in a prospective payment system with outpatient elders. Subsequently, when the prospective payment system is instituted, his hours are cut back due to decreases in reimbursement. What could John have done differently?

Scenario 2: Melissa works in acute care practice with people who have a variety of diagnoses. On the oncology floor she is working with a middle-aged woman who seems very depressed. This woman indirectly hints of suicide. What should Melissa do?

Scenario 3: Mimmi works in an interdisciplinary rehabilitation department. She is a certified hand therapist and has over 10 years working with that population. Lately, a new secretary in the department has been assigning the clients as the orders are processed. The secretary is now assigning clients with hand concerns to all the therapists, not primarily to Mimmi's caseload. Mimmi would like to follow more of the hand patients. What should she do?

Scenario 4: Melvin is the director of a small outpatient clinic. Lately he has noticed that his client load has decreased. He ignores the situation, thinking that it is temporary. Finally, he attempts to figure out what is wrong. By then it is too late, because he didn't realize that his primary admitting physician was unhappy with the care provided by one of the therapists in the department and is admitting elsewhere. How should Melvin have handled the situation differently?

Scenario 5: You are the administrator of a therapy department. You find out that Medicaid is not reimbursing for a key therapy service in your state. Describe the steps that you will take to obtain reimbursement.

Scenario 6: You become aware that one of your state senators is supporting some Medicare concerns of elders but not concerns related to therapy. Describe the steps that you would take to work with this senator.

Exercise 15–3   Self-Reflection

Identify a situation in which you were an advocate. Reflect about the following questions:
Were you successful? Why or why not?
Did you take a proactive stance in the advocacy effort? Why or why not?
What did you learn from the experience? What would you do differently?

Source for some of the above resources:
  http://www.apha.org/legislative/advocacylinks.htm

Internet Advocacy Resources

Related to Organizations

Agency for Health Care Policy and Research (AHCPR) *http://www.ahcpr.gov* which is part of the Public Health Service in the U.S. Department of Health and Human Services, supports efficacy and cost research.

American Association of Retired Persons (AARP) *www.aarp.org* has many resources for Americans age 50 and older. Strongly involved in policymaking.

American Chiropractic Association *www.amerchiro.org*

American Health Care Association (AHCA) *http://www.ahca.org/* deals with the concerns of those in the long-term care community.

American Medical Association *www.ama-assn.org/*

American Medical Student Association *http://www.amsa.org/* has many advocacy resources, including an advocacy tool kit.

American Occupational Therapy Association *http://www.aota.org/*

American Physical Therapy Association *http://www.apta.org/*

American Psychological Association *http://www.apa.org/*

American Public Health Association *http://www.apha.org/* has advocacy resources.

Center for Medicare Advocacy *http://www.harp.org/* private nonprofit organization, focuses on Medicare and other issues for those with chronic conditions.

Health Administration Responsibility Project *http://www.harp.org/* helps with advocacy issues related to managed care.

Joint Commission on Accreditation of Healthcare Organizations *http://www.jcaho.org/* evaluates and accredits health care organizations.

National Conference of State Legislatures *http://www.ncsl.org/* helps legislatures and staff of state legislatures with resource information.

National Information Center for Children and Youth with Disabilities (NICHCY). *http://www.nichcy.org/*

National Rehabilitation Organization: *http://nationalrehab.org/*

National Senior Citizens' Law Center. *www.nclc.org/* helps with advocacy for people with low incomes.

Quackwatch, Inc. *http://www.quackwatch.com/* provides resources for dealing with medical quackery.

National Organizations for Disease and Disability Conditions

Most of these organizations have policy sections. Consider networking with them about mutual concerns.

Alzheimer's Disease
Alzheimer's Association *http://www.alz.org*

Arthritis
Arthritis Foundation *www.arthritis.org*

Brain-Injured
Family Caregiver Alliance *http://www.caregiver.org*
Brain Injury Association *http://www.biausa.org/*

Cerebral Palsy
United Cerebral Palsy (UCP) *http://www.ucpa.org/*

Diabetes
American Diabetic Association *http://www.diabetes.org/*

Emphysema
National Emphysema Foundation *http://www.emphysemafoundation.org/*

Epilepsy
Epilepsy Foundation *http://www.efa.org/*

Heart/Stroke
American Heart Association *http://www.americanheart.org/*
American Stroke Association *http://www.strokeassociation.org/*

Hospice
Hospice Foundation of America *http://www.hospicefoundation.org/*
National Hospice and Palliative Care Organization *http://www.nho.org/*

Mental Illness
National Alliance for the Mentally Ill (NAMI) *http://www.nami.org/*
National Mental Health Association *http://www.nmha.org*

Muscular Dystrophy
Muscular Dystrophy Association *http://www.mdausa.org*

Multiple Sclerosis
Multiple Sclerosis *http://www.msfacts.org/*

Osteoporosis
National Osteoporosis Society *http://www.nos.org.uk/*

Parkinson's Disease
American Parkinson Disease Association *http://apdaparkinson.com/*

Spinal Cord
National Spinal Cord Injury Association *http://www.spinalcord.org/*

Vision
Glaucoma Research Foundation (GRF) *http://www.glaucoma.org/*
Macular Degeneration International *http://www.maculardegeneration.org/*

Some of these references found on *http://www.patientadvocacy.org/links.html*

CHAPTER REVIEW QUESTIONS

1. Define the ethical responsibility of a therapist to be involved in advocacy.
2. Relate the basic skills of advocacy:
   a. Self-reflection
   b. Knowledge
   c. Assertive communication
3. Provide an example of therapist advocacy on each of the following levels:
   a. client
   b. professional
   c. organizational
4. Relate the features of an effective legislative lobbying campaign.
   a. legislative visit
   b. letter writing
   c. testimony provision

CHAPTER DISCUSSION QUESTIONS

1. Until relatively recently, therapists have not had to be seriously involved in advocacy efforts. Discuss how the advent of managed care and federal budget reform is making therapists rethink the importance of advocacy skills in professional practice.

2. Reflection has been emphasized as an important component of effective advocacy. Why is self-motivation important to advocacy over the long term?
3. Discuss an experience you have had in trying to effect reform or bring about institutional change. What did you learn from this experience?

REFERENCES

Alberi, R. E. and M. L. Emmons. 1978. *Your Perfect Right: A Guide to Assertive Behavior,* 3rd ed. San Luis Obispo CA: Impact Publishers.

AOTAction Network. 2000. *Helping to Ensure the Future of OT Through Congressional Action.* Bethesda MD: American Occupational Therapy Association.

American Physical Therapy Association. 1999. Right to care: A physical therapist's guide to creating positive change in managed care. *PT Magazine* 7(1): insert.

American Occupational Therapy Association. 2000a. Occupational Therapy Code of Ethics. *American Journal of Occupational Therapy,* 54(6): 614–16.

———. 2000b. How a bill becomes a law. In *Public policy 101,* ed. C. Metzler and C. Willmarth. Bethesda MD: American Occupational Therapy Association.

———. 2000c. Guidelines for a site visit for members of the U.S. Congress. In *OT Advocate Packet.* Bethesda MD: American Occupational Therapy Association.

———. 2000d. Tips for writing a letter to your member of Congress. In *OT Advocate Packet.* Bethesda MD: American Occupational Therapy Association.

———. 2000e. Tips for meeting with your members of Congress. In *OT Advocate Packet.* Bethesda MD: American Occupational Therapy Association.

———. 2000f. What is the RA? URL *http://www.aota/org*

———. 2000g. AOTA expands your influence. *http://www.aota/org/*

American Physical Therapy Association. 2002a. APTA Code of Ethics. *https://www.apta .org/PT_Practice/ethics_pt/code_ethics*

———. 2002b. Guide for professional conduct. *https://www.apta.org/PT_Practice/ ethics_pt/pro_conduct*

———. 2002c. PT advocacy. *http://www.apta.org/Advocacy,*

———. 2002d. House of Delegates Policies. *http://www.apta.org/Home/Members/ governance/governance*

American Public Health Association. 2000. Face to face meetings with policymakers. *http://www.apha.org/legislative*

Callahan, S. 2000. Educational innovations: Incorporating a political action framework into a BSN program. *J Nurs Ed* 39(1): 34–36.

Coile, R. C. 2000. Health care 2000: Top 10 trends for the new century. In *Russ Coile's Health Trends 2000,* Special Report, pp. 1, 4–12 (January).

Connolly, J. 1999. APTA battles the BBA. *PT Magazine* 7(7): 46–55.

Davis, C. M. 1998. *Patient Practitioner Interaction: An Experiential Manual for Developing the Art of Health Care,* 3rd ed. Thorofare NJ: Slack.

Evert, M. M. 1995. Presidential address: Our journey together. *Am J Occupa Ther* 49 (10): 1065–67.

Foose, D. 1999. Elder abuse: Stepping in and stopping it. *PT Magazine* 7(1): 56–62.

Griffith, D. 1999. Capital watch: Take action in your state. *PT Magazine* 7(3): 16–17.

Loukas, K. M. 1999. Representing you! *OT Pract* 4(11): 9–10.

Lozano, P., V. M. Biggs, B. J. Sibley, T. M. Smith, E. K. Marcuse, and A. B. Bergman. 1994. Advocacy training during pediatric residency. *Pediatrics* 94(4): 532–36.

Namerow, M. J. 1982. Implementing advocacy into the gerontological nursing major. *J Geront Nurs* 8(3): 149–51.

Sachs, D. and R. Linn. 1997. Client advocacy in action: Professional and environmental factors affecting Israeli occupational therapists' behavior. *Can J Occupa Ther* 64 (4): 207–15.

Scott-Lee, S. J. 1999. Lobbying for occupational therapy, *OT Pract* 4 (8): 5, 12.

Vermithrax, D. 2000. Lobbying/advocacy techniques. *http://www.trytel.com/~aberdeen /techniq.html*

Wynn-Gilliam, K. 2000. APTA mobilizes on manipulation: Association at work series. *PT Magazine* 8(2): 34–38.

Learn to write to your congressperson. *http://www .learn2.com/*

Tips on writing a letter to a legislator. *http://www.propeople.org/advocate.htm*

Glossary

Access   The ability to obtain a health care service when you need it.

Accreditation   A voluntary quality-assurance and improvement process whereby an organization is rated against accepted standards of performance.

Actuarial analysis   The insurance process that predicts the risk of covered events in the risk pool and calculates a premium for pool members called actuarial adjustment.

Advocacy   The process of identifying issues and participating in policymaking and policy change.

Allied health profession   A federal labor classification for certain non-medicine, non-nursing, health-assessment and treating and technical health occupations, including physical therapy and occupational therapy.

Allopathic medicine   Traditional medicine, with a focus on the source of disease from external agents. Associated with the biomedical model; graduates have the M.D.

Assignment of benefits   The process whereby a patient transfers insurance benefits directly to the provider from the insurer.

Assistive technology   Equipment, software, and devices that enable persons with disabling conditions to access and become more independent in their environments.

Barriers   Physical, social, and attitudinal obstructions to full participation in society for persons with disabling conditions.

Benchmarking   The measurement and comparison of performance over time or against a known standard.

Beneficiary   The recipient of the benefits from an insurance contract.

Benefit period   The length of time from day of admission to the hospital to 60 days post-hospital or SNF discharge. Used in determining deductible and co-insurance payments for the Medicare program.

Biomedical model   A perspective on disablement that locates the problem in the person with the disabling condition and the solution in medical care services.

Bundling   A term for the collation of fees for individual but related services into one new fee category.

Capitation   Payment mechanism for health care whereby a provider is paid a flat fee for each covered member in a health plan per month.

Carrier   Medicare Part B claims processor and reviewer.

Case-based payment   Payment mechanism for health care whereby a provider is paid for an entire episode of care. Typically paid as a per diem (day), per visit, or per episode payment.

Case management   The process of eligibility determination and coordination of services for a person receiving multiple health care services.

Case mix adjustment   A system of classifying patients for payment purposes by clinical characteristics and anticipated resource utilization.

Categorical eligibility   One of the methods to qualify for Medicaid; mandated in all states. Includes low-income women and children, wards of the state, and persons with disabilities (receiving SSI payments).

Chiropractic   A form of manipulative and body-based alternative medicine centered on the nervous system's role in health maintenance.

Clinical practice guideline   A statement of the process of care based on the best available evidence of the effectiveness and efficiency of care.

Clubhouse model   The use of the social model in community-based settings as a form of mental health treatment.

Coalition   A group of individuals or organizations that come together to participate in advocacy; a prerequisite for effective advocacy.

Community rating   A process of actuarial adjustment that assigns a premium rate based on people living in a geographic region.

Consolidated billing   The requirement for SNF to bill for all Medicare Part A services that prevents contractual providers (e.g., therapists) from independently billing for their care.

Cost-based reimbursement   A retrospective method of health care financing whereby a provider reports costs of providing care and is paid by an insurer.

Cost limits   Payment mechanisms utilized in insurance contracts to share/limit costs of health care. Includes plan limit, first-dollar coverage, co-insurance, co-payment, and deductible.

Cost shifting   Associated with underpayment of the true costs of caring for Medicare beneficiaries, which are then paid by private insurers who pay artificially high prices for care.

Credentialing   A process used by insurers and some health care organizations to ensure that providers achieve minimum standards of education and experience.

Custodial care   A facility that provides long-term residential and skilled health care services.

Defined benefit plan   The sponsor of the insurance plan predetermines the benefits for a health insurance plan. Typical of most forms of health insurance today.

Defined contribution plan   The sponsor of the insurance plan (e.g., business or government) predetermines the level of funding for a health insurance plan offered to eligible beneficiaries. Benefits are provided based on this funding and excess beneficiary contributions.

Deinstitutionalization   The predominant philosophy guiding mental health treatment since the early 1960s.

Direct access   The ability of a patient to obtain physical therapy and occupational therapy services without requiring referral from another provider.

Disablement   A process whereby a person who experiences an illness or injury develops a set of impairments, functional limitations, and disabilities. Associated with the medical rehabilitation model.

Dual eligibility   Persons who qualify for both Medicare and Medicaid coverage. Typically low-income elderly or persons with disabilities.

Dualism   Two sources of health policymaking in the United States government and private enterprise. A unique feature of the U.S. health care system.

Empowerment   A social attitude and philosophy that provides an environment and skills that enable people with disabling conditions to make and act upon individual choices.

Enabling factors   System characteristics that predispose a person to be able to access health care services (e.g., availability of insurance, provider location).

Entitlement   A statutory guarantee to a set of benefits for eligible persons.

Epidemiology   The science of public health; the systematic monitoring and investigation of disease and injury.

Fee for service   Payment mechanism for health care whereby a provider is paid an amount of money for each procedure performed.

Fee schedule   A list of procedures with an associated payment amount for each service.

Financing   The methods of paying for health care. Broadly speaking, includes private insurance, out-of-pocket payments, and government insurance programs.

Formal care   The personal health care system consisting a mix of acute, sub-acute, and long-term care facilities and related health care personnel.

Gatekeeper   A primary care provider in a health maintenance organization, usually a physician, who provides primary care and coordinates/controls access to the rest of the health care system.

Global budgeting   Payment mechanism for health care whereby a provider is given a lump sum of money to care for a population for a period of time, usually a year.

Gross Domestic Product   Total output of goods and services in the United States in a year.

Health services   Related policy and systems that organize, finance, and deliver health care.

Holism   An integrated philosophy including mind, body, and spirit for the treatment of persons with mental illness

Homeopathy   A form of alternative medicine that uses small amounts of substances that produce pathological symptoms in normal persons to treat patients with similar symptomatic disease states.

Humane philosophy   A movement that began at the beginning of the twentieth century that described the need to provide care and services for persons with mental illness.

Inclusion   A social philosophy that minimizes barriers and empowers persons with disabling conditions to achieve full participation in society.

Independent living   A social movement that promotes employment, access to adequate housing, education, and employment, and acts against discrimination for persons with disabling conditions.

Informal care   Personal health care that is provided by nonprofessional workers, primarily family and friends.

Integrated delivery system   A combination of primary care, secondary care, tertiary care, and quaternary care providers through a process of vertical or horizontal integration.

Intermediary   Medicare Part A claims processor and reviewer.

Intermediate care: A facility that provides residential services and a minimum level of professional care focusing on periodic monitoring and basic personal care.

Level of care   A description of a stage of the informal or formal care system; often considered to be part of a "continuum of services."

Leverage   A position of dominance in an economic market that forces other players to negotiate on terms favorable to the person in the dominant position.

Lobbying   The process of redressing grievances to elected representatives; a First Amendment right in the United States.

Marginalization   A social process that isolates and stigmatizes persons with disabling conditions from the general population.

Markets   An interaction between buyers and sellers involved in the exchange of economic resources (i.e., money, goods, and services).

Means-tested   Pre-qualification process for Medicaid and SCHIP that requires eligible beneficiaries to meet certain income and asset requirements.

Medical negligence   An act (or failure to act) by a health care professional that causes an injury or other adverse event to a patient.

Medically necessary   Sometimes termed medical "necessity." The determination by a provider with physician status that a health care intervention is required. A prerequisite for all forms of health care insurance reimbursement. Associated with the certification and recertification process in Medicare.

Medically needy eligibility   A state-option qualification for Medicaid based on demonstrated medical need and, in some cases, income/asset level.

Medicare assignment   An agreement between a provider and Medicare to accept (participate) the fee schedule as payment in full for services (minus the appropriate deductible and co-insurance).

Medigap   A term for private supplemental insurance plans that provide benefits for services not covered by traditional Medicare.

Moral hazard   Financially irresponsible behavior regarding insurance experienced as favorable selection and adverse selection.

Naturopathy   A form of alternative medicine that uses nutrition, herbalism, detoxification, and acupuncture to treat illness and disease.

Need factors   The presence of a medical condition that predisposes a person to access health care services.

Osteopathic medicine   A form of manipulative medicine that was largely incorporated into the allopathic medicine model in the twentieth century.

Outcome   The results of a health care intervention.

Panel   A group of providers selected by a managed care organization to provide services to plan members. May be open or closed.

Patient-focused care   Developed initially in hospitals, a redesign process of health care services from the perspective of the patient.

Peer review   A process whereby therapist activity is examined and compared to accepted standards of practice.

Peer review organizations   Medicare-sponsored organizations that perform quality-control, investigatory, and patient-education functions.

Penetration   The percentage of the insurance market that is controlled by managed care.

Personal care services   Home-based attendant care for persons with disabilities that assist with community integration (e.g., bathing, dressing).

Physician-hospital organization   An integration of physician practices and the hospital to create leverage and compete with managed care organizations.

Policy   A plan or course of action that organizes and allocates power (i.e., financial, physical, and human resources) to achieve a desired goal.

Predisposing factors   Demographic variables (e.g., age, gender) that help predict access and utilization of health care services.

Presumptive eligibility   Used in the Medicaid program to provide temporary benefits until permanent eligibility can be determined.

Primary care   The most common form of health care in the United States. Care for common, episodic illnesses. Occurs primarily in outpatient settings.

Process   The delivery of health care services, including physical therapy and occupational therapy. It has two components: technical excellence and interpersonal excellence.

Product-line teams   The reorganization of patient care services away from traditional discipline-specific services to patient-focused teams (e.g., a joint replacement team).

Professional regulation   A voluntary or mandatory process of ensuring the competence of health care providers. It has three levels: registration, certification, and licensure.

Prospective payment   A form of health care payment whereby providers are paid a set fee or rate prior to the delivery of services. Case-based payment, capitation, and Medicare Part A payment mechanisms are examples of prospective payment schemes.

Quality   Health care services that are efficient and effective.

Quaternary care   High-technology health care for uncommon, acute, and chronic disorders (e.g., organ transplantation). Associated with academic medical centers.

Reflection   A process of self-examination that is critical in understanding the personal motivations that affect the advocacy process.

Safety-net provider   A health care provider that provides care to a large or predominantly uninsured or underinsured population.

Secondary care   Care for common, chronic-type disorders (e.g. diabetes mellitus, hypertension).

Social disability model   A perspective on disablement that locates the problem in the policies, systems, and attitudes of those who are not experiencing disablement.

Social insurance   A form of government-sponsored health insurance whereby people paying premiums (taxes) are not eligible for benefits. Benefits are paid to those who have a defined social need. Examples are Medicare and Medicaid.

Spend-down   A process whereby a person with potential Medicaid eligibility "spends down" his or her assets to a certain level in order to gain eligibility for the program.

Standard   An accepted or, in some cases, optimal level of practice or performance.

State option   Eligibility criteria for Medicaid that can be included or excluded by the states (e.g., medically needy eligibility).

Structure   The stable elements of the health care system (e.g., physical structures, human resources).

Swing bed unit   A sub-acute care ward, typically in a hospital, for patients recovering from an acute illness or injury.

System   The organization and structure of physical and human resources to meet a need identified and addressed by policy.

Tertiary care   A technologically sophisticated level of care associated with inpatient hospital stays.

Testimony   Providing information to public policymakers in verbal and written form as well as in response to questions.

Underwriting   The insurance process that examines individual characteristics to determine eligibility and cost of insurance.

Uninsured   People who have impaired access to health care due to lack of health insurance.

Universalism   A philosophy on disablement that emphasizes the common experience of disability and advocates policies that reduce barriers and reinforce inclusion.

Utilization review   A process of peer review of provider documentation to determine the appropriateness of health care services.

Vested   After payment of taxes into the Medicare trust fund for 40 quarters, a person is eligible for Part A benefits upon reaching retirement age, experiencing permanent disability, or develping end-stage renal disease.

Vocational rehabilitation   A process of assessment, education, training, and support for persons with disabling conditions to prepare them for the workforce.

Voluntary agency   Not-for-profit organization that provides advocacy, education, and limited personal health care for persons with illness or disease. For example, the National Multiple Sclerosis Society.

Waiver program   The process that allows states to apply to the federal government in order to establish new and innovative Medicaid programs.

Index

AAMC. See Association for Academic Medical
    Centers
Access
    affordability, as greatest barrier, 18–19
    defined, 14
    demographic makeup, effect of, 16
    direct, 24–26. See also Direct access
    factors affecting, 15–18
    gatekeeper role, 24
    health insurance, relationship to, 19–23
    health status, perception of, 16
    Medicare/Medicaid, 19, 21
    Penchansky and Thomas's concepts, 17–18
    SCHIP, 21
Accreditation, 51
Activities of daily living (ADL), 97
Actuarial analysis/adjustment, 89
Acute medical delivery system, 172, 173
ADA. See Americans with Disabilities Act of 1990
ADL. See Activities of daily living
Adverse selection, 90
Advocacy
    appearing at hearings and preparing testimony,
        266, 269
    assertive communication, 258–59
    client advocacy skills, 259–61
    DESC communication model, 259
    and ethics, 256–57
    Internet resources, 271–75
    legislative, 263
    legislative visit, 265
    professional, 261–62
    with professional organizations, 262–63
    reflective questions, 258
    regulatory, 263
    sequential steps, 264–71
    skills, 256, 257–58
    on the state level, 269
    themes, 256
AFDC. See Aid for Families with Dependent Children
    program
Affirmative action, 74
African Americans
    and access, to health services, 16
    sickle cell anemia, 16
    uninsured population, percentage of,
        22

under utilization, of post-acute institutional care,
    188
Agency for Healthcare Research and Quality, 19, 51
AHA. See American Hospital Association
Aid for Families with Dependent Children program
    (AFDC), 161
Allied health professions, 212
Allopathic medicine, 217
Alzheimer's disease, 197, 231, 237
AMA. See American Medical Association
American College of Sports Medicine, 219
American Corrective Therapy Association, 220
American Council on Exercise, 220
American Heart Association, 191
American Hospital Association (AHA), 179, 181
American Kinesiotherapy Association, 220
American Massage Therapy Association, 222
American Medical Association (AMA), 223
*American Medical Association Guide to the Evaluation of
    Permanent Impairment*, 99
American Nurses Association (ANA), 218, 223
American Occupational Therapy Association
    (AOTA), 5, 61, 70, 234, 260, 262–63
American Physical Therapy Association (APTA), 5,
    61, 222, 260, 262
American Speech Therapy Association (ASTA), 260
Americans with Disabilities Act of 1990 (ADA), 4, 61,
    62, 234, 260
    barriers and concerns, 77–78
    history, 76
    purpose, 77
    Titles I, II, III, and IV, 77
ANA. See American Nurses Association
AOTA. See American Occupational Therapy
    Association
APTA. See American Physical Therapy Association
Assignment of benefits, 96, 97
Assisted Living Federation of America, 197
Assistive technology, 79–81
Assistive Technology Act (ATA)
    barriers and concerns, 81
    history, 80
    purpose, 79
    technology, defined, 79
    and therapy, 81
    Titles I, II, and III, 79–80
Association for Academic Medical Centers (AAMC),
    178

ASTA. *See* American Speech Therapy
  Association

Balanced Budget Act of 1997 (BBA), 31, 32,
  137, 146, 200
Barden-LaFollette Act, 73
Barrier-free environment, 61
BBA. *See* Balanced Budget Act of 1997
Benchmarking, 111
Beneficiary, 88
Benefit period, 129
Biomedical model, 8–9
Bundled payment system, 109
Bureau of the Census, 20
Buyer-sponsored organizations, 95–96

Canadian Seniors' Health Promotion Project,
  252
Capitalism, 5
Capitation, 37, 93, 110
CARF. *See* Commission on the Accreditation of
  Rehabilitation Facilities
Carriers, 127, 150
Case management, 117, 118
Case mix adjustment, 136, 144
Case-based payment, 37, 93, 109–10
Categorical eligibility, 158–59
Center for Medicare and Medicaid Services
  (CMS), 125, 127, 134, 149, 247
Certification, 54, 149
Children's Defense Fund, 164
Chiropractic medicine, 221
Civil Rights Act of 1964, 76
Clinical practice guidelines, 51
CMS. *See* Center for Medicare and Medicaid
  Services
Coalitions, 264
COBRA. *See* Consolidated Budget Reconcilia-
  tion Act of 1985
Coercive government power, 4
Co-insurance, 92–93, 96
Commission on the Accreditation of
  Rehabilitation Facilities (CARF), 53
Commonwealth Fund, 20
Community Mental Health Act of 1963, 235
Community rating, 90
Confidentiality, 54
Consolidated billing, 145
Consolidated Budget Reconciliation Act of 1985
  (COBRA), 101
Co-payment, 92
Cost shifting, of Medicare underpayment, 136
Cost-based reimbursement, 135

COTH. *See* Council of Teaching Hospitals and
  Health Systems
Council of Teaching Hospitals and Health Systems
  (COTH), 178–79
CPT. *See* Current Procedural Terminology
Credentialing process, 91, 108
*Crossing the Quality Chasm: A New Health System for the
  21st Century* (Institute of Medicine), 45
Current Procedural Terminology (CPT), 146

Deductible, 92
Defensive medicine, 35
Defined benefit plan, 152
Defined contribution plan, 152
DESC communication model, 259
Developmental Disabilities Act (DDA)
  barriers and concerns, 69–70
  history, 66–69
  and therapy, 62, 70
  Titles I, II, and III, 69
Diagnosis-Related Groups (DRGs), 37, 136–37, 188
Direct access
  effects of, 26
  states permitting, listed, 25
  to therapists, 24–26
Disability rights movement, 61
Disablement. *See also* Disablement, public policy
  ability to work, 7–8
  biomedical model, 8–9
  defined, 7
  disenfranchisement, 5
  historical/societal perspectives, 60–61
  inclusion, 61
  marginalization, 10, 11
  medicalization, 8
  Nagi model, 9
  negative stereotypes, 10
  paradigm shift (1968-1988), 61, 62
  power, lack of, 3
  scope and history, 7
  social disability model, 9–10, 60
  social response, 7
  theoretical models, 2, 8–11
  universalism, 10–11
Disablement, public policy
  ADA, 76–79. *See also* Americans with Disabilities
    Act of 1990
  affirmative action plan, 74
  ATA, 79–81. *See also* Assistive Technology Act
  barriers and controversies, 82–83
  children and youth, 63–70
  DDA, 66–70. *See also* Developmental Disabilities
    Act
  focus, of major policies, 63

IDEA, 63–66. *See also* Individuals with Disabilities Education Act
    independent living, 74
    RA, 70–76
    societal perspectives, codified, 61, 68
    and therapy, 61–62, 65–66, 70, 75–76, 78–79, 81
    working with, 81–83
    work-related, 70–79
Discounted fee schedule, 109
Disenfranchisement, 5
DNR (do not resuscitate), 54
Donabedian, Avedis
    quality of health care framework, 49–53
    seven pillars of quality, 48
Dualism, 2, 89
Durable power of attorney, 54

Education for Handicapped Act (EHA), 63, 69, 76
Employee Retirement Income Security Act of 1974 (ERISA), 100–101
Employer-based health care insurance
    declining trends, in benefits and enrollment, 19–20
    and eligibility, 90–91
Empowerment, 3, 69, 76
Enabling factors, 16
Entitlement program, 127
EOC. *See* Equal Opportunity Commission
Epidemiology, 248–49
Equal Opportunity Commission (EOC), 77
ERISA. *See* Employee Retirement Income Security Act of 1974
ERISA exemption, 95, 100, 106
Evidence-based practice, 51

Favorable selection, 90, 110
Fee schedule, 146
Fee-for-service (FFS), 36–37, 93, 96
First-dollar-coverage limit, 92, 96
Focus on Therapeutic Outcomes (FOTO), 52
Formal care. *See also* Skilled nursing facilities (SNFs)
    adult day services, 196–97
    appropriate level of care, determining, 191–92
    assisted living, 197–98
    home health care, 192–94
    hospice, 194–96
    sub-acute care, 200–201
Functional Independence Measure (FIM), 52, 141

Gag clause, 100
Gatekeeper role, 24, 108–09, 183
Gender
    and access, to health services, 16
    females, as informal caregivers, 190

Global budgeting, 37
Government
    coercive power, reasons for use of, 4
    power, distribution of, 4
    regulatory role, 3
Great Society Program, 158
Group model, 114
Group practice without walls model (GPWW), 183
Guide for Professional Conduct, 256

Hahnemann, Samuel, 222
HCFA. *See* Health Care Financing Administration
Health care expenditures
    cost containment efforts, 36
    gross domestic product, percentage of, 30
    hospital expenditures, 32–33
    increasing growth, reasons for, 34–35
    national, 30
    payment structures/mechanisms, 36–37
    per capita, 30
    physician expenditures, 33
    prescription drug expenditures, 33–34
    quality perspectives, effects of, 49
Health care financing
    in Canada, 38
    Medicare/Medicaid, 31–32, 38
    private health insurance, 30–31
    sources, 30–32
    in Sweden, 38–39
    in the United Kingdom, 39
Health Care Financing Administration (HCFA), 149, 150, 161
Health care insurance
    access, relationship to, 18–19
    actuarial analysis/adjustment, 89
    beneficiary, 88
    continuation issues, 101
    contracts, 90–94. *See also* Health care insurance, contracts
    credentialing process, 91
    moral hazard, 89–90
    national comprehensive program, lack of, 124–25
    premium, 88
    purpose, 88–89
    regulation, 100–101
    risk pool, 88–89
    selection, adverse and favorable, 90
    state regulation, of private companies, 89
    types. *See* Health care insurance, types
    uninsured population, 19–24. *See also* Uninsured
Health care insurance, contracts
    basic features, 91
    beneficiary cost limits, 92–93
    covered events, 91–92

Health care insurance, contracts (*continued*)
covered services, 92
eligibility, 90–91
explained, 90
provider cost limits, 93
underwriting, 91
Health care insurance, types
casualty insurance, 99–100
classification categories, 94–95
direct contracting, 95–96
indemnity insurance, 96
long-term-care insurance, 97
private/commercial insurance, 95
self-insurance, 95
service benefit plans, 96–97
workers' compensation, 97–99. *See also* Workers'
compensation
Health care personnel
allied health professions, 212
classification categories, U.S. Department of
Labor, 211–12
complementary/alternative medicine providers,
220–22
exercise-related occupations, 219–20
future trends and changes, 222–23
nurses, 218–19
occupational therapist assistants and aides, 213
occupational therapists, 212
physical therapist assistants and aides, 214–15
physical therapists, 213–14
physicians, 216–18
the rehabilitation team, 215–16
size and scope, of the labor force, 211, 211–12
technology, effect on demand, 210
Health care policy. *See also* Disablement, public policy
dualism, effect of, 3
empowerment, and the powerless, 3
ethical considerations, 5–7
foundational principles, 2
government authority, 4–5
Long's ethical principles, 6
presidential reforms, 19
and private enterprise, 5
Health Insurance Portability and Accountability Act
of 1996 (HIPAA), 101, 150
Health Maintenance Organization (HMO) Act of
1973, 106
Health maintenance organizations (HMOs), 112
Health Plan Employer Data and Information Set
(HEDIS), 51
Health Resources Services Administration, 50
Health services
accessibility, 14–26. *See also* Access
defined, 1–2

expenditures, 32–37. *See also* Health care
expenditures
funding, sources of, 30–32. *See also* Health care
financing
lack of uniformity, 2
quality, 44–56. *See also* Quality health care
Healthy People Initiative, 249–50, 251
HEDIS. *See* Health Plan Employer Data and Information Set
HIPPA. *See* Health Insurance Portability and Accountability Act of 1996
Hispanics, percentage of uninsured population, 22
HMOs. *See* Health maintenance organizations
Home Health Resource Group (HHRG), 142
Homeopathy, 222
Horizontal integration, 181–82
Hospice Foundation of America, 194
Hospitals
acute care versus long-term care, 178
general versus specialty, 178
historical development, 172–73
integrated delivery systems, 181–82
levels of care, 179–80
ownership, 177–78
Physician-hospital organizations (PHOs), 182
Physician–hospital relationship, 183–84
size, 176–77
structure, 174–75
teaching hospitals, 178–79
Human Services, 247

IDEA. *See* Individuals with Disabilities Education Act
IEP. *See* Individualized Education Program
Inclusion, 61, 76, 82
Independent practice associations (IPAs), 114, 183
Independent-living philosophy, 61, 74
Individualized Education Program (IEP), 65–66
Individuals with Disabilities Education Act (IDEA)
barriers and concerns, 65
history, 63–65
and therapy, 61, 65–66, 81
Informed consent, 54
Institute of Medicine, 44, 45, 48, 51, 180, 243
Integrated health care systems, 173, 181–82
Intermediaries, 127, 150
Interpersonal excellence, 51, 52
IPAs. *See* Independent practice associations

JCAHO. See Joint Commission on the Accreditation
of Health Care Organizations
Job lock, 101
Johnson, Lyndon B., 158
Joint Commission on the Accreditation of Health
Care Organizations (JCAHO), 53, 149

Kaiser Commission on Medicaid and the Uninsured, 165
Kaiser Family Foundation, 20
Kaiser of California, 113
Kinesiotherapist, 219

Legislative advocacy, 263
Levels of care, in post-acute care system, 188
Leverage, 108
Licensure, 54
Living will, 54
Lobbying, 263
Long's ethical principles, 6

Mainstreaming, 61
Managed care
    adapting to changes, 116
    benefits and concerns, for therapists, 114–16
    case managers, 118
    communication, importance of, 116–18
    defined, 107
    ethical concerns, 110
    growth, reasons for, 106
    and HMOs, difference between, 106
    limited access, to providers, 107–09
    payment mechanisms, 109–10
    principles, 107–11
    products, 111–13
    provider panels, open and closed, 107–08
    provider structures, 113–14
    quality improvement monitoring, 110–11
    referrals, by primary care physicians, 108–09
    shared risk, between provider and insurer, 109
Managed indemnity, 111
Management services organizations (MSOs), 183
Marginalization, 10, 11
Massage therapy, 221–22
Matrix system, 175–76
MDS, 131–32, 138
Means-tested programs, 157
Medicaid
    benefits, 161–63
    cost, of program, 158
    defined, 157
    demographic makeup, of insured, 158
    eligibility. *See* Medicaid, eligibility
    history, 158
    managed care plans, 163–64
    personal care services, 162
    provider participation, 163
    shared participation, federal-state, 158
    waiver program, 162–63

Medicaid, eligibility
    categorical eligibility, 158–59, 161
    dual eligibility, 160–61
    immigrants, 161, 162
    medically needy eligibility (state-option criteria), 159–60
    spend-down programs, 159–60
Medical necessity, 9, 128
Medical negligence, 54
Medical Outcome Study–Short Form (SF-36), 53
Medicalization, of disablement, 8, 9
Medically needy eligibility, 159–60
Medically underserved communities, 50
Medicare
    characteristics, of program, 126
    fraud and abuse, 150
    future challenges, 151
    history, 124
    hospital insurance. *See* Medicare, Part A: Hospital Insurance
    managed care options, Part C, 148–49
    medical insurance. *See* Medicare, Part B: Supplementary Medical Insurance (SMI)
    Medigap policies, 149
    policy and procedures, 127
    quality assurance and monitoring, 149–50
    reform proposals, 151–52
    resulting changes, in health care system, 125–26
    rising costs and long-term viability, 125
    solvency, of trust funds, 151
    three-tier cake, 124, 127
Medicare assignment, 148
Medicare Integrity Program, 150
Medicare, Part A: Hospital Insurance
    benefit period, 129–30
    benefits, 128–29
    cost shift, 136
    Diagnosis-Related Groups, 136–37
    eligibility, 128
    home health agency prospective payment, 141–44
    home health care benefit, 132–34
    hospice benefit, 134–35
    hospital prospective payment, 136–37
    inpatient rehabilitation facility prospective payment, 141
    prospective payment, and reform, 144
    skilled nursing facility (SNF) benefit, 131–32
    skilled nursing facility (SNF) prospective payment, 137–41
    skilled occupational therapy, defined, 133
    skilled physical therapy, defined, 132
    transfer rule, 137

Medicare, Part B: Supplementary Medical Insurance
(SMI)
  benefits, 144–45
  comprehensive outpatient rehabilitation facilities
    (CORF), 146
  eligibility, 144
  fee schedule, 146–48
  Medicare assignment, accepting or declining, 148
  outpatient hospital programs, 145–46
  physical and occupational therapists, in private
    practice, 146
  provider participation, 148
  provider types, 145
Medicare Skilled Nursing Facility Manual, 131
Medigap policies, 149
Mental Health Centers Act of 1963, 232
Mental Health Parity Act, 234
Mental health practice, and public policy
  arts and crafts movement, 230
  biomedical model, 230
  deinstitutionalization, 232–33
  historical and policy aspects, 230–34
  holistic approach, and pragmatism, 230
  institutionalization, 230–31
  Medicare/Medicaid, effects of, 232
  medicine, growth and influence of, 231–32
  movement away from mental health practice,
    233–34
  nontraditional practice, 234
  World Wars, effects of, 231
Mental health practice sites
  adult day-care programs, 236–37
  clubhouse models, 236
  community health centers, 235–36
  geriatric psychiatric units, 237
  home-care programs, 237
  hospitals, 235
  nontraditional settings, 237–38
  nursing homes, 237
  state institutions for mentally ill, 234–35
MHS. *See* Multihospital systems
Minimum Data Set for Nursing Home Resident As-
    sessment and Care Screening (MDS). *See*
    MDS
Multihospital systems (MHS), 179

Nagi model, 9
National Adult Day Services Association, 196
National Athletic Trainers' Association Board of Cer-
    tification, 219
National Center for Complementary and Alternative
    Medicine (NCCAM), 220
National Certification Board for Therapeutic Mas-
    sage and Bodywork, 222

National Committee of Quality Assurance (NCQA),
    53–54
National Council on Disabilities, 77, 81
National Governors Association, 165
National Institute of Health, 220
National Institute of Mental Health (NIMH), 231
National Mental Health Act (NMHA) of 1946, 231
National Multiple Sclerosis Society, 191
National Strength and Conditioning Association, 220
National Sub-acute Care Association, 200
Naturopathy, 222
NCCAM. *See* National Center for Complementary
    and Alternative Medicine
NCQA. *See* National Committee of Quality Assurance
Need factors, 16
Network model, 114
NIMH. *See* National Institute of Mental Health
NMHA. *See* National Mental Health Act (NMHA) of
    1946
Nursing Home Reform Act of 1987, 200

OASIS. *See* Outcome and Assessment Information Set
Occupational Health and Safety Act of 1970
    (OSHA), 98
Occupational Therapy Code of Ethics, 256, 257
ORYX, 53
Osteopathic medicine, 217
Outcome and Assessment Information Set (OASIS),
    133–34, 142
Outcomes, 52–53

PACE. *See* Program of All-Inclusive Care
Palliative care, 195
Patient-focused care, 175
Patient's Bill of Rights, 5, 6, 55
Peer review, 51
Peer review organizations (PROs), 149
Penchansky and Thomas's access factors
  acceptability, 18
  accessibility, 17
  accommodation, 17–18
  affordability, 18
  availability, 17
Penetration, managed care, 108
Personal care services, 162
Personal Responsibility and Work Opportunity Rec-
    onciliation Act, 161
Personal-based perspective, 48, 49
Pew Healthcare Trust, 223
Physiatrists, 217
Physical Therapy Code of Ethics, 256–57
Physician-hospital organizations (PHOs), 182, 183
Point of service (POS) plans, 112–13
Population-based perspective, 46–48, 49

Post-acute care health system, 172, 173
   common services, 202
   financing, 188–89
   formal care. *See* Formal care; Formal care
   historical development, 188
   informal care, 189–91
   organization, 202
   treatment alternatives (levels of care), 188
   voluntary agencies, 191
Power
   economic (private enterprise), 5
   government authority, 4–5
   moral/ethical values, 5–7
   and policy making, 2, 3
   sources, in U.S., 3, 6–7
PPOs. *See* Preferred provider organizations
Predisposing factors, 16
Preferred provider organizations (PPOs), 111–12
Premium, insurance, 88
Presumptive eligibility, 165
Primary care, 179–80
Primary physician care, 180
Private enterprise
   economic power, 5
   symbiotic relationship, with government, 5
Process, 49–50, 51–52
Product-line teams, 175
Professional regulation, 54
Program of All-Inclusive Care (PACE), 196
Prospective payment systems, 109, 125, 135
Protection and Advocacy Technology (PAAT) program, 80
Provider panels, 96–97, 107–08
Provider-service organizations, 95–96
Public health
   agencies, 247–48
   assurance, 250–51
   challenges, 245–46
   defined, 243–46
   epidemiological assessment, 248–49
   expenditures, compared with private health, 244–45
   major achievements, 243–44, 245
   organization, 246–48
   policy development, 249–50
   population-based perspective, 47
   and therapy services, 251–52
Public Health Functions Steering Committee, 243
Public Health Service, 247

Quality health care
   accreditation, 51, 53–54
   health status, of U.S. citizens versus comparable industrialized countries, 45–46
   legal issues, 54
   legal mandates, 48–49
   medical error, 44–45
   medical interventions, discrepancies in outcomes, 45, 50
   outcomes, 52–53
   Patient's Bill of Rights, 55
   peer review, 51
   personal-based perspective, 48, 49
   population-based perspective, 46–48, 49
   process, 49–50, 51–52
   quality of health care framework (A. Donabedian), 49–53
   quality pyramid, 55–56
   report cards, 51–52
   seven pillars of quality (A. Donabedian), 48
   structure, 49–50
Quarternary care, 180

Race/Ethnicity
   and access, to health services, 16
   disability classifications, cultural insensitivity of, 74
   disabled minorities, discrimination against, 77–78
   health insurance coverage, 22
RAPS. *See* Resident Assessment Protocols
Registration, 54
Regulatory advocacy, 263
Rehabilitation Act of 1973 (RA), 10, 62, 69
   barriers and concerns, 75
   history, 70, 72–76
   section 103, 75
   sections 501, 503, and 504, 74–75
   and therapy, 75–76, 82
Report cards, 51–52, 111
Resident Assessment Instrument (RAI), 131
Resident Assessment Instrument (RAI), 200
Resident Assessment Protocols (RAPS), 132
Resource Based Relative Value Scale (RBRVS), 146
Resource Utilization Groups (RUGS), 138–39
Respite care, 195
Restorative care, 199
Retrospective payment systems, 109, 125, 135
Risk pool, 88–89
Robert Wood Johnson Foundation, 249
RUGS. *See* Resource Utilization Groups
Rural communities
   and access, to health services, 17
   home health care, utilization of, 192
   medical underservice, 50
   post-acute health care, inaccessibility of, 188

Safety-net providers, 164
SCHIP. *See* State Children's Health Insurance Program

Secondary care, 180
Service Employees International Union, 223
Sheltered workshops, 74
Sickle cell anemia, 16
Skilled nursing facilities (SNFs)
    demographic information, 198–99
    growth, in the last two decades, 198
    Medicare benefits, 131–32
    physicians, lack of care by, 200
    quality of care concerns, 200
    reaction/adjustment, to residential life, 200
    services provided, 199
Slagle, Eleanor Clark, 212
Smith-Fess Act of 1920, 70
Social conscience, 4
Social disability model, 9–10
Social insurance, 127
Social justice, 6
Spend-down programs, 159
SSI. *See* Supplemental Security Income
St. Christopher's Hospice, 194
Staff model, 113
Standards, 51
Starfield, B., 45–46
State Children's Health Insurance Program (SCHIP)
    age demographics, for uninsured, 21
    benefits, 165
    enrollment, 165
    history, 164
    presumptive eligibility rules, 165
State-option criteria, 159
Stop-loss coverage, 95
Strong for Life program, 252
Structure, 49–50
Supplemental Security Income (SSI), 19
Swing bed units, 201

TANP. *See* Temporary Assistance to Needy Families
    (TANP)
Technical excellence, 51
Temporary Assistance to Needy Families (TANP), 19,
    31–32, 161
Tenet Healthcare, 177
Tertiary care, 180
Testimony, 269

Ticket to Work, 76
Title XIX of the Social Security Act, 158
To Err is Human: Building a Safer Health System (Institute of Medicine), 44
Tort system of law, 48–49
Tracy, Susan, 212
Trialliance for Health Rehabilitation Professions, 260
Turning Point program, 249

Underwriting, 91
Uniform Data System for Medical Rehabilitation, 52
Uninsured
    children, 21–22
    demographic makeup, 21–23
    family income and employment, 22–23
    health status, 23–24
    increasing trend, factors influencing, 19–20
    minorities versus white Americans, 21–22
    number of, in population, 19–21
Universalism, 10–11
Urban Institute, 164
U.S. Department of Health and Human Services, 247
Utilization review, 149, 150

Vertical integration, 182
Vested, 128
Veterans Administration and Military Health Insurance Programs
Veterans Administration and Military eligibility, 165,
    166
    TRICARE, 167
Vitalism, 222
Vocational rehabilitation, 73
Voluntary agencies, 191

Waiver program, 162–63
Work Incentives Improvement Act of 1999, 76
Workers' compensation
    benefit programs, 98
    disability classifications, 98–99
    payment of benefits, 99
    purpose, 97
    rising costs, 99
Workers' compensation laws, 70, 98
World Health Organization (WHO), 195, 246